Practice
Guidelines for
Obstetrics &
Gynecology

Practice Guidelines for Obstetrics & Gynecology

Second Edition

Geri Morgan, CNM, ND
Nurse–Midwife
Planned Parenthood of Central
and Northern Arizona
Phoenix, Arizona

Carole Hamilton, BSN, MA, CNM
Nurse–Midwife
Beal and Constantino, PC
Tucson, Arizona

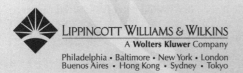

LIPPINCOTT WILLIAMS & WILKINS
A **Wolters Kluwer** Company

Philadelphia • Baltimore • New York • London
Buenos Aires • Hong Kong • Sydney • Tokyo

Acquisitions Editor: Jennifer E. Brogan
Assistant Editor: Susan Barta Rainey
Senior Project Editor: Rosanne Hallowell
Senior Production Manager: Helen Ewan
Managing Editor / Production: Erika Kors
Art Director: Carolyn O'Brien
Manufacturing Manager: William Alberti
Indexer: Lynne McCabe
Printer: R.R. Donnelley & Sons

Second Edition

9 8 7 6 5 4 3 2 1

Library of Congress Cataloging-in-Publication Data

Morgan, Geri
  Practice guidelines for obstetrics and gynecology / Geri Morgan, Carole Hamilton.--2nd ed.
    p. ; cm
  Rev. ed. of: Practice guidelines for obstetrics and gynecology / Janet Scoggin, Geri Morgan. c1997.
Includes bibliographical references and index.
ISBN 0-7817-3867-9
  1. Obstetrics Outlines, syllabi, etc. 2. Gynecology--Outlines, syllabi, etc. 3. Women--Health and hygiene--Outlines, syllabi, etc. I. Hamilton, Carole, MA. II. Scoggin, Janet. Practice guidelines for obstetrics and gynecology. III. Title.
  [DNLM: 1. Obstetrics--Handbooks. 2. Genital Diseases, Female--Handbooks. 3. Pharmaceutiocal Preparations--Handbooks. WQ 39 M848p 2003]
RG101 .S3577 2003
618--dc21

2002017862

Care has been taken to confirm the accuracy of the information presented and to describe generally accepted practices. However, the authors, editors, and publisher are not responsible for errors or omissions or for any consequences from application of the information in this book and make no warranty, express or implied, with respect to the content of the publication.

The authors, editors, and publisher have exerted every effort to ensure that drug selection and dosage set forth in this text are in accordance with the current recommendations and practice at the time of publication. However, in view of ongoing research, changes in government regulations, and the constant flow of information relating to drug therapy and drug reactions, the reader is urged to check the package insert for each drug for any change in indications and dosage and for added warnings and precautions This is particularly important when the recommended agent is a new or infrequently employed drug.

Some drugs and medical devices presented in this publication have Food and Drug Administration (FDA) clearance for limited use in restricted research settings. It is the responsibility of the health care provider to ascertain the FDA status of each drug or device planned for use in his or her clinical practice.

LWW.com

To Janet Scoggin and all the others
who have touched our lives —
without them, this book would
not have been possible

Reviewers

Linda C. Andrist, PhD, RNC, WHNP
Associate Professor and Coordinator, Adult/Women's Health Nurse
Practitioner Program
MGH Institute of Health Professions
Boston, Massachusetts

Linda Evinger, RN, MSN, C-OGNP
Instructor of Nursing
School of Nursing and Health Professions
University of Southern Indiana
Evansville, Indiana

Terry A. Fulcher, RN, BSN, R-ACCE, IBCLC
Perinatal Nurse Educator
Catholic Health System
Sisters Hospital
Buffalo, New York

Anita Jaynes, RN, BSN, MA
Staff RN, Labor and Delivery
Saint Joseph Hospital
Omaha, Nebraska

Marva M. Price, DrPH, MPH, FNP, RN
Faculty - Clinical Assistant Professor
Family Nurse Practitioner Program
Duke University School of Nursing
Durham, North Carolina

Mary C. Sobralske, PhD (c), MSN
Assistant Professor of Nursing
Department of Nursing
Gonzaga University
Spokane, Washington

Rosemary Theroux, PhD, RNC
Assistant Professor, Nursing
University of Massachusetts
Lowell, Massachusetts;
Women's Health Private Practice
Framingham, Massachusetts

Laura B. Willsher, RN, MSN
Clinical Coordinator
Family Nurse Practitioner Program
Grambling State University
Grambling, Louisiana

Preface

The guidelines in *Practice Guidelines for Obstetrics and Gynecology*, 2nd edition, are presented in outline form. They were developed to provide a quick clinical reference and to aid in a uniform quality of care for advance practice nurses, residents, interns, physician assistants, midwives, those doing telephone triage, and students who care for women.

Part I is an overview of well woman care throughout the life cycle. It outlines basic care in obstetrics as well as gynecology, and contains history-taking information, physical exam procedures, lab work recommendations, and teaching information needed for both situations. Included in this section are discussions of screening tests, contraceptive methods, preconceptual counseling, the initial prenatal visit, and return prenatal visits. For nurse-midwives and other practitioners who will be attending deliveries, guidelines for intrapartum and postpartum care are included. Part I concludes with a description of perimenopause, menopause, hormone replacement therapy, and Kegel exercises.

Part II features common discomforts of pregnancy. These discomforts have been organized alphabetically in a convenient table format for quick reference. The table includes etiologies, differential diagnoses, relief measures, and danger signs.

Part III is a discussion of abuse, domestic violence, and sexual coercion or assault, which may apply to a significant number of patients. This section describes how to recognize and treat a patient who has been abused.

Parts IV and V were difficult to separate. Both are concerned with the management of common problems and procedures; Part IV describes common gynecologic issues, while Part V focuses on obstetric issues. Most topics begin with a definition of the condition, followed by its etiology, clinical features (including history, signs, and symptoms), and management. Within Part IV, if management of the patient is different during pregnancy, that information appears in Part V. The topics in these sections are listed in alphabetic order for ease of reference.

Part VI is concerned with complementary and alternative therapies. An overview presents various therapies used in women's health and wellness. The remainder of Part VI discusses herbal therapies that are growing in popularity and have been used by more than one in three Americans this year as an adjunct or alternative to other medical therapies.

Part VII is a concise review of drugs referred to in the book and commonly used in women's health care. The drugs suggested in this book for the treatment of various conditions are recommended in the medical literature and conform to accepted medical practice. Because the type and dosage of therapeutic regimens often change, it is recommended that practitioners check updated literature and package inserts for revised recommendations. The drug index specifies dosages, pregnancy category classifications, indications, adverse reactions, drug interactions, precautions, and the form in which the drug is supplied.

Part VIII describes topical agents, including adrenocorticoids, anesthetics, antibiotics, antifungals, antipsoriatics, antiseborrheics, antivirals, emollients, keratolytics, lotions and solutions, and pediculicides and scabicides. The information is presented in an alphabetized table that specifies recommended dosages and other considerations.

Geri Morgan, CNM, ND
Carole Hamilton, BSN, MA, CNM

Contents

PART 5: Management of Common Problems and Procedures Specific to Pregnancy, 217

Geri Morgan and Carole Hamilton

PART 6: Complementary Therapies, 289
Geri Morgan

PART 7: Drug Index, 307
Geri Morgan and Carole Hamilton

PART 8: Topical Agents, 357
Geri Morgan

Bibliography, 365

Index, 373

PART 1

Guidelines for Well Woman Care

Geri Morgan, CNM, ND

GYNECOLOGIC CARE

For many women, visits to gynecologic care providers are their sole source of preventive health care. Therefore, these visits must be comprehensive and accomplish the following three purposes: (1) detection, diagnosis, and treatment of gynecologic problems; (2) screening for other health problems; and (3) general health maintenance and prevention of illness.[1] To accomplish these purposes, the practitioner must take a detailed history and perform a thorough physical exam. The proper understanding and use of screening tests is also necessary.

I. History Taking

    A. Identification information

    B. Reason for visit: Why has the woman sought care?

    C. Menstrual history: First day and duration of the last menstrual period; age at menarche; usual interval, duration, and amount of menses; spotting or cramps midcycle; any significant problems, such as cramping, nausea, or depression

    D. Gynecologic history: Past and current gynecologic problems, genitourinary disorders, vaginitis, sexually transmitted diseases (STDs), infertility

    E. Obstetric (OB) history: Gravidity (number of pregnancies), parity (number of viable pregnancies), abortions (spontaneous, elective), course of pregnancies and labor, problems with pregnancies, labor, deliveries, or postpartum occurrences

    F. Contraceptive history: Types of and satisfaction with current and previously used contraceptives

    G. Medical history: Complete medical history including substance use, allergies, any previous transfusions, exposure to diethylstilbestrol

    H. Surgical history: Circumstances of any previous surgeries

    I. Family history: Chronic diseases of first-degree family members, such as diabetes, cancer, cardiac disease, or osteoporosis

    J. Social or cultural history: Cultural background, support system, living situation, current or a history of abuse and domestic violence

    K. Occupational history: Possible exposure to toxic substances, heavy lifting, standing or sitting too long, night work

    L. Sexual history: Sexually active, sexual preference, number of partners in the last year, any problems with intercourse, any history of sexual violence or rape

    M. Nutritional history: 24-hour diet recall, caffeine, usual weight, recent weight changes, eating disorders

    N. Activity and exercise history: Activities of daily living, regular exercise

II. Physical Exam

    A. General: Record height, weight, blood pressure, pulse, and temperature.

---

[1]Litchtman & Papera, 1990

    B. Head and neck: Inspect eyes, ears, nose, mouth, oropharynx, tongue, and thyroid gland.

    C. Lymph nodes: Palpate and inspect anterior and posterior cervical, submental, supraclavicular, axillary, epitrochlear, and inguinal nodes.

    D. Back: Inspect straightness and palpate for costovertebral angle tenderness.

    E. Lungs: Inspect, percuss, and auscultate.

    F. Heart: Auscultate for rate, rhythm, regularity, murmurs, and extra heart sounds.

    G. Breasts

        1. Inspect in three positions: arms at side, over the head, and pressed against hips with elbows extended laterally. Look for symmetry, nipple alignment, abnormal venous pattern, coloration and skin appearance, and changes including dimpling and puckering.

        2. Palpate all four quadrants of each breast with patient lying down and arm over her head on the side being examined. Use radial or transverse techniques. Note size, shape, consistency, tenderness, and nodularity.

        3. Inspect nipples for eversion; note any discharge following expression.

        4. Palpate subclavicular area, noting masses or tenderness.

    H. Abdomen: Inspect for contour, scars, and masses. Palpate for masses, liver, spleen, or kidney enlargement and tenderness.

    I. Lower extremities: Inspect and palpate, noting varicosities, lesions, edema, erythema, warmth, and pain.

    J. Pelvis

        1. Inspect external genitalia for lesions, scars, and configurations.

        2. Palpate Bartholin's and Skene's glands and note urethral discharge.

        3. Perform speculum exam to observe vagina and cervix.

            a. Note color of the cervix, any erythema, irregularities, lesions, ectropion or friability, configuration of the os, and discharge. Obtain Papanicolaou (Pap) smear and any necessary cultures.

            b. Inspect the vagina. Note the color, rugae, and presence of any abnormality or discharge.

        4. Perform bimanual exam to evaluate uterus and adnexa, noting contour, nodularity, position, size, and tenderness.

        5. Perform rectal exam if indicated.

III. Recommendations for Preventive and Screening Tests for Women. Clinicians often see women whose medical problems could have been avoided with proper prevention and screening. Despite the benefits, preventive services should be used selectively. One should be confident that the benefit of the tests' ability to detect disease will be greater than the disadvantages of any harm done or excessive cost incurred. The efficacy of the preventive and screening tests shown in Table 1-1, Preven-

Table 1-1. Prevention and Screening Recommendations for Women

Intervention	Health Condition	Target Group	Recommendations
Blood Pressure Measurement	CHD, cerebrovascular disease, renal disease	*Routine:* 18 yr+ *High risk:* 18 yr+, diastolic BP is 85–90 mm Hg, 1 or more CHD risk factors present	Every 1–2 yr Every yr
Mammography	Breast cancer	*Routine:* 50–75 yr+	Every yr (ACP, CTF, ACOG)
		40–50 yr	Every 1–2 yr (USPSTF, ACOG)
		High Risk: 10 yr prior to the onset of breast cancer in a first-degree family member	Every yr (ACS)
Papanicolaou Smear	Cervical cancer	*Routine:* 18 yr+, no other risk factors	Every 1–3 yr
		High Risk: 18 yr+ with presence of risk factors	Every yr
Hemocult	Colorectal cancer	40 yr+ (ACOG)	Every yr
Sigmoidoscopy	Colorectal cancer	*Routine:* 50 yr+ (ACP)	Every 3–5 yr (ACP)
		High Risk: 40 yr+ (CTF), 50 yr+ (USPSTF), history of one first-degree family member with colon cancer or personal history of endometrial, ovarian, or breast cancer	Every 3–5 yr (CTF, USPSTF)
Colonoscopy	Colorectal cancer	*Very High Risk:* More than one first-degree family member with colon cancer, especially if younger than 40 years at diagnosis; familial polyposis	Every 3–5 yr (ACP, CTF, USPSTF)

(continued)

Table 1-1. Prevention and Screening Recommendations for Women *(Continued)*

Intervention	Health Condition	Target Group	Recommendations
		coli; personal history of colon cancer; ulcerative colitis, 10 yr of adenomatous polyps	
Nonfasting Cholesterol	CHD	*Routine:* 18 yr+ (ACP, USPSTF)	Every 5 yr
		High Risk: 18 yr+, 1 or more CHD risk factors	More frequently (ACP, USPSTF) individual clinical judgment (CTF)

ACOG = American College of Obstetricians and Gynecologists; ACP = American College of Physicians; ACS = American Cancer Society; CHD = congenital heart disease; CTF = Canadian Task Force; and USPSTF = United States Preventive Services Task Force

(Adapted with permission from Lemcke D.P., Pattison J., Marshall L.A., & Crowley D.S. [Eds.]. [1995]. *Primary care of women* [pp. 51–52]. Norwalk, CT: Appleton & Lange.)

tion and Screening Recommendations for Women, has been thoroughly evaluated by the Canadian Task Force (CTF), the United States Preventive Services Task Force (USPSTF), the American College of Physicians (ACP),[2] the American College of Obstetricians and Gynecologists (ACOG), and the American Cancer Society (ACS). The table emphasizes services for which the evidence of prevention is the strongest.

 CONTRACEPTION

I. **Discussion of Contraception.** Discuss contraception with patients
   A. At the annual exam.
   B. When the patient comes to the office for a pregnancy test.
   C. During the last trimester of pregnancy.
   D. During the first few days postpartum.
   E. At the postpartum office visit, usually at 6 weeks.
   F. At any other time the patient requests it.

II. **Method Desired.** Unless the patient is absolutely sure which contraceptive method she desires (or if she desires not to use contraception), include the following in the patient visit:

---

[2]Eddy, 1991

A. Contraceptive history
1. What methods has the patient used in the past?
2. How long did she use each method?
3. Were there any complications from any method?
4. What was her level of satisfaction with each method?
5. Why did she discontinue using each method?
6. Would she consider using a method she has used in the past? Why or why not?

B. Health history

C. Physical exam if not done within the past year

D. Lab work
1. Pap smear
2. Hematocrit, if indicated
3. Gonococcus (GC) and chlamydia screening, if indicated

E. Counseling: Offer information about methods the patient has not used and give her a handout comparing methods. Factors that may influence her selection include the following:
1. Social and cultural trends
    a. Interest in a method that is currently popular
    b. Family background
    c. Lifestyle
    d. Partner cooperativeness with contraception
2. Religion: Prohibition of some, or all, methods
3. Psychological factors
    a. Negative or positive feelings about certain methods
    b. Recent negative publicity about a certain method
    c. Unfavorable past experience with a certain method
4. Technicalities
    a. Ease of use (may or may not be an important consideration)
    b. Ability to master the technique involved in using certain methods
    c. Access to medical care
5. Frequency of sexual intercourse and number of partners
    a. If sex is infrequent, a barrier method may be preferable to the upkeep and potential complications of other methods.
    b. If the patient has multiple partners, she is at greater risk for STDs and pelvic inflammatory disease (PID). An intrauterine device (IUD) would not be an ideal choice, but barrier methods may provide some protection.
6. Ability to comply with the requirements of a contraceptive method. Examine whether the patient is likely to use a coitus-related method or remember to take a pill every day.
7. Length of anticipated use of a contraceptive method. If needed for only a few months, an IUD or Norplant may not be the best choice.

8. Possible side effects and questions of safety related to the method

   a. The patient must decide what risks she is willing to take.

   b. Both positive and negative side effects should be discussed.

9. Effectiveness of a contraceptive method. This would be a high priority if a subsequent pregnancy would be unacceptable and if abortion is not an option.

10. Cost of contraceptive method: Will her insurance company pay for this method?

11. Reversibility of a contraceptive method:

    a. Some methods require a longer waiting period before fertility returns.

    b. Sterilization can sometimes be reversed with surgery but should be considered permanent.

 ## CONTRACEPTIVE METHODS

I. Abstinence

  A. Definition: Abstinence is the lack of genital contact that could prevent pregnancy.

  B. Effectiveness: 100%

  C. Advantage: If personal choice, can increase self-esteem

  D. Disadvantages

    1. Sexual frustration may occur.

    2. Partner may disapprove.

    3. Patient may be unprepared if decision is to have intercourse.

    4. Adolescents may need counseling, support, and a firm belief system to comply.

II. Cervical Cap

  A. Definition: The cervical cap is a barrier method of contraception, similar to the diaphragm, except that it fits over just the cervix to prevent sperm from entering the uterus.

  B. Effectiveness: The effectiveness rate is about 90%. Effectiveness increases with the length of time a person has used this method. Older women report a higher success rate.

  C. Advantages

    1. It can be left in place from 24 to 36 hours.

    2. It does not require oral or injectable hormones.

  D. Disadvantages

    1. There are only four sizes, with internal diameters of 22, 25, 28 and 31 cm, making it difficult to fit.

    2. Because of cervical position, size, and so on, only 50% of women can be fitted.

    3. Manual dexterity is needed to properly place the cervical cap.

    4. After 12 to 24 hours in place, the cervical cap may cause an increased incidence of foul-smelling discharge.

    5. It should not be used on heavy flow days of the menstrual period because this may cause menstrual regurgitation into the fallopian tubes and predispose the patient to endometriosis. It should be removed 6 to 8 hours after intercourse on lighter flow days.

    6. It has been implicated in cervical ulcers and spread of human papilloma virus (HPV).

    7. It may provide less protection from STDs than a diaphragm.

E. Management

    1. After the patient has been fitted, she needs to demonstrate an ability to insert the cap, check for correct position, and remove it.

    2. Patients who have had an abnormal Pap smear or history of HPV on the cervix with treatment by cryosurgery, laser, or loop electrosurgical excision procedure (LEEP) are not good candidates for the cervical cap.

F. Teaching

    1. Proper care of the cap is the same as for the diaphragm.

    2. Pregnancy or a weight loss or gain over 30 pounds may change the cervix. Refitting may be necessary.

III. Combined Monthly Contraceptive Injection (Lunelle)

A. Definition: Lunelle (25 mg medroxyprogesterone acetate and 5 mg estradiol cypionate) is a once-a-month intramuscular (IM) injectable suspension with actions similar to those of oral contraceptives.

B. Effectiveness: 99% to 99.6%

C. Advantages

    1. Is not affected by antibiotics and other medicines because it uses a different pathway

    2. Has a safety and side effect profile similar to birth control pills (BCPs)

    3. Provides immediate contraception; requires no backup method

    4. Is convenient and private; does not require daily pill taking

    5. Provides quick return to fertility in 2 to 4 months after last injection

    6. Allows return to regular menstrual cycle one to two cycles after discontinuation

D. Disadvantages

    1. May cause increased spotting, especially during the first month

    2. Requires an injection every 28 days, plus or minus 5 days

    3. Causes side effects similar to those for BCPs

    4. Does not protect against STDs

E. Management

    1. Questions and contraindications are similar to those for BCPs.

2. The initial injection must be within 5 days of start of menses.
3. The patient should be informed that no backup method is necessary.
4. The patient must return to the office or inject herself every 28 days, plus or minus 5 days.
   a. The injection should not be given before 23 days.
   b. If the patient returns after 33 days, consider the following:
      (1) If the patient was not sexually active during the previous 2 weeks, do a sensitive pregnancy test and, if negative, give an injection.
      (2) If the patient has been sexually active during the previous 2 weeks, advise her to abstain for the next 2 weeks (some policies allow sexual activity if a condom is used) and then return for a sensitive pregnancy test. If the test is negative at that time, an injection may be given.

IV. **Combined Oral Contraceptives**
   A. Definition: Birth control pills (BCPs) are synthetic steroids similar to the estrogens and progestins that are natural female sex hormones. These steroids are used in doses and in combinations that provide contraception by inhibiting ovulation, implantation, or both.
   B. Effectiveness
      1. Theoretical: 99.5% to 100%
      2. Use: 90% to 96%, probably resulting from errors in usage
   C. Advantages
      1. Provide menstrual benefits
         a. Less dysmenorrhea and premenstrual tension
         b. Lighter periods, resulting in less anemia
         c. Regularity of menstrual periods
      2. Are totally self-reliant; do not require partner cooperation
      3. Are not coitus related; allow for spontaneity
      4. Afford protection from illnesses
         a. Decreased risk of PID after being on the pill for 1 year
         b. Decreased risk of endometrial and ovarian cancer
         c. Decreased incidence of ovarian cysts
         d. Decreased incidence of fibroadenomas of the breast and fibrocystic breast disease
      5. Can be used to manipulate timing and frequency of menses
      6. Can be used in the treatment of menstrual irregularities, acne, ovarian cysts, anemia, and hirsutism, as well as many other conditions
   D. Disadvantages
      1. Memory requirement to take the pill daily
      2. Psychological side effects, such as decreased libido, mood changes, irritability, fatigue, and increased premenstrual syndrome (PMS)

3. Physical side effects

   a. Nausea and vomiting: may disappear after two to three cycles

   b. Breast tenderness: may also improve after two to three cycles

   c. Headaches: may increase in frequency and intensity

   d. Spider veins: varicosities may increase

4. Medical complications

   a. Deep vein thrombosis (DVT): There is an association between estrogen and DVT; however, the risk of DVT is very low with BCPs because the estrogen dose is low.

   b. Myocardial infarction (MI) and stroke[3]

   (1) Low-dose BCPs rarely increase the risk of acute MI in healthy women less than 35 years of age—3 per million nonsmokers and 35 per million smokers.

   (2) Smokers over 35 should not use BCPs; they should be encouraged to stop smoking. They have an increased risk of MI or stroke at a rate of 396 occurrences per million versus 88 per million in nonsmokers over 35 years of age.

   c. Hypertension with birth control initiation in 1% of patients. This is reversible, in most cases, after discontinuation.

E. Contraindications

   1. Absolute contraindications

      a. Known or suspected carcinoma of the breast

      b. Known or suspected estrogen-dependent neoplasia

      c. Thromboembolic disease or thrombophlebitis, cerebral vascular disease, coronary artery disease, or history of these conditions

      d. Undiagnosed uterine bleeding

      e. Known or suspected pregnancy

      f. Impaired liver function or hepatic disease

   2. Relative contraindications

      a. Hypertension

      b. Migraine headaches

      c. Diabetes or prediabetes

      d. Epilepsy or convulsions

      e. Active gallbladder disease

      f. Active-phase mononucleosis

      g. Sickle cell trait or disease

      h. Age 35 to 40 and heavy smoker (>10 cigarettes per day)

      i. Breast-feeding (may decrease milk supply)

F. Management

   1. Initiation of the pill

      a. The patient should be a candidate for BCPs, as determined by her history and physical exam.

---

[3]Nelson & Hatcher, 2000

    b. The most appropriate BCP should be selected.

       (1) The majority of women will be able to take most, if not all, combined oral contraceptives (BCPs).

       (2) In general, a BCP should be prescribed with 35 μg of estrogen or less and a low-potency progestin.

       (3) If the patient has previously taken a particular BCP that worked well, it should be prescribed again when possible.

       (4) Table 1-2, Oral Contraceptives: Complicating Factors and Recommendations, provides information for selecting the most appropriate pill based on the patient's history and known medical complications.

2. Instructions for starting BCPs

    a. If the patient is having menstrual cycles, she should take her first pill on the first Sunday or any day that is no more than 6 days after her period starts.

    b. If the patient is postpartum, she should start the pills on the second to sixth postpartum week to minimize the chance of thrombophlebitis. Cesarean section patients should start the pills at 6 weeks postpartum.

    c. If the patient is less than 12 weeks postpartum but still amenorrheic because of breast-feeding, she may start the pill anytime.

    d. If the patient is postabortion (spontaneous or induced), she should start the pills within 7 days.

    e. If the patient is going to take BCPs, she should consider the following guidelines:

       (1) 28-day pack—Take one pill every day, preferably about the same time every day. When one pack has been completed, start a new pack.

       (2) 21-day pack—Take one pill every day, preferably about the same time. When one pack has been completed, take no pills for 7 days. On the eighth day, start a new pack.

       (3) Continuous dosing—This practice may be recommended for social reasons or for menorrhagia, dysmenorrhea, menstrual migraines, endometriosis, anorexia, or severe anemia. Use either a 21- or 28-day pack, taking only the 21 days of active pills. Discard nonactive pills from the 28-day pack. After completing the active pills in a pack, start a fresh pack the next day. This practice may be repeated for two to three cycles. It is recommended that withdrawal bleeding be allowed by the end of the third cycle; the patient will have a "free" week from pills. After no more than 1 week, restart BCPs as before. Some recommend stopping for 4 days and then restarting the active pills.[4]

(text continues on page 18)

---

[4]Hatcher et al., 1998

Table 1-2. Starting Oral Contraceptives: Complicating Factors and Recommendations

Complicating Factors	Comments	Recommendations	Brands
Acne	Increased androgen levels increase serum production, leading to pimples and acne as well as increased hair growth.	Give pills with moderate to high estrogen and with low progestins.	Ortho Tri-Cyclen—received FDA approval* Alesse—pending FDA approval† Others: Ortho-Cyclen, Ovcon 35, Tri-Levlen
Breakthrough Bleeding and Spotting	If it occurs on days 1–10 of active pills, suspect estrogen deficiency. If it occurs on days 10–21 of active pills, suspect progestin deficiency.	Use a continuous dose (35 mcg of estrogen) of a monophasic agent. Use a pill that has low endometrial effect with high progestin. Triphasic pills with moderate estrogen and low progestin have been found to work well.	Lo/Oval Ortho-Cyclen Levlen Estrostep Fe Ortho Tri-Cyclen Triphasil Tri-Levlen
Breast Feeding	A small amount of hormone passes through the milk; this is not significant.‡ Progestin-only pills have the least effect on breast-fed babies. There is a potential for suppression of the milk supply with combined BCPs.	Reassure the mother, and if she is still concerned, consider another method. Offer a depot medroxyprogesterone acetate (DMPA) injection or progestin-only BCPs. Consider starting pills 4–6 weeks postpartum after milk has been established; low dose is preferred.	Micronor Nor-QD Alesse Tri-Norinyl

(continued)

Table 1-2. Starting Oral Contraceptives: Complicating Factors and Recommendations (*Continued*)

Complicating Factors	Comments	Recommendations	Brands
Depression	Depression may be exacerbated by a possible progestin excess.	Start patient on pill with low progestin/androgen content.	Ortho Tri-Cyclen Triphasil Tri-Levlen Ortho-Cyclen
Diabetes and Glucose Intolerance	BCP use slightly increases insulin resistance.

There is no evidence that BCP use increases cardiovascular or renal complications in women with insulin-dependent diabetes.§

Women with diabetes who use BCPs have a slightly higher risk of MI or stroke than women without diabetes who use BCPs. | Start low dose, low progestin and low androgen pill. | Alesse Loestrin 1/20 Brevicon Nelova 0.5/35 Tri-Norinyl |
| *Endometriosis* | In patients with endometriosis, the aim is to create a pseudopregnancy state when using BCPs. | Recommend monophasic BCPs with high progestins.

Consider continuous use of active pills without a break. Pill use may stop for 4–7 days when breakthrough bleeding occurs. | Loestrin 1/20 Loestrin 1.5/30 |
| *Headache— Premenstrual, Migraine (without focal neurologic symptoms)* | Headaches have many different causes. | Explore possible causes such as current medications. If there is a prior headache history, give low-dose monophasic pills and monitor patient carefully for an increase in severity or frequency of headaches. | Loestrin 1/20 |

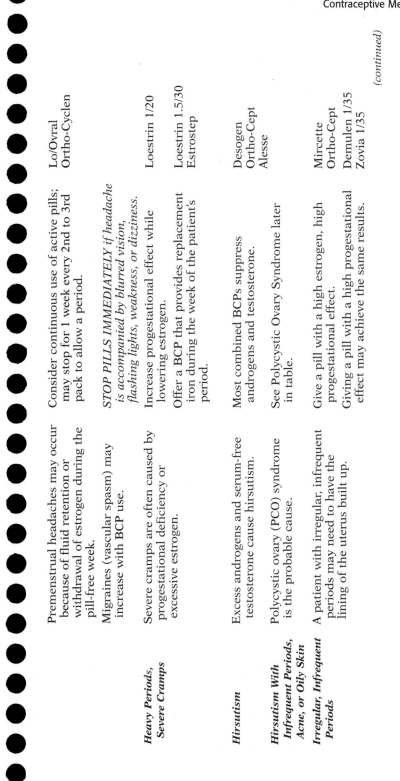

Condition	Explanation	Management	Pills
	Premenstrual headaches may occur because of fluid retention or withdrawal of estrogen during the pill-free week.	Consider continuous use of active pills; may stop for 1 week every 2nd to 3rd pack to allow a period.	Lo/Ovral Ortho-Cyclen
	Migraines (vascular spasm) may increase with BCP use.	*STOP PILLS IMMEDIATELY if headache is accompanied by blurred vision, flashing lights, weakness, or dizziness.*	
Heavy Periods, Severe Cramps	Severe cramps are often caused by progestational deficiency or excessive estrogen.	Increase progestational effect while lowering estrogen.	Loestrin 1/20
		Offer a BCP that provides replacement iron during the week of the patient's period.	Loestrin 1.5/30 Estrostep
Hirsutism	Excess androgens and serum-free testosterone cause hirsutism.	Most combined BCPs suppress androgens and testosterone.	Desogen Ortho-Cept Alesse
Hirsutism With Infrequent Periods, Acne, or Oily Skin	Polycystic ovary (PCO) syndrome is the probable cause.	See Polycystic Ovary Syndrome later in table.	
Irregular, Infrequent Periods	A patient with irregular, infrequent periods may need to have the lining of the uterus built up.	Give a pill with a high estrogen, high progestational effect.	Mircette Ortho-Cept
		Giving a pill with a high progestational effect may achieve the same results.	Demulen 1/35 Zovia 1/35

(continued)

Table 1-2. Starting Oral Contraceptives: Complicating Factors and Recommendations (*Continued*)

Complicating Factors	Comments	Recommendations	Brands
Medications: Antibiotics, especially PCN and sulfa Anticoagulants Antidepressants Antihistamines Carbamazepine Dilantin Griseofulvin Primidone Rifampin St. John's Wort Tegretol Topiramate	Medications may decrease the effectiveness of BCPs. The drugs listed at left change how the liver works or lower the body's ability to absorb the hormones.	If the patient is on medication for a short period of time, recommend a backup method. If the patient is using medication on a long-term basis, consider a high-dose pill. Use active pills only on a continuous 2- to 3-cycle basis; monophasic works best in this situation.	Condoms, foam Oral Ogestrel Zovia 1/50 Ovcon 50
History of Nausea or Vomiting in Pregnancy or With Prior Pill Use	Nausea or vomiting is related to estrogen. It often gets better after three cycles of BCPs. It can also occur when pills are restarted after a hormone-free week.	Take pill with food or at night. Determine which pill caused nausea and change the pill. Choose a pill with low estrogen and endometrial acitivity.	Alesse Levlite Mircette Estrostep Loestrin 1/20
Perimenopausal Signs in Nonsmoker Over Age 35	Hormones in BCPs will regulate the menses and can also relieve signs and symptoms of menopause (e.g., hot flashes, anxiety).	Choose a low-dose pill	Loestrin 1/20 Alesse

Condition	Description	Recommendation	Products
Polycystic Ovary Syndrome (PCO)	Suppression of the menstrual cycle through use of BCPs can counteract polycystic ovary syndrome.	Use a high-dose pill. Consider continuous use of active pills.	Ovral Ogestrel Demulen 1/50 Zovia 1/50
Premenstrual Syndrome (PMS)—Anxiety, Irritability, Moodiness	All pills can cause PMS symptoms; the primary cause is usually progestin excess. Improper estrogen amounts can also result in MS symptoms. Changing the amount of hormones taken on a weekly basis may increase the problem.	A monophasic pill is the best alternative. The patient may be placed on a continuous dose regimen. See instructions on how to take BCPs.	Lo/Ovral Ortho-Cept Ovcon
Smoker Younger Than 35	Smoking increases a woman's risk for deep venous thrombosis, MI, and stroke.	Counsel the patient regarding smoking; suggest alternate methods of birth control. If the patient insists on taking BCPs, give her low-dose estrogen.	DMPA, IUD Loestrin 1/20 Alesse Levlite Mircette
Smoker Older Than 35	If a woman smokes and is older than 35, the risk of disease outweighs the benefits of BCP use.	Do not give combined BCPs. Counsel the patient to use other methods of birth control.	See Progestin Only Pills in Part I Tubal ligation, DMPA, IUD, barrier method
Weight Gain	Excessive progesterone or androgen may be the cause.	Suggest a pill low in progesterone and androgen.	Ortho Tri-Cyclen Ortho-Cept

*Redmond GP, Olson WH, Lippman JS, Kafrissen ME, Jones TM, Jorizzo JL. (1997). Norgestimate and ethinyl estradiol in the treatment of acne vulgaris: A randomized placebo-controlled trial. *Obstetrics and Gynecology, 89* (4), 615.

†American Health Consultants. (2001, April). *Contraceptive Technology Update, 22* (4).

‡American Academy of Pediatrics / American College of Obstetricians and Gynecologists. (1992). *Guidelines for perinatal care* (3rd ed.). Elk Grove Village, IL: American Academy of Pediatrics.

§Dickey, R. (2000). *Managing contraceptive pill patients* (10th ed.). New Orleans: EMIS Medical Publishers.

(4) Missed-pill instructions

(a) If one active pill is missed, take it as soon as it is remembered. Take the rest of pills at their normal time. Use a backup contraception method for 7 days.

(b) If two active pills are missed, take one as soon as the missing pills are remembered. Take one later that day, one the next morning, and one later the next evening. Take the rest of the pills at their normal time. Use a backup contraception method for the rest of the pack.

(c) If three or more pills are missed and the patient has had sex during that time, consider emergency contraceptive pills (ECPs).

(d) If three or more active pills are missed, follow these guidelines:[5]

(i) Tell Sunday pill starters to keep taking one pill each day until the following Sunday. On Sunday, they should throw out the rest of the pack and start a new pack of pills that day.

(ii) Tell Day 1 starters to throw out the rest of the pack immediately and start a new pack that day.

(iii) Counsel the patient that she may not have a period this month. However, if she misses her period 2 months in a row, a pregnancy test is needed.

(e) According to the "Seven Day Rule" developed by British family planning providers, women are most likely to become pregnant when they start a pill pack late (more than 7 days without an active pill) or miss pills in the third week of the active pills. If two or more pills are missed during the third week of active pills, the next pack of active pills should be started the next day.[6] This prevents the patient from having more than 7 days without an active pill.

3. Printed instructions: Give the patient printed instructions that include

a. The importance of using an alternate method of contraception for the first 7 days that active pills are taken.

b. A description on how to take the BCPs, including how to manage common errors in administration.

c. An explanation that any side effects she experiences will depend on how her particular body responds to the certain BCP that she is taking. Many side effects resolve after the second and third cycles.

d. A list of medications that affect hormone metabolism of the BCP, including both over-the-counter (OTC) and prescribed medications.

---

[5]Physician's Desk Reference, 2001
[6]American Health Consultants, April 2001

    e. Instructions to inform other caregivers that she is taking BCPs, prior to receiving any other prescribed or OTC medications.

    f. Signs indicating when to call the office. Be sure the patient is aware of the cardinal warning signs of BCP complications, as listed in Display 1-1.

    g. The date to return for a follow-up visit.

    h. A copy of the signed BCP consent form.

4. Follow-up

    a. Between the first 6 to 12 weeks of BCP usage, the patient should be checked for the following:

        (1) Weight: An unexplained gain or loss of 10 pounds or more in 1 month requires further investigation.

        (2) Blood pressure: If blood pressure is abnormal, 135/85 or higher, and the patient is not on medication, she needs close follow-up.

    b. Breakthrough bleeding should be managed as follows:

        (1) Because the bleeding may resolve spontaneously within 3 months, advise patient to wait unless very heavy bleeding is noted.

        (2) If breakthrough bleeding is still present in fourth cycle, the pill needs to be switched:

            (a) Bleeding early in the cycle may be caused by an estrogen deficiency. Change to a pill with increased estrogen potency.

            (b) Bleeding late in the cycle may be caused by estrogen or progesterone. See Table 1-2.

    c. Management of amenorrhea

        (1) Pill-induced amenorrhea

            (a) Do a pregnancy test to confirm or rule out pregnancy.

            (b) Remember-any discharge, including brown spotting, is a period.

            (c) Try switching pills to another brand, preferably one with an increased estrogen effect.

            (d) Add 1 to 2 mg of Estrace or another estrogen to days 1 to 21 of the BCPs for one to two cycles.

DISPLAY 1-1   Cardinal Warning Signs of BCP Complications

Severe abdominal pain
Severe chest pain
Shortness of breath
Severe headaches
Blurred vision
Leg pain (calf or thigh)
Liver disease or hepatitis

(2) Postpill-induced amenorrhea

   (a) Consider that this condition is usually limited to 6 months or less.

   (b) Reassure the patient.

   (c) If more than 6 months have passed since the last pill was taken, see Amenorrhea in Part IV.

V. Condom—Female

A. Definition: The female condom is a single-use polyurethane sheath with a movable inner ring at closed end, which is inserted into the vagina. The large fixed ring remains outside to cover part of the introitus.

B. Effectiveness: 80%

C. Advantages

   1. Provides significant protection against STDs and viral infections such as hepatitis. May decrease the risk of herpes simplex virus 2 (HSV2), HIV, and HPV.

   2. Does not require a prescription

D. Disadvantages

   1. High pregnancy rate

   2. Cost

   3. Noise—extra lubrication may help

E. Management

   1. Place condom carefully and correctly.

   2. If breakage occurs, consider ECPs. If available, also consider immediately placing foam, film, or suppository in vagina.

VI. Condom—Male

A. Definition: The male condom is a latex, polyurethane, or natural membrane sheath worn over the penis in coitus to prevent impregnation or infection.

   1. Ninety-nine percent of condoms are made of latex, which provides protection against pregnancy because sperm cannot penetrate the condom. Organisms that cause STDs, HPV, and HIV do not penetrate latex condoms but may penetrate condoms made from intestine (e.g., Natural Skin).

   2. Some condoms come with spermicide, which increases their effectiveness.

B. Effectiveness: 85% to 89%

   1. Inconsistent use accounts for most failures.

   2. Breakage has been reported from as low as 1 to as high as 12 per 100 episodes of vaginal intercourse.

   3. Because leakage of sperm may occur with arousal, the condom must be worn before sexual contact.

C. Advantages

   1. Provide significant protection against STDs and viral infections such as hepatitis. May decrease the risk of HSV2, HIV, and HPV.

2. Are cheap

3. Are easily available—sold OTC

D. Disadvantages

1. There are more effective methods to prevent pregnancy.

2. Condoms must be applied to penis just before intercourse.

3. Up to 5% of the population have an allergic response to either the latex or the spermicide.

E. Management

1. Condoms must be used every time before sexual intercourse.

2. Use with spermicide is recommended because effectiveness is increased by 5% to 7%.

3. Directions for each individual spermicide need to be read and followed exactly concerning time of insertion, length of effectiveness, and so on.

4. Breakage or slippage

    a. Prevent problems by using the correct size and by careful, correct application.

    b. If available, immediately place foam, film, or suppository in vagina.

    c. Consider ECPs.

VII. Depo-Provera Contraceptive Injection

A. Definition: This injection consists of a depot medroxyprogesterone acetate (DMPA) suspension.

B. Effectiveness: Less than 1% of patients using Depo-Provera will become pregnant provided they receive their injection every 12 weeks.

C. Advantages

1. Does not contain estrogen

2. Protects for 12 weeks with one injection of 150 mg IM

3. Is convenient

4. Is reversible: 66% of former Depo-Provera users can be expected to become pregnant within 1 year of their last injection. Ninety-three percent will be pregnant within 24 months.

5. Can be used by nursing mothers

6. Does not tend to increase blood pressure, frequency of seizures, and most migraines

7. Is recommended for patients who smoke more than 10 cigarettes per day, especially if over 35 years of age

D. Disadvantages

1. Irregular or unpredictable bleeding

    a. Bleeding usually lessens over time but continues to be irregular.

    b. Amenorrhea may result in 60% to 80% of users by 1 year.

    c. Heavy bleeding occurs in 0.5% of users.

      d. Users experience a slow return to fertility; discourage use by those desiring pregnancy within 1 to 2 years.

   2. Decreased calcium and minerals stored in bones; this effect is reversible upon discontinuation.

   3. Other side effects

      a. Increased appetite (may gain weight)

      b. Headaches

      c. Temporary hair loss

      d. Stomach cramps: Often noted within the first 2 weeks of the injection and tend to decrease until the next injection

      e. Fatigue

      f. Decreased sex drive

   4. No protection against STDs

E. Contraindications

   1. Pregnancy

   2. Allergy to Depo-Provera

   3. Current liver disease

   4. Undiagnosed uterine bleeding

F. Management

   1. Use

      a. Administer 150 mg of DMPA IM every 12 weeks.

      b. Start medication within 5 days of a menstrual cycle or within 4 weeks after delivery if patient is not breast-feeding. Counsel the patient that DMPA is not effective for 24 hours after receiving the injection.

      c. If the patient has amenorrhea, suggest she receive a pregnancy test before her next injection.

      d. If the patient is overdue for her injection by 6 or more days (some policies suggest 14 days), advise patient that she needs to have abstained from sexually activity (or have used another form of protection) for the previous 2 weeks. A negative pregnancy test after this period will allow a restart of Depo-Provera.

      e. Counsel patient to increase calcium to 1000 to 1200 mg daily. Dietary intake is preferred, but two Tums per day will suffice.

      f. Warn patient that her first period after discontinuation of DMPA may be lighter, heavier, or longer than her previous periods. Bad cramping, bloating, and gas are common.

   2. Side effects

      a. For breakthrough bleeding, the following may be helpful:

        (1) Take 600 to 800 mg of Motrin (ibuprofen) orally three times a day for 5 to 7 days.

        (2) Consider one to two cycles of low-dose BCPs.

        (3) If breakthrough bleeding only occurs 2 to 3 weeks prior to the next injection, give the injection early.

(4) Many patients on seizure medication experience breakthrough bleeding at 10 to 11 weeks because of increased clearance of DMPA. Suggest routinely giving DMPA every 10 weeks to these patients.

b. For post-Depo-Provera amenorrhea (6 months after last injection), the following may be helpful:

(1) Before 6 months, reassure the patient that it sometimes takes awhile for her periods to restart.

(2) After 6 months, consider BCPs after ruling out pregnancy. If the patient does not have withdrawal bleeding after the second cycle, adding 1 to 2 mg of estradiol (Estrace) or other estrogen to the first 3 weeks of the BCP may prime the endometrium.

VIII. Diaphragm

A. Definition: A diaphragm is a small rubber cup with a rim stabilized by a rubber-covered steel spring. It fits in the vaginal vault, forming a barrier between the sperm and the cervix. It is used with spermicidal jelly or cream to increase effectiveness.

B. Effectiveness

1. Theoretical: 97%
2. Use: 85%

C. Advantages

1. Minimal side effects
2. Protection against STDs

D. Disadvantages

1. Discomfort from poorly fitted diaphragm
2. Perceived interference with spontaneity of lovemaking
3. Perceived messiness
4. Potential source of bladder infections
5. Professional fitting required
6. Refitting necessary after a baby, pelvic surgery, or a weight loss or gain of more than 20 pounds

E. Contraindications

1. Absolute

   a. Allergy to rubber, spermicide, or both
   b. Inability of patient or partner to learn correct insertion technique
   c. Recurrent urinary tract infections (UTIs)
   d. Inability to achieve satisfactory fitting
   e. History of toxic shock syndrome
   f. Severe uterine prolapse, anteversion, or retroversion
   g. Severe cystocele
   h. Rectal or vaginal fistulas

2. Temporary

    a. Postpartum involution incomplete: Wait at least 6 weeks after delivery before fitting and longer if involution did not occur normally.

    b. Pelvic infection or surgery (e.g., PID, spontaneous): Wait until condition resolves, usually about 1 month.

    c. Inability of the patient to feel comfortable touching genitals

F. Management

  1. Diaphragm fitting

    a. Determine if the patient is a candidate for a diaphragm, by using the screening process outlined above.

    b. Select the most appropriate type of diaphragm.

      (1) ALL-FLEX arcing spring diaphragm (Ortho)

        (a) Provides the most support and, therefore, is useful for a patient with less than adequate vaginal or uterine support (almost any woman who has had a vaginal delivery)

        (b) May be used by all women except those with exceptionally firm vaginal tone and those who find the arcing spring uncomfortable

      (2) Flat spring diaphragm (Ortho)

        (a) Requires strong vaginal support

        (b) Is useful for patients with a shallow arch behind the symphysis pubis

      (3) Coil spring diaphragm (Ortho)

        (a) May have average vaginal support

        (b) Is useful for patients with a deep arch behind the symphysis pubis

      (4) Wide seal arcing diaphragm (Milex)

        (a) Is useful for most patients

        (b) Claims to make a more effective seal

    c. Fit the patient with the diaphragm, using the following technique:

      (1) During bimanual exam, introduce the third finger into the posterior fornix and tilt the wrist upward to mark where the index finger makes contact with the back of the symphysis. Use the measurement from the tip of your middle finger to the contact point on the index finger as a guide to select the size of diaphragm to use.

      (2) Place cream in the diaphragm to use as a lubricant and place it into the vagina. Lodge the diaphragm behind the symphysis and check to ensure that it completely covers the cervix.

      (3) Have the patient bear down and cough while feeling the diaphragm to ensure that it does not move from behind the pubic arch.

    d. If this is the first time the patient has used a diaphragm, show her where her cervix is and have her practice inserting and removing the diaphragm. Check for proper placement.

    e. Give the patient printed instructions, which include information on

      (1) How to insert, remove, and care for the diaphragm.

      (2) How to use the diaphragm.

      (3) How to avoid toxic shock syndrome:

        (a) Do not wear the diaphragm during menses.

        (b) Avoid leaving the diaphragm in place longer than 24 hours.

        (c) If the cardinal warning signs of toxic shock syndrome appear, as listed in Display 1-2, call the health care provider or seek other medical help immediately.

2. Follow-up: If this is the first time the patient has used a diaphragm, instruct her to return in 2 to 4 weeks with the diaphragm in place. Check for proper placement and ask her about any problems she may have encountered. Instruct the patient to return at any time if she has difficulty with the diaphragm or

    a. She experiences any discomfort.

    b. Her diaphragm is damaged, deteriorating, or more than 2 years old.

    c. Her diaphragm needs to be refitted

      (1) After having a baby.

      (2) After any pelvic surgery.

      (3) After gaining or losing 20 pounds or more.

      (4) If the diaphragm was initially fitted before the patient had experienced at least 20 acts of coitus.

    d. She desires a different method of contraception.

IX. Emergency Contraception (ECPs)

A. Definition: Emergency contraceptives are true contraceptives in that they prevent pregnancy, by thickening cervical mucus, supressing ovulation and thinning the endometrium to inhibit implantation. ECPs will not cause an abortion or hurt the fetus if the patient is already pregnant.[7]

B. Effectiveness: ECPs should be given within 72 hours of unprotected sex. The effectiveness decreases the later the ECPs are given from exposure. Combined oral contraceptives, at 92% to 96%, are slightly less effective than progestin-only pills, which are 95% to 98% effective.

DISPLAY 1-2   **Cardinal Warning Signs of Toxic Shock Syndrome**

Fever (temperature of 101°F or more)
Diarrhea
Vomiting
Muscle aches
Sunburn-like rash

---

[7]American Health Consultants, April 2001, p. 4

C. Advantage: Prevention of pregnancy
D. Disadvantages
    1. Changed menses: The next cycle may be early, light, or heavy.
    2. Similar side effects or complications as those of BCPs: While ECPs will act on a shorter duration, the side effects are similar.
E. Management
    1. ECPs cannot be given if the patient has contraindications to BCPs.
    2. ECPs should be taken no later than 72 hours after unprotected sex.
    3. Table 1-3 should be consulted for the number and timing of pills by brand.
    4. If the patient has a history of nausea with BCPs, she should take 25 to 50 mg of Dramamine or Bonamine 1 hour prior to taking the ECPs. They should not be taken on an empty stomach.
    5. If contraception is desired, the patient should consider the following factors:
        a. A DMPA injection may be given the same day. A sensitive pregnancy test is required 2 to 3 weeks later. Some policies require that the patient wait for menses and then initiate DMPA within 5 days.
        b. BCPs may be started the following day. She should use a backup method for 7 days. Some policies require that the patient wait for menses and then initiate BCPs within 7 days.
        c. If the patient has missed several BCPs, she may restart her BCPs the next day without the need to make up for missed pills. She should use a backup method for 7 days.
        d. If the patient desires an IUD, is a candidate, and guidelines do not require prior chlamydia or gonorrhea testing, an IUD may be inserted up to 5 days after unprotected sex.
    6. Counseling
        a. If her period does not start within 3 to 4 weeks or the week after her inactive pills, urge the patient to return for a pregnancy test. Give her the signs and symptoms of pregnancy.

Table 1-3. Emergency Contraception

Brand Name	No. of Pills to Swallow ASAP	No. of Pills to Swallow 12 hr later
Plan B (progestin only)	1	1
Levlen	4	4
Lo/Ovral	4	4
Nordette	4	4
Ovral	2	2
Preven	2	2
Tri-Levlen (yellow pills only) Triphasil	4	4

    b. If the patient has been exposed to STDs, encourage condom use.

    c. Encourage consideration of a more effective birth control method.

X. Intrauterine Device (IUD)

    A. Definition: An IUD is a contraceptive device made of plastic with barium sulfate (for visibility on x-rays or sonography) and either copper (Cu T 380A ParaGard by Ortho), progesterone (Progesterone T Progestasert System by the ALZA Corporation), or levonorgestrel (Mirena by Berlex). It is introduced into the endometrial cavity through the cervical canal and has a monofilament nylon tail that protrudes from the cervix into the vagina. The IUD works primarily by preventing sperm from fertilizing the ova. All three IUDs do this by creating a local infection and increasing uterine and tubal fluids that alter transportation of sperm and ova. In addition, Mirena and Progestasert thicken cervical mucus and alter the endometrial lining, interfering with sperm motility.

    B. Effectiveness

      1. 97% to 99% effective

      2. Length of effectiveness

        a. ParaGard—Approved for 10 years of use

        b. Mirena—Approved for 5 years of use

        c. Progestasert—Approved for 1 year of use

    C. Advantages

      1. Relatively carefree method

      2. Highly effective

      3. Mirena

        a. Decreased bleeding over time: 20% will have amenorrhea after 1 year.

        b. Adjunct therapy possibilities for perimenopausal therapy

    D. Disadvantages

      1. Heavier menstrual bleeding or intramenstrual spotting (more likely with ParaGard than Mirena)

      2. Pain and cramping (decreases with time)

      3. Possible expulsion, especially during the first 6 months of use

      4. Possible embedding or perforation of uterus

      5. Increased risk of PID

      6. Higher risk of HIV infection (with IUD users)

    E. Contraindications

      1. Absolute

        a. Active pelvic infection (acute or subacute), including known or suspected gonorrhea or chlamydia

        b. Known or suspected pregnancy

      2. Strong relative

        a. Nulliparity

      b. Multiple sexual partners or strong likelihood that the woman will have multiple partners during the time that the IUD is in place

      c. Multiple sexual partners by the partner of an IUD user

      d. Postpartum endometritis or infected abortion within the year

      e. Acute or purulent cervicitis

      f. Bleeding disorders not yet definitively diagnosed

      g. History of ectopic pregnancy or conditions that predispose a woman to it

      h. Single episode of pelvic infection if patient desires subsequent pregnancy

      i. Immunosuppression—AIDS, diabetes, corticosteroid treatment, and so forth

      j. Blood coagulation disorders

      k. Previous pregnancy while using the IUD

      l. History or current diagnosis of HPV on the cervix

  3. Other conditions that may contraindicate IUD insertion

      a. Valvular heart disease (potentially making the patient susceptible to subacute bacterial endocarditis)

      b. Endometrial or cervical malignancy

      c. Severe cervical stenosis

      d. Small uterus that sounds to less than 6 cm

      e. Endometrial polyps

      f. Congenital uterine abnormalities or fibroids that prevent proper placement

      g. Allergy to copper

      h. Inability to check for IUD string

      i. Past history of gonorrhea, chlamydia, herpes, syphilis, or PID

      j. Genital actinomycosis

      k. Previous problems with IUD expulsion

      l. Vaginal discharge or infection

F. Management

  1. A complete history and physical, including recent Pap smear, should be in the patient's chart.

      a. Any possibility of STDs or pregnancy should be ruled out.

      b. The IUD may be inserted at the postpartum checkup.

      c. Patients who have never been seen need an initial visit, a Pap smear if one was not performed within 1 year, a chlamydia culture, and a gonorrhea culture. The IUD will be inserted at the second visit.

  2. All patients must have read, discussed, and signed the IUD consent form.

  3. Insertion at any time of the menstrual cycle is acceptable. However, the following factors should be considered when timing the IUD insertion:

    a. The infection and expulsion rate are higher when the IUD is inserted with the menses.

    b. The cervix is as dilated at midcycle as during menses; therefore, the IUD can be inserted as easily at midcycle but with a lower rate of infection and expulsion.

    c. Insertion after day 18 of the cycle may result in more pain and bleeding in the short term.

    d. If the patient has had unprotected sex since her last menses or delivery, pregnancy should be ruled out.

4. The following procedure should be performed when inserting the IUD:

    a. Move slowly and gently during all phases of IUD insertion. *Always read the manufacturer's instructions for the specific IUD you are inserting.*

    b. One-half hour before the procedure, consider giving a prostaglandin inhibitor, such as ibuprofen, for discomfort.

    c. Explain the procedure to help patient relax.

    d. Show and describe the IUD.

    e. Perform a bimanual exam to ascertain the position of the uterus. Perforations occur most often in a retroflexed uterus that was not diagnosed before the IUD was inserted.

    f. View the cervix and wash the cervix with an antiseptic solution, such as a 1:2500 solution of iodine. If iodine is present in the antiseptic solution, rule out an allergy to iodine.

    g. Consider injecting an intracervical local anesthesia at this point in the insertion process or using Hurricaine Spray.

    h. Grasp the anterior lip of the cervix with a tenaculum about 1.5 to 2.0 cm from the os if the uterus is anteverted. If the uterus is retroverted, then grasp the posterior lip of the cervix. Use of a tenaculum is not always necessary, but it is generally recommended.

    i. Sound the uterus slowly and gently. Place a cotton swab at the cervix when the sound is in all the way. Remove the sound and swab at the same time. This step permits measurement of the depth of the fundus to within 0.25 cm.

    j. Load the IUD into the inserter barrel under sterile conditions.

    k. Apply steady gentle traction on the tenaculum and introduce the inserter barrel through the cervical canal into the fundus.

    l. Insert the IUD into the cavity according IUD instructions.

    m. Exercise caution when inserting IUDs in parous women who have not been pregnant for several years. They are more likely to experience vasovagal attacks and postinsertion pain. These problems are also more common in women who are anxious or who have a narrow cervical canal, a small uterine cavity, an empty stomach, or a past history of syncopal attacks.

    n. If using a tailed IUD, clip the string. Leave about 5 cm. It is always possible to trim the string at a later date. Always document the length of the string in the patient's chart.

      o. Have the patient feel for the IUD string before leaving the examining room. She should be instructed to feel for the IUD string after each menses.

    5. A follow-up visit after the first menses is recommended or the patient should be rechecked after 2 weeks, if postpartum.

G. Side effects and complications

    1. Spotting, bleeding, hemorrhage, and anemia: Approximately 15% of women will have their IUDs removed because of increased menstrual flow, menstrual cramping, spotting, or bleeding.

    2. Cramping and pain

      a. Mild to moderate cramping immediately after insertion and for a few days: Control with medication.

      b. Severe cramping

        (1) If it occurs after insertion, consider removal.

        (2) Rule out PID.

    3. IUD expulsion (partial or complete): The patient should be alert for signs and symptoms of IUD expulsion, such as lengthening or absence of IUD string, increased cramps, intermenstrual or postcoital spotting, dyspareunia, or increased vaginal discharge.

      a. A partially expelled IUD must be removed.

      b. A missing IUD string may indicate expulsion or uterine perforation, or the string may have been pulled into the cervical canal or uterus. The cervical canal can be explored for the string. *Never* explore the uterus before ruling out pregnancy.

        (1) The string may become visible when placing the Cytobrush in the cervix and twisting.

        (2) An ultrasound or radiograph will show placement.

        (3) When the IUD is in the uterus, the endometrial cavity may be probed with alligator forceps, uterine packing forceps, or a Novak curette.

    4. Uterine perforations: confirm and consult.

    5. Pregnancy

      a. Pregnancy should be confirmed, and an ultrasound should be ordered to rule out ectopic pregnancy and check for intrauterine pregnancy, gestation, placement of IUD, and placement of placenta. Consult as necessary.

      b. The IUD should be removed as soon as possible after an intrauterine pregnancy is diagnosed.

      c. There is a higher incidence of spontaneous abortion, septic abortion, and ectopic pregnancy with an IUD in place.

      d. If the patient desires an elective abortion, the IUD may be removed at the same time.

    6. Genital Actinomycosis: Actinomycetes species are normally found in the gastrointestinal (GI) tract. They have been implicated in endometritis, PID, and pelvic and abdominal abscesses. Actinomycetes on a Pap smear suggests a genital infection.

     a. No signs and symptoms—Inform patient and monitor carefully for signs or symptoms of PID. Consider an antibiotic such as 100 mg of doxycycline twice a day for 14 days. Order another Pap smear in 1 to 2 months. If it is positive for actinomycetes, discuss the findings with the patient and then remove the IUD or have her watch for signs and symptoms of PID.

     b. Symptoms of PID—Preload with an antibiotic according to Centers for Disease Control and Prevention (CDC) guidelines. Then remove the IUD and aggressively treat the PID.

  7. PID

     a. Remove the IUD as soon as PID is diagnosed.

     b. Treat aggressively. The CDC recommends the following:[8]

       (1) Regimen A—Ofloxacin 400 mg orally twice daily for 14 days, *plus* metronidazole (Flagyl) 500 mg orally twice daily for 14 days

       (2) Regimen B—Ceftriaxone (Rocephin) 250 mg IM or cefoxitin 2 g IM *and* probenecid, 1g orally concurrently, *plus* doxycycline 100 mg orally twice daily for 10 to 14 days

H. Removal

  1. Removals during menses are somewhat easier.

  2. Procedure for removal is as follows:

     a. Avoid breaking the string by applying gentle, steady traction and removing the IUD slowly. If the IUD does not come out easily, sound the uterus and then slowly rotate the sound 90°.

     b. If gentle traction does not now lead to IUD removal, consult for dilation and curettage.

XI. Natural Family Planning

A. Definition: Natural family planning is a contraceptive method based on the concept of fertility awareness: the woman's ability to identify certain physiologic changes that occur during her menstrual cycle that indicate fertile and infertile phases. Abstinence is recommended for the fertile period if pregnancy is not desired.

B. Effectiveness

  1. When used to prevent pregnancy, effectiveness varies from 60% to 90%.

  2. When used to become pregnant, effectiveness has not been reported.

C. Advantages

  1. Is a natural method

  2. Promotes communication between couple

  3. Can be used if pregnancy is desired

  4. Can easily be combined with other methods

---

[8]CDC, 1998, p. 84

D. Disadvantages

1. Often fails to prevent pregnancy unless used correctly and consistently
2. Requires good record keeping
3. Requires abstinence during the woman's fertile period
4. Does not work well when menstrual cycles are more than 40 days, less than 20 days, irregular, or changed by stress, illness, travel, and so on

E. Contraindications: If pregnancy should be avoided, another more effective method needs to be considered.

F. Methods

1. Basal body temperature (BBT)

   a. BBT is the temperature of the body at complete rest.

   b. The BBT method is based on the following facts:

      (1) Estrogen and progesterone, while present throughout the menstrual cycle, rise sharply after ovulation.

      (2) Progesterone causes the BBT to rise several tenths of 1° over what it was before ovulation. This may be a sharp rise in 1 day or a stair-step rise over 2 to 3 days.

      (3) If pregnancy is not desired, safe days begin 4 days after ovulation.

   c. To calculate the safe and fertile days, follow these steps:

      (1) The temperature needs to be taken every day before rising.

      (2) Ovulation has occurred when the recorded temperatures are 0.3° higher for 3 consecutive days than the temperatures recorded for the 6 days before the rise.

   d. Patient teaching is as follows:

      (1) To avoid pregnancy, do not have intercourse until the fourth day after ovulation.

      (2) It's easier to determine when ovulation has occurred than to know when it will occur. Therefore, it is safer to have sex only after ovulation has occurred.

      (3) This method is more effective when combined with the cervical mucus method.

      (4) If pregnancy is desired, intercourse should occur before and at the time of ovulation.

2. Cervical mucus

   a. The cervical mucus method is based on the following facts:

      (1) Mucus produced by the cervical cells changes during the menstrual cycle.

      (2) After the period, when estrogen is low, mucus is scant. If present, it is sticky and opaque with cellular matter.

      (3) As estrogen levels increase, the mucus increases in amount. It becomes thinner and milkier.

      (4) Just before ovulation, estrogen peaks. The mucus is high in volume and clear. High elasticity is demonstrated by

gers; this is called spinnbarkeit. The mucus forms a fern-like pattern when dried on a slide.

(5) As progesterone rises, the mucus volume decreases. It becomes thick and cloudy white to white yellow, with a large amount of cellular matter. This infertile mucus acts as a barrier to sperm ascending the cervical canal.

b. Patient teaching should include the following points:

(1) To be absolutely safe, it is best to abstain from intercourse until after ovulation, when infertile mucus is present.

(2) Intercourse is probably safe during menses and after until the presence of any mucus.

(3) This method is more effective when combined with the BBT method.

3. Rhythm

a. The rhythm method is based on the following facts.

(1) The egg once released from the ovary will live 12 to 24 hours.

(2) Sperm may remain alive in the uterus and fallopian tubes for 72 hours. The time before ovulation may vary considerably. The time after ovulation is more consistent at 14 days, plus or minus 2 days before menses begins.

b. To optimize the chance of pregnancy, coitus should occur every day for several days before ovulation. This allows sperm to be in the fallopian tube when ovulation occurs.

c. Used alone, the rhythm method is unreliable and not recommended.

4. Ovulation kits

a. While expensive, they have the advantage of letting the patient know ovulation has occurred.

b. If pregnancy is not desired, intercourse may begin on day 4 after ovulation.

XII. Norplant

A. Definition: The Norplant consists of subdermal implants of six non-biodegradable Silastic rods that release levonorgestrel gradually over 4 to 5 years.

B. Effectiveness

1. Approximately 99% effective the first year of use

2. In the fifth year of use, 96% to 97.5% effective

C. Advantages

1. Because they contain progestin only, they have no estrogen side effects.

2. The low effective dose causes few alterations in carbohydrate metabolism, blood coagulation factors, blood pressure, or body weight.

3. Postpartum women who are breast-feeding can use them.

D. Disadvantages

1. Irregular bleeding: Occurs in 60% to 80% of patients the first 1 to 3 months after insertion. With continued use, this decreases to 12% to 17% after the first year. BCPs, preferably with levonorgestrel, can be used for 2 to 3 months to help with the adjustment.

2. Depression and mood swings

3. Weight gain: Progestin does not cause weight gain directly. It has been implicated in increasing appetite. Diet counseling may help.

4. Hair loss: Progestin changes the cycle of hair growth. Time will resolve this problem.

5. Amenorrhea: Normally occurs in a small percentage of users. Pregnancy needs to be ruled out.

6. Scarring: A small scar may be left at insertion or removal site.

E. Contraindications

1. Pregnancy

2. Desire to be pregnant within 1 to 2 years

3. Undiagnosed abnormal uterine bleeding

F. Complications

1. Infection at the site: Treat with antibiotics.

2. Pregnancy: If pregnancy occurs, the Norplant needs to be removed. There are no known fetal problems caused by progestins.

G. Management

1. Insertion

   a. The patient needs good counseling.

   (1) If pregnancy is desired within 3 to 5 years, another method may be a better choice.

   (2) Irregular bleeding is a common problem. Sixty to seventy percent of Norplants are removed for this problem.

   b. The patient should be having her period, be 4 to 6 weeks postpartum, or have been practicing abstinence or using condoms for 2 to 3 weeks with a negative sensitive pregnancy test to receive the Norplant.

   c. The Norplant kit contains everything needed except lidocaine, to be used for local anesthesia.

   d. Norplant directions for insertion should be followed.

   e. The patient should receive the following counseling after insertion:

   (1) Keep the site dry for 24 hours.

   (2) Loosen the gauze if it is too tight.

   (3) Watch for signs or symptoms of infection.

   (4) Note that the arm over the implants may be sensitive for 1 to 2 months.

    2. Removal

       a. Counsel the patient regarding alternate family planning methods if pregnancy is not desired.

        (1) The patient may be started on BCPs or an IUD before removal.

        (2) Depo-Provera 150 mg IM may be given the day of removal.

       b. Refer to Norplant directions for removal.

       c. Instruct the patient in these removal guidelines:

        (1) Keep the arm dry for 24 hours.

        (2) Watch for signs or symptoms of infection.

        (3) Return in 5 to 7 days to check operation site for infection and healing.

XIII. Progestin-Only Pills

  A. Definition: Progestin-only pills contain a low dose of progestin that thickens cervical mucus, suppresses ovulation, and thins the endometrium to inhibit implantation.

  B. Effectiveness: 95% to 99.5%

  C. Advantages

    1. Offer good alternative if unable to take estrogen

    2. Decrease blood loss and menstrual cramps

    3. Provide rapid return to fertility

    4. Are better for breast-feeding women than combined BCPs, as BCPs may suppress lactation

  D. Disadvantages

    1. Higher failure rate than combined BCPs

    2. Increased spotting and irregular periods

    3. Amenorrhea in 10% of patients, which may concern some women

    4. No STD protection

    5. Possible side effects, such as irritability, depression, increased PMS, and increased headaches

  E. Management

    1. May use for smokers over 35 years of age and patients with migraine headaches, a history of thrombosis, and elevated blood pressure.

    2. Teach the importance of taking the pill at the same time of day to decrease failure rate.

    3. Provide information on medications that may decrease the pills effectiveness (see Table 1-2).

    4. Consider the following information when a pill is missed:

       a. The chance of pregnancy is greater while taking progestin-only pills than with combined BCPs.

       b. See Combined Oral Contraceptives (BCPs) for management of missed pills.

5. Amenorrhea

   a. *Rule out* pregnancy.

   b. If patient is not pregnant, reassure her that amenorrhea is a known side effect of the pill.

6. Heavy bleeding

   a. Rule out other causes: STDs, cervical problems, pregnancy, uterine fibroids, and cancer.

   b. If all normal, offer ibuprofen (Motrin) 600 to 800 mg orally three times a day for 5 days.

   c. Consider changing to a combined BCP or other form of contraception.

XIV. Spermicides

A. Definition: Spermicides are chemical agents that inactivate the sperm in the vagina. Spermicides come in many forms, from jellies, creams, sponges, and suppositories to foams and thin film sheets that look like plastic wrap.

B. Effectiveness: Common failure rates of 20% to 30% per year

C. Advantages

   1. Can be bought OTC

   2. Provide some protection against STDs, including HIV

   3. Have a low cost

D. Disadvantages

   1. They require application 10 to 30 minutes before sexual intercourse.

   2. Jellies, creams, and foam remain effective for 6 to 8 hours, while suppositories lose effectiveness in 1 hour.

   3. Reapplication is necessary for each coital episode.

   4. Up to 5% of the population have an allergic response, which may be as mild as an unpleasant feeling, stinging, or increased discharge to major edema, pain, and the inability to urinate.

E. Management

   1. Use with a condom is recommended to increase effectiveness.

   2. Directions for each individual spermicide need to be read and followed exactly concerning time of insertion, length of effectiveness, and so on.

XV. Tubal Ligation (TL)

A. Description: A portion of the two fallopian tubes are cut, cauterized, clipped, and removed to prevent the sperm from fertilizing the ova.

B. Effectiveness: 99.6%

C. Advantages

   1. Permanent

   2. Long-term method

   3. Cost effective over the long term

D. Disadvantages

1. With all the risks of surgery and post-op infections, patients are more likely to regret having a TL.

2. Nulliparous women and patients under 25 are more likely to regret having had a TL—13% as compared to 6% after 5 years.

3. Good counseling is a must.

   a. Present other methods of contraception.

   b. Caution that this procedure must be considered irreversible; hence, the women must desire no more children in the future.

   c. Discuss the surgery itself, including the procedure and complications.

   d. Include the husband or significant other, if applicable. Ask if he has considered a vasectomy.

   e. Warn of possible menstrual changes, which could be irreversible.

   f. Provide safe sex information, if applicable.

XVI. Withdrawal

A. Definition: The man withdraws his penis from the vagina prior to ejaculation. This significantly reduces the amount of sperm placed inside the vagina.

B. Effectiveness: 70% to 80%

C. Advantages

1. Readily available

2. No cost

3. Possible psychological preference

D. Disadvantages

1. It has a high rate of failure.

2. It may reduce pleasure for one or both partners.

3. Those who ejaculate prematurely are not good candidates.

4. Two acts of sexual intercourse close together will increase the chance of pregnancy because of residual sperm.

5. It does not protect against STDs.

XVII. New Methods Not Yet Approved

A. Etonogestrel implant

1. Definition: The implant is a single rod, 3-year subdermal implant that releases initially 60 to 70 mg of etonogestrel per day, decreasing to 25 to 30 mg per day by the end of the third year.

2. Effectiveness: Highly effective. In one European study of 200 women, the 2-year cumulative pregnancy rate was 0%.

3. Advantages

   a. It consists of a single, easily implanted, easily removed rod.

   b. Fertility returns within a few days of removal.

    4. Disadvantages

      a. It needs to be surgically implanted and removed.

      b. Side effects include the following:

        (1) It affects bleeding patterns.

        (2) It is associated with headaches, nausea, breast pain, and depression.

B. Contraceptive patch (brand name EVRA)

    1. Definition: EVRA is a sustained-release patch the size of a matchbook cover that releases a progestin and estrogen (ethinyl estradiol). The common dose is 250 μg per day of progestin and 25 μg per day of estrogen. FDA approval is pending.

    2. Effectiveness: Unavailable

    3. Advantages

      a. Easy administration; worn 3 weeks out of 4

      b. Different pathways from oral contraceptives

    4. Disadvantages: Side effects similar to BCPs

C. Vaginal ring (brand name NuvaRing)

    1. Definition: NuvaRing is a hormone vaginal ring providing daily doses of 120 μg of etonogestrel and 15 μg of ethinyl estradiol.

    2. Effectiveness: Data unavailable

    3. Advantages

      a. One size fits all.

      b. It remains in place for 3 weeks and is then removed for a week.

    4. Disadvantages

      a. It is a foreign body in the vagina.

      b. It may be expelled without the patient being aware.

      c. The partner may dislike it.

 PRECONCEPTUAL PLANNING

Good preconceptual planning enhances optimum pregnancy outcome. Provider-initiated preconceptual planning should be addressed whenever possible during the childbearing years, because it facilitates lifestyle changes and maintains healthy options prior to conception.

I. **Timing of Preconceptual Advice.** Offer preconceptual advice at

    A. Annual exams.

    B. Whenever a woman comes in for a pregnancy test that is negative.

    C. Any visit if the woman is sexually active and not using effective contraception.

    D. Health education classes.

II. **Aspects of Preconceptual Care**

    A. Nutrition to enhance healthy outcomes

      1. Advise her to eat healthy meals.

2. Make vegetarians aware of combination meals to create complete proteins.

3. Advise women who have a history of or current eating disorders to seek the care of a specialist.

   a. Anorexia

   b. Bingeing and purging

   c. History or current practice of frequent fasting

   d. Severe obesity

4. Counsel patient if she is not close to the proper weight for her height.

5. Advise her that taking a vitamin with folic acid will reduce risk of neural tube defects by up to 70%.

B. Lifestyle issues that are detrimental to good pregnancy outcomes

1. Smoking more than five cigarettes a day can directly influence fetal and infant health.

2. Alcohol is the leading teratogen in the western world.[9] Excessive and chronic ingestion of alcohol is likely to produce fetal maldevelopment, commonly referred to as fetal alcohol syndrome. It is not known just how much alcohol is considered safe in pregnancy. Advise none.

3. Employment hazards such as exposure to lead, solvents, x-rays, or other chemicals can cause birth defects prior to the woman even knowing that she is pregnant. Investigate and avoid these hazards prior to conception.

4. STDs can adversely influence a pregnancy outcome. Advise the patient to avoid multiple sexual partners, bisexual partners, those who use intravenous (IV) drugs, and partners who have other partners.

5. Cats can be carriers of toxoplasmosis, which is passed in the feces and can cause birth defects in children. While outdoor cats and those who eat meat are more prone to carry this disease, consider all cats carriers. Advise the patient to find someone else to change the litter box.

C. Prescription, OTC, recreational, or illicit drugs: Some of these medications can cause birth defects, preterm labor, or addiction in the unborn child.

1. Prescription drugs should be reviewed with those planning pregnancy and those who are at increased risk for pregnancy.

   a. Antiepileptic drugs are known to increase the risk of certain birth defects. Monotherapy causes fewer problems than polytherapy. Patients should be advised not to stop taking or adjust their medication without first reviewing the situation with their neurologist to find the medication(s) that will work best for them and a possible pregnancy.

   b. Many chemotherapeutic drugs are known to be teratogenic. If the woman desires pregnancy after finishing her course of

---

[9]Cunningham et al., 2001, p. 567

therapy, she should discuss ova salvage prior to starting therapy.

   c. Drugs for treating acne should be avoided during pregnancy as they can cause serious defects. These drugs include Accutane and tetracycline.

   d. Anticoagulation medication such as Coumadin

   e. Hormones, especially androgenic hormones

2. OTC medications are thought to be safe by the general public and by many clinicians. Because they are readily available and not subject to medical advice, they can cause problems. Advise women taking OTC medications to consider these to be drugs. They should avoid them or use them with caution and always tell their care providers what they are taking.

3. Illicit "street" drugs are known to cause fetal growth restriction, neonatal addiction syndrome, miscarriage, fetal loss, or ongoing learning and behavior problems in children. Strongly advise the patient to seek and continue with substance abuse programs prior to attempting pregnancy.

4. Alcohol ingestion is the most commonly identified cause of mental retardation. The baby is born with distinct facial characteristics. They often have fine and gross motor function and speech impairments. Suggest substance abuse counseling, Alcoholics Anonymous, and support groups.

5. Women should be advised to start taking a normal-dose multivitamin with folic acid of at least 0.4 mg daily. They should not take megadoses of any fat-soluble vitamin, especially vitamin A, which is teratogenic in high doses. If anemic, women should build up their iron stores with iron supplementation prior to conception.

6. While oral contraceptives have not been shown to cause birth defects, it is best to stop taking them about 3 months prior to pregnancy, so that she can have 2 normal menses. This will assist in dating the pregnancy.

D. Medical History

   1. Personal history: If the woman has a personal history of gonorrhea, chlamydia, herpes, syphilis, or condyloma, there should be a thorough examination to observe for lesions, masses, or abnormal discharge. Screen and counsel the patient as necessary.

   2. Epilepsy (past or current)

      a. Ask when she had her last seizure

      b. Verify medication; check folate levels and antiepileptic medication levels to see if they're at therapeutic levels.

      c. Refer for evaluation by a neurologist; polymedications are more teratogenic than one medication.

      d. Ensure the woman continues her medication, because tonic-clonic convulsions carry more risk to the fetus and mother than most antiepileptic medications.

3. Diabetes
   a. Check the patient's hemoglobin A_{IC}.
   b. If the patient is on insulin, refer her to an endocrinologist for evaluation of and possible adjustment of insulin dose.
   c. If the patient has juvenile diabetes, refer her to an ophthalmologist for evaluation.

4. Hypertension
   a. Check blood pressure; if within normal range and normal weight for height, discuss diet and exercise.
   b. Refer patient to internist if blood pressure is high and check baseline metabolic profile.

5. Heart disease: Refer patient to internist for cardiac evaluation prior to pregnancy.

6. Lupus
   a. Pregnancy is not contraindicated with lupus that has been stable longer than 6 months.
   b. Lupus activity in one pregnancy does not predict the course of successive pregnancies.
   c. Check autoantibodies. Anti-SS-A can cause congenital heart block; anticardiolipin antibodies (ACAs) can cause fetal loss and preeclampsia. Lupus anticoagulant can cause fetal loss, preeclampsia, or thrombosis; there can be a false-positive serology. Anti-SS-B antibody can cause fetal rash.

7. Other diseases, such as asthma, kidney disease, or thyroid disease, should be stabilized prior to pregnancy.

E. Genetic History
   1. If the woman is Black, offer a screen for sickle cell disease or trait.
   2. If she is Jewish, especially of Eastern European background, then offer to test hexosaminidase levels for Tay-Sachs disease carrier status.
   3. If there is a family history of cystic fibrosis, refer her for genetic testing.
   4. If there is a family history of muscular dystrophy, offer to test creatine phosphokinase (CPK) levels.
   5. If there is a family history of thalassemia, check a complete blood count (CBC) with indices.

F. Other
   1. Check the rubella titer. If the patient is nonimmune, then immunize her and have her postpone pregnancy for 1 month.
   2. If there are issues of sexual abuse or physical abuse, refer for counseling, as abuse can increase during pregnancy.
   3. If hobbies or employment expose woman to lead or other toxic chemicals, stop exposure prior to pregnancy.
   4. Advise patient to avoid hot tubs, saunas, and tanning booths that raise body temperature; temperature exposure should be no higher than 100°F for 20 minutes.

CARE DURING PREGNANCY

I. Philosophy

    A. Every childbearing family has a right to the following care during pregnancy:

        1. A safe, satisfying experience with respect for human dignity and worth

        2. Variety in cultural forms

        3. Self-determination

    B. Comprehensive maternity care, including educational and emotional care throughout the childbearing years, is a major means for intercession into the improvement and maintenance of the health of the nation's families. Comprehensive maternity care is most effectively and efficiently delivered by interdependent health disciplines.

II. Objectives

    A. To foster the delivery of safe, satisfying, and economic maternity care

    B. To recognize that childbearing is a family experience and encourage the active involvement of family members in the care process

    C. To uphold the right to self-determination of women and their families, within the boundaries of safe care

    D. To focus on health and growth as developmental processes during the reproductive years

    E. To use the reproductive experience as an opportunity to promote good health habits

    F. To stimulate community awareness and responsiveness to the need for alternatives in childbearing

III. Initial Antepartum Visit

    A. Purpose

        1. Conduct the initial visit, including a complete medical, OB, and family health history.

        2. Conduct a complete physical exam.

        3. Order and evaluate appropriate lab work and additional diagnostic procedures.

        4. Establish an estimated date of confinement.

        5. Identify deviations from the normal course of pregnancy.

        6. Delineate a plan of care, mutually agreed upon with the patient.

        7. Provide instruction and education to patients on the following topics related to normal pregnancy:

            a. Nutrition and weight gain

            b. Normal anatomic and physiologic changes

            c. Exercise and stress management

            d. Danger signs and when to contact the care provider

            e. Referral to appropriate community services

B. History: Initial history to be completed as outlined under Gynecologic Care in the beginning of Part I. Also include in the OB history:

   1. Any exposure to the following:

     a. Tobacco or alcohol

     b. Prescription or street drugs taken during pregnancy

     c. Aspirin or ibuprofen use

     d. X-rays during pregnancy

     e. Extreme heat during pregnancy, such as fever, hot tubs, or saunas

     f. Toxoplasmosis

       (1) Exposure to cat feces by emptying the cat's litter box. This is most critical when the cat has access to wild birds or animals.

       (2) Ingestion of rare or raw meat

     g. Herpes genitalis: a history or pattern of recurrent lesions

   2. History of past pregnancies with outcomes and problems

   3. Current pregnancy history

     a. Contraceptive use before this pregnancy

     b. First day of last *normal* menstrual period and any bleeding since then

     c. Signs and symptoms of pregnancy to date

     d. Date of positive pregnancy test

C. Physical exam: As outlined under Gynecologic Care. In addition, it should include the following:

   1. Abdominal exam

     a. Assess for progressive abdominal and uterine enlargement.

     b. Measure fundal height.

     c. Auscultate the abdomen for fetal heart tones; these should be heard by Doppler at 10 to 12 weeks' gestation.

     d. Assess fetal position (using Leopold's maneuvers) after 28 weeks.

   2. Pelvic exam

     a. Palpate the size, shape, and position of the uterus.

     b. If pregnancy is advanced, check for dilation and effacement.

     c. Evaluate pelvic type and size.

D. Lab work

   1. Initial lab work

     a. At the initial visit, all patients should have the following lab work done, unless they can produce evidence that it has been done elsewhere during the present pregnancy:

       (1) CBC

       (2) Serology

       (3) Blood type and Rh factor

       (4) Antibody titer

        (5) Rubella titer

        (6) Hepatitis B and C screen

        (7) Urinalysis

    b. At the initial physical exam, a Pap smear, GC, and chlamydia culture should be done on all patients.

    c. Additional lab work may be ordered as indicated.

        (1) Alpha-fetoprotein (AFP) or AFP-Plus at 15 to 18 weeks

        (2) Antinuclear antibody (ANA) test if previous fetal loss occurred

        (3) Sickle cell screen

        (4) HIV screen

        (5) Baseline liver function test (LFT) and kidney function test, if there is a history of pregnancy-induced hypertension (PIH)

        (6) Group B streptococcus (GBS) culture—CDC recommends a rectal and vaginal swab at 35 to 37 weeks on all women with a prior infant with GBS or GBS found in urine during pregnancy[10]

        (7) Herpes culture

        (8) Thyroid screen

        (9) Fasting blood sugar (FBS) or 1-hour postprandial (1°PP) glucose test

        (10) Clotting time, prothrombin time (PT), partial thromboplastin time (PTT), platelet count, and fibrinogen level

        (11) Wet mount

  2. Routine lab work during the antepartum course includes the following:

    a. Dipstix of urine at each prenatal visit for

        (1) Glucose.

        (2) Protein.

        (3) Blood.

        (4) Nitrites.

        (5) Ketones.

    b. CBC and 1-hour test with a 50-g loading dose of glucola at 24 to 28 weeks

    c. Antibody titer on all Rh(D)-negative patients at initial visit and at 24 to 28 weeks. If a patient registers for care after 30 weeks and has not received the prophylactic RhoGAM, it is usually given until 36 weeks.

    d. Additional lab work that might be indicated: See Laboratory Studies in Pregnancy.

E. Ultrasonography: Can be done when indicated. If only one is ordered, it is best done between 18 to 22 weeks. Indications for ordering include

---

[10]CDC, 1996, p. 20

    1. Unsure dates.

    2. Size-date discrepancy.

    3. Question of abnormality.

        a. Placenta previa

        b. Multiple gestation

        c. Fetal anomaly

        d. Maternal abnormality

IV. Return Antepartum Visit

  A. Schedule for return visits

    1. 1 to 28 weeks' gestation: every 4 weeks

    2. 28 to 36 weeks' gestation: every 2 weeks

    3. 36 weeks gestation until term: every week

    4. If the patient is allowed to go past 40 weeks, see her twice a week with appropriate testing (e.g., nonstress tests [NSTs], fetal movement count)

  B. Teaching and counseling

    1. Provide opportunity for patient to discuss questions, concerns, and needs.

    2. Review checklist for topics to be discussed and procedures to be done at the appropriate weeks of gestation.

    3. Provide individualized health instruction, counseling, and guidance.

    4. Review recent laboratory reports.

    5. Provide relief for minor discomforts or physical complaints.

    6. Refer patient for other needed services.

        a. Dietitian

        b. Dentist

        c. Social services

        d. Childbirth education

        e. Physical therapist

        f. Counseling or mental health

    7. Form and revise plan of care after discussing options with patient.

  C. Physical assessment

    1. Weeks of gestation: Review dates if necessary.

    2. Weight

    3. Blood pressure

    4. Fundal height

    5. Fetal heart rate

    6. Presenting part

    7. Urine dipstix

    8. Vaginal exams: Perform at the following times:

        a. The initial physical exam

      b. At 36 to 37 weeks if unsure of presentation

      c. At 40 weeks and beyond

      d. At other times as appropriate:

         (1) To check for labor

         (2) History of threatened premature labor

         (3) History of cone biopsy or other cervical surgery

         (4) Twin gestation—examine every 2 weeks after 24 weeks

         (5) Any other medical indication

         (6) At the patient's request, as long as membranes are intact

V. Obstetric Pearls of Wisdom ("Geri's" Gems)

  A. Clinical signs of pregnancy noted on exam

    1. Piskacek's—When the ovum implants, the uterine cornu softens, and an almost tumorlike enlargement may occur.

    2. Goodell's—At 6 weeks, the cervix softens, and congestion occurs.

    3. Chadwick's—At 6 weeks, a bluish or purplish discoloration of the vulva and vaginal mucosa occurs.

    4. Hegar's—At 6 weeks, the uterine isthmus softens and is compressed by the enlarging body of the uterus. The result is the exaggeration of uterine anteflexion during the first 3 months of pregnancy. The increased pressure on the bladder causes urinary frequency.

  B. Fundal height

    1. Rule: After 18 weeks, the measurement of fundal height using a centimeter tape should equal the patient's gestation in weeks.

    2. Table 1-4 shows an expected growth scale.

Table 1-4. Fundal Height Scale

Gestational Age	Fundal Height
4 weeks	Similar to nonpregnant
6 weeks	Small orange, tennis ball
8 weeks	Baseball
10 weeks	Small grapefruit
12 weeks	Small cantaloupe—at symphysis pubis
16 weeks	Halfway between symphysis and umbilicus
18 weeks	May be at umbilicus area but not full bodied
20 weeks	At umbilicus and full bodied
24 weeks	2–3 finger widths above umbilicus
28 weeks	Halfway to xiphoid
32 weeks	Three-quarters way to xiphoid
36 weeks	At xiphoid
40 weeks	2–3 finger widths below xiphoid

C. Haase's rule: Provides guideline for crown-to-heel length of the embryo in centimeters

   1. During the first 5 months, square the number of lunar months of pregnancy.

   2. After 5 months, multiply the lunar months of pregnancy by 5.

D. McDonald's rule: Predicts the length of pregnancy

   1. The height of the fundus in centimeters times 2/7 equals the duration of the pregnancy in lunar months.

   2. The height of the fundus in centimeters times 8/7 equals the duration of pregnancy in weeks.

E. Recommendations for management of nausea during pregnancy

   1. Before rising in the morning, eat a few crackers, a handful of dry cereal, or a piece of dry toast or bread.

   2. Get up slowly, avoiding sudden movements.

   3. Consume small, frequent meals and avoid long periods without food.

   4. Drink fluids between rather than with meals.

   5. Try small amounts of apple juice, grape juice, or carbonated beverages when nausea develops between meals.

   6. Avoid greasy and fried foods.

   7. Eat lightly seasoned foods; avoid excessive use of pepper, garlic, chili, or other strong spices.

   8. Drink peppermint tea or eat peppermint candies.

   9. Take 5 mL of Emetrol every 15 minutes but no more than five doses.

   10. Take 50 to 100 mg of vitamin B_6 (pyridoxine) twice a day.

   11. Take 20 mg of Unisom twice a day.

   12. Take 1/2 tablet of Unisom and 25 mg of vitamin B_6 together (Bendictin) twice a day.

   13. Take 800 to 1000 mg of ginger root (Zingiber) twice a day and as necessary.

   14. Use Sea-Band for motion sickness—applies pressure to wrist at acupressure sites.

VI. Collaborative Care and Referral

A. The following conditions may be considered for collaborative management:

   1. History of seizure disorder or epilepsy controlled by medication

   2. Two or more consecutive spontaneous abortions

   3. More than five previous deliveries

   4. Acute pyelonephritis or frequent UTIs

   5. Primipara over 35 years or multipara age 40 or older

   6. Failure to gain weight

   7. Abnormal presentation before labor

   8. Postdates

   9. Gestational diabetes

10. Prior fetal or neonatal death
11. Genital herpes
12. Uterine bleeding or history of postpartum hemorrhage
13. Polyhydramnios or oligohydramnios
14. Fetal growth retardation
15. Premature rupture of membranes; more than 12 hours without regular uterine contractions
16. Twin pregnancy
17. Alcohol and drug abuse
18. Anemia (hemoglobin less than 10, hematocrit less than 30%)
19. Positive purified protein derivative (PPD) test for tuberculosis (TB) but negative chest radiograph
20. Uterine myomata
21. Preeclampsia
22. Asthma
23. Hypothyroidism
24. Hepatitis carrier
25. Pap smear of class III or greater (indicating severe dysplasia or cancer-in-situ [CIS])
26. Persistent vomiting
27. Severe recurrent headaches
28. Absence of fetal heart tones or fetal movement after 28 weeks' gestation
29. Concern or request of patient to see a physician
30. Previous cesarean section

B. Conditions that necessitate referral to a physician include the following:

1. Previous classical cesarean section
2. Chronic hypertension, poorly controlled
3. Heart disease, class II to IV
4. Active tuberculosis or other lung disease
5. Rh(D) negative with positive antibody titer
6. Hydatidiform mole
7. Renal disease, moderate to severe
8. Diabetes mellitus greater than Type 2
9. Hepatitis during pregnancy
10. Severe psychiatric disorders
11. Uncontrolled seizure disorder
12. Acute or chronic neurologic disorder
13. History of severe preeclampsia or eclampsia
14. Bleeding disorders
15. Placenta previa
16. Positive test for HIV

NUTRITION AND WEIGHT GAIN IN PREGNANCY

I. **Good Nutrition.** It is important to emphasize good nutrition in pregnancy and while breast-feeding.
  A. Calories: Pregnant and breast-feeding women have increased calorie needs.
    1. Pregnancy: Increase intake by 300 calories.
    2. Breast-feeding: Increase intake by 500 calories.
  B. Protein: From 80 to 100 g of protein are needed daily.
    1. Reasons
      a. To enable the body to lay down new tissue
      b. To promote fetal growth
      c. To prevent edema
    2. Daily requirement
      a. 1 quart milk (32 g)
      b. Three servings of meat, fish, chicken, or rice and beans (60 to 90 g)
  C. Twins: Women pregnant with twins need
    1. An extra 30 g of protein a day.
    2. An extra 200 calories a day.
  D. Whole grains
    1. Reasons
      a. They help prevent constipation.
      b. They are a good source of B vitamins.
      c. They provide complex carbohydrates for energy.
    2. Daily requirement: Four servings of whole grain breads, pasta, cereals, or legumes
  E. Milk and other dairy products
    1. Reason: They are a good source of protein and calcium.
    2. Daily requirement: Four servings of low-fat milk, cheese, or cottage cheese
  F. Fruits and vegetables
    1. Reasons
      a. They provide many vitamins and minerals.
      b. Citrus varieties are high in vitamin C.
      c. They help prevent constipation.
    2. Daily requirement: Five servings. (Lettuce should be the dark green variety.)
  G. Water
    1. Reasons
      a. To keep up with expanding blood volume
      b. To avoid constipation
    2. Daily requirement: Two quarts of fluid

    H. Substances to avoid

        1. Artificial sweeteners, especially aspartame, which can be associated with headaches and dizziness

        2. Caffeine

        3. Drinks and foods with a high sugar content

II. **Appropriate Weight Gain**

    A. Discuss appropriate weight gain at the initial OB visit.

    B. Determine normal weight for patient's height by using the following method or any other weight-height table:

        1. One hundred pounds for the first 5 feet of height. Then add 5 lb for every additional inch.

        2. Small frame, subtract 10%

        3. Large frame, add 10%

    C. Determine patient's prepregnancy weight.

    D. Inform patient that she should gain 25 to 40 lb, depending on her body build and prepregnancy weight.

    E. Weight Gain

        1. Expected weight gain

            a. Trimester 1—Two to 4 lb total

            b. Trimester 2—¾ lb per week

            c. Trimester 3—One pound or less per week

        2. Problems with weight gain or loss

            a. If the patient is gaining more than 2 lb per week, check for problems.

            b. The patient can gain 10% of her original body weight before there is clinical evidence of edema.

            c. Weight loss is most significant in the first trimester, because the baby grows rapidly and needs nutrients.

            d. Weight loss of more than 5 lb in 2 weeks requires a diet history, lab tests, and consultation with a physician.

            e. Any weight lost during the first trimester of pregnancy should be gained back by 20 weeks of estimated gestational age (EGA).

            f. A gain of less than 2 pounds per month after the first trimester increases the risk of infants born small for gestational age (SGA).

III. **Management**

    A. Loss of weight or failure to gain appropriately: try to determine the reason and treat the patient accordingly.

        1. Nausea or vomiting

        2. Heartburn: lack of room in stomach

        3. Fear of gaining weight

            a. Counsel and reassure patient. Explain distribution of weight gained during pregnancy.

    b. Emphasize the importance of weight gain. Explore the body image and acceptability of a large body to the patient, partner, or others.

    c. Offer the patient a referral to a dietitian or mental health counselor.

B. Excessive weight gain: try to determine the reason and treat the patient accordingly.

    1. Multiple gestation: Suspect this if there is a sudden or continuous large gain, out of proportion to the woman's body build and eating habits.

    2. Diabetes

    3. Edema: Check for other signs of preeclampsia.

    4. Idiosyncratic weight gain: For example, consider a history of large weight gain with previous pregnancies, which was lost after delivery.

    5. Uncontrolled intake of food

        a. Counsel patient on diet, explaining that the baby needs nutritious food in moderate amounts, not junk foods and fats.

        b. Stress the importance of regular exercise in controlling weight gain.

        c. If the patient desires, suggest a self-help, weight-control group, such as the TOPS Club (Take Pounds Off Sensibly), Overeaters Anonymous, and so forth. Give her a copy of the 1800-calorie diabetic diet to follow. If she loses weight on 1800 calories or if ketones are present in the urine, increase her diet to 2200 to 2400 calories until weight gain is within the normal range.

 ## LABORATORY STUDIES IN PREGNANCY

Initial prenatal lab work includes a CBC with differential, blood type and Rh factor, antibody titer, serology, rubella titer, and chlamydia and GC screens. Optional tests, if indicated, include HIV, drug screen, hepatitis panel, and TB and GBS screening.

I. **CBC With Differential**

    A. Order the test routinely at the initial prenatal visit.

    1. If the hemoglobin is less than 10 or the hematocrit is less than 30%, treat with extra iron and foods high in iron.

    2. If there are any other abnormal values, repeat lab work, if necessary, to confirm a problem, and consult a physician if needed.

    B. Order test if there is any sign of systemic infection or bleeding.

II. **Hematocrit and Hemoglobin.** Assess values as part of the CBC at the initial visit and the 26- to 28-week lab work.

III. **Blood Type and Rh Factor**

    A. Order antibody titer for all pregnant patients at the initial visit.

    1. If the test is positive, ask the patient if she has had RhoGAM.

2. Repeat the test for antibody identification. Consult a physician if the factor may be harmful to the fetus.

B. Repeat the antibody titer at 26 to 28 weeks' gestation for all Rh(D)-negative patients.

C. Give RhoGAM prophylactically to all Rh(D)-negative pregnant patients at 28 to 30 weeks' gestation. No further antibody screen needs to be done. If a patient has not previously received prophylactic RhoGAM, it may be given until 36 weeks' gestation.

IV. Serology

A. Rapid plasma reagent (RPR) test—Ordered for all pregnant patients unless they have a previous record of negative RPR or Venereal Disease Research Laboratory (VDRL) test during their present pregnancy. If the test is positive, order a *Treponema pallidum* antibodies (TP-PA) test. Treat the patient according to CDC guidelines.

B. VDRL test

1. The VDRL test is a titer, which can become positive through infection by any number of febrile diseases as well as syphilis. Once the VDRL, RPR, or fluorescent treponemal antibody absorption become positive, they remain positive for life. The RPR is more sensitive than the VDRL, and therefore is useful for diagnosis of early syphilis—but only if the patient was previously RPR-negative. If previously positive, diagnosis *must be made on the basis of rising VDRL titers. A fourfold increase in titer indicates an active infection.* Serial titers may be necessary to confirm or rule out infection.

2. After treatment, order follow-up VDRL tests monthly during pregnancy, and at 3, 6, and 12 months. If the syphilis infection lasted more than 1 year, repeat the VDRL test 24 months after treatment.

V. Rubella Titer

A. Order titer for all pregnant patients at the initial visit.

B. If a negative titer is less than 1:10, recommend immunization after delivery.

C. If the titer is greater than 1:1000, repeat it to rule out a lab error.

1. If it is still elevated, repeat the titer in 3 weeks for potential convalescent serum.

2. If it has decreased, consult a physician concerning possible rubella in pregnancy.

D. If the titer is negative and possible exposure occurred during pregnancy, consider serial titers.

VI. HIV

A. Encourage all women to take an HIV test.

B. Counsel patient and obtain written or verbal consent prior to withdrawal of blood.

VII. Hepatitis B Screen

A. Order the screen at the initial visit.

    B. Obtain another screen at any time during the pregnancy if the clinical picture is suggestive. Consider screen if nausea and vomiting, malaise, pruritus, or jaundice persists.

    C. If screen is positive, see Hepatitis guidelines in Part IV.

VIII. Serum AFP or AFP-Plus

    A. Administer test by 15 to 18 weeks' gestation.

    B. Offer AFP-Plus to all patients.

    D. If test is positive, consider the potential increased risk of a baby with a neural tube defect or Down's syndrome.

        1. Check the estimated date of confinement with an ultrasound. If the blood was drawn between 15 and 20 weeks' gestation, have the lab recalculate AFP using the corrected EGA. If the blood was not drawn at the correct time, redraw the blood when the gestational age is correct.

        2. If the risk remains elevated, refer the patient for genetic counseling and possible amniocentesis.

IX. Dipstix Urine Test

    A. Perform test at each prenatal visit.

    B. If positive for ketones, review food intake.

    C. If positive glucose is greater than +2 twice, see Diabetes Mellitus in Pregnancy in Part V.

    D. If more than a trace of protein is present, follow these procedures:

        1. Obtain a clean-catch or catheterized urine specimen and recheck it.

        2. If protein is still present, rule out preeclampsia and pregnancy-induced hypertension.

        3. If no hypertension exists, obtain a urine culture and sensitivity to rule out an asymptomatic UTI.

        4. If there is no UTI, order kidney function tests and consult a physician as necessary.

    E. If the test is positive for blood, follow these procedures:

        1. Obtain a clean-catch or catheterized urine.

        2. If urine remains positive for more than a trace of blood, consult a physician; it may indicate a kidney stone or other problems.

    F. If the test is positive for nitrites, treat the patient for infection and send the urine for culture and sensitivity.

X. Urinalysis, and Urine Culture and Sensitivity

    A. Order tests for all patients at initial visit and at 26 to 28 weeks. Urine test results that indicate a UTI include the following:

        1. Culture and sensitivity bacteria colony count greater than 100,000

        2. Clean-catch urinalysis with the following indications:

            a. Bacteria

            b. Nitrites

            c. Red blood cells

      d. Possible proteinuria secondary to bacteriuria

      e. White blood cells greater than 50/mL or greater than 25 per HPF of spun urine

B. If patient has no history of frequent UTIs and the initial culture is positive, treat her and repeat the culture for test of cure following medication.

C. If the patient has a history of frequent UTIs, follow these procedures:

    1. With an initial negative culture, repeat the culture at 27 to 28 weeks.

    2. With an initial positive culture, treat the patient and repeat the culture 1 week after treatment and at 24 and 32 weeks.

D. If signs and symptoms of a UTI develop at any time during the pregnancy, order a urinalysis and urine culture and sensitivity.

E. If frequent UTIs occur during the pregnancy:

    1. Consider screening for:

      a. Glucose-6-phosphate dehydrogenase (G6PD) anemia if the patient is African American, Asian, or of Mediterranean descent.

      b. Diabetes.

    2. Consider tests of kidney function, such as blood urea nitrogen, creatinine, or 24-hour urinary creatinine clearance.

    3. Consider prophylactic treatment, such as 50 mg of Macrodantin orally every day until delivered, if treated two or more times this pregnancy.

F. For urine test results that indicate GBS, follow these procedures:

    1. Treat the patient as recommended per protocol.

    2. Note results in a visible place on the history and physical for labor and delivery.

    3. Teach patient the significance of the finding.

XI. Pap Smear

A. Perform Pap smear on all pregnant patients at new OB exam, unless one is documented within 6 months of exam.

B. Perform Pap smear on all patients presenting for exam who have not had one within a year.

XII. Gonorrhea Culture

A. Perform the culture at the new OB exam.

B. Perform at any time during the pregnancy that a patient presents with

    1. Signs and symptoms.

    2. A concern that she might have an STD.

    3. A diagnosis with another STD.

C. If the gonorrhea culture is positive, follow these steps:

    1. Order a VDRL test and perform a chlamydia culture, if not already done.

2. Consider recommended treatment involving 125 mg of Rocephin IM plus 1 g of Zithromax orally in a single dose.[11]

3. Repeat the culture:

   a. One week after treatment.

   b. At 36 weeks, if treated during pregnancy.

   c. At the 6-week postpartum visit, if treated during pregnancy.

D. If the patient is still positive after treatment, follow these steps:

   1. Re-treat the patient.

   2. Reinstruct the patient regarding importance of taking all the medicine, mode of transmission, partner(s) treatment, and abstaining from intercourse until the patient and her partner have a negative culture.

XIII. Chlamydia Culture

A. Obtain a culture for all new OB patients.

B. Obtain a culture at any time during the pregnancy that a patient presents with

   1. A clinical picture that is suggestive of chlamydia.

   2. A diagnosis of syphilis or gonorrhea.

C. If the patient is positive and pregnant, treat her with 500 mg of amoxicillin three times a day for 7 days.[12] Zithromax 1 g orally is preferred because it is a one-dose treatment. Repeat the culture 2 to 3 weeks after treatment. If she is still positive:

   1. Re-treat her.

   2. Reinstruct the patient about the importance of taking all the medicine, mode of transmission, partner(s) treatment, and abstaining from intercourse until the patient and partner(s) have a negative culture.

D. Notify the pediatrician at delivery.

XIV. Herpes Simplex Culture

A. Obtain the culture any time suggestive lesions appear or if a Pap smear suggestive of herpes is obtained.

B. If the culture is positive or the patient has history of herpes, see Herpes Simplex guidelines in Part IV.

XV. Thyroid Screen

A. Obtain thyroid-stimulating hormone if

   1. The patient has been on thyroid medication.

   2. There is any abnormality of the thyroid on exam.

   3. There are signs or symptoms of thyroid disease.

   4. The patient has poor weight gain or depression.

B. If the screen reveals abnormal results, perform a thyroid panel and consult as necessary.

---

[11]CDC, 1998, p. 61
[12]CDC, 1998, p. 54

XVI. Blood Sugar Tests

A. Order a 1-hour post 50-g glucola load.
1. Administer test preferably between 24 and 28 weeks.
2. Check institution or office guidelines to see if a 3-day high-glucose diet is required before this test.
3. Do immediately if the patient has the following:
   a. History of stillbirth or unexplained neonatal death
   b. History of gestational diabetes
   c. Sibling or parent with insulin-dependent diabetes
   d. Two consecutive episodes of glycosuria unrelated to carbohydrate intake
   e. Strong suspicion of diabetes, based on two or more predisposing factors

B. If any of the values obtained are abnormal, perform a 3-hour glucose tolerance test (GTT). Results are considered abnormal if the following values are met or exceeded:
1. Fasting blood sugar is greater than 105 mg of glucose/100 mL of plasma.
2. Two-hour PP fasting blood sugar is greater than 140.
3. One-hour post 50-g glucola is greater than 140.
4. If one-hour glucose is more than 200 mg of glucose/100 mL of plasma, a presumptive diagnosis of gestational diabetes should be made. A 3-hour GTT need not be done. See Diabetes Mellitus in Pregnancy in Part V.
5. The following GTT upper limits of normal:
   a. Fasting blood sugar of 105
   b. One-half or 1-hour blood sugar of 190
   c. Two-hour blood sugar of 165
   d. Three-hour blood sugar of 145

C. If any two GTT values are above normal, see Diabetes Mellitus in Pregnancy in Part V.

XVII. Clotting Time, PT, PTT, Platelet Count, and Fibrinogen Level

A. Obtain values if the patient has the following:
1. History of abnormal clotting, severe anemia, or unusually long or heavy menstrual periods
2. Platelet count of less than 100 on CBC
3. Potential disseminated intravascular coagulation (see Bleeding in Pregnancy Over 20 Weeks' Gestation in Part V)

B. Consult with physician if abnormal results occur.

XVIII. ANA, or ACA if there is a history of stillbirth or multiple miscarriages

XIX. Wet Mount. Obtain if the patient has the following:

A. Unusual or suspicious discharge seen on routine exam
B. Complaints of vaginal discharge or itching, burning, or irritation

XX. Cervical Culture. Obtain if the patient has the following:

A. Abortion, threatened or complete

   B. Prolonged rupture of membranes
   C. A history of premature labor, previous GBS history, or GBS in the urine during this pregnancy (obtain at 35 to 37 weeks' gestation)
   D. Endometritis

XXI. Stool For Ova and Parasites
   A. Obtain sample if the patient has the following:
      1. Diarrhea, unrelieved for 48 hours despite treatment
      2. Severe anemia or anemia that does not respond to treatment
   B. Also obtain guaiac results.

XXII. Serum Pregnancy Test
   A. To determine pregnancy
   B. To use as a preoperative precaution
   C. To check the viability of the fetus, using a serial quantitative beta human chorionic gonadotropin test, which can be ordered every 2 to 3 days

XXIII. Sickle Cell Screen
   A. Order screen for all pregnant African American patients.
   B. If positive, order hemoglobin electrophoresis.
      1. If homozygous, the patient has sickle cell disease. Refer her to a physician for care.
      2. If heterozygous, consider ordering electrophoresis to test the blood of the baby's father. If he is heterozygous, there is a chance that the baby could inherit sickle cell disease.

 CARE DURING LABOR AND DELIVERY

I. Initial Assessment
   A. Determine if the patient is in labor.
      1. Uterine contractions
         a. Time of onset
         b. Intensity
         c. Frequency
         d. Duration
      2. Status of membranes
         a. If ruptured, time of rupture
         b. Color
         c. Amount of fluid
      3. Presence of show
         a. Amount
         b. Consistency
         c. Color (rule out frank bleeding)
      4. Quality of fetal movement
   B. Ascertain estimated date of confinement

    C. Review antepartum course.
        1. Determine if size equals EGA.
        2. Review history of HSV, GBS, or placenta previa.
    D. Review history.
        1. Family history
        2. Medical and surgical history
        3. Past OB history
        4. History of present pregnancy
    E. Perform physical exam.
        1. Observe mother's reaction to labor.
        2. Note vital signs.
        3. Palpate the abdomen for the following:
            a. Uterine contractions
            b. Fundal height
            c. Condition of abdominal wall
            d. Fetus
                (1) Position
                (2) Presentation
                (3) Attitude
                (4) Estimated fetal weight
        4. Monitor fetal heart rate.
        5. Perform pelvic evaluation.
            a. Cervical dilation and effacement
            b. Fetal presentation, position of presenting part, and station
            c. Status of membranes
        6. Perform speculum exam as indicated for
            a. Diagnosis of spontaneous rupture of membranes.
            b. Culture of the cervix.
            c. Visualization of the vagina and cervix for any lesions (i.e., history of herpes).
            d. Identification of the source of vaginal bleeding.

II. **Ongoing Management**
    A. First stage of labor
        1. Observe and guide the physical progress of labor and birth.
        2. Continue assessment of labor.
            a. Monitor maternal blood pressure and temperature according to hospital/institution guidelines.
            b. Evaluate uterine contractions for frequency, duration, and intensity.
            c. Perform cervical exams for dilation, effacement, station, and position of fetus.
            d. Monitor fetal heart rate for 20 minutes before or after three consecutive contractions; then monitor heart rate for 10 minutes before or after two consecutive contractions every hour.

e. Perform vaginal exams as necessary to assess labor. Limit exams for a patient with ruptured membranes.

3. Encourage ambulation to facilitate labor. Do *not* encourage ambulation if the patient's membranes are ruptured and the vertex is high.

4. Encourage the patient to drink or hydrate with IV fluids. IV infusion is necessary for

   a. Clinical signs of dehydration.

   b. Prolonged vomiting or an inability to drink or retain oral fluids.

5. Insert a buff cap or IV with keep vein open (KVO) status for the following conditions:

   a. Greater than para V

   b. Hemoglobin and hematocrit below 9.0 and 27%, respectively

   c. History of bleeding disorder or previous postpartum hemorrhage

   d. Breech presentation

   e. Twin gestation

   f. Hypertension or other medical conditions

   g. Prolonged labor

6. Amniotomy

   a. Indications

      (1) To induce labor

      (2) To stimulate labor

      (3) To check for the presence of meconium if fetal distress or maternal complications occur, such as hypertension or prolonged labor

   b. Criteria

      (1) Vertex presentation with head at 2 station or lower

      (2) Term pregnancy

      (3) Ripe cervix, with a Bishop's score of at least 8 (a score of 9 is almost fail proof)

7. Provide pain relief as desired by the patient and according to approved guidelines.

8. Assist the patient and her family to cope with labor and birth by providing support and comfort measures.

9. Identify deviations from normal.

   a. Manage frequently encountered problems according to approved guidelines.

   b. Consult or refer the patient when indicated.

10. Document the progress of labor, deviations from normal, and any consultations.

B. Second stage of labor

   1. Teach the patient the proper bearing-down technique.

   2. Provide emotional support.

   3. Auscultate the fetal heart rate every 5 minutes or with continuous electronic monitoring.
   4. Catheterize the patient if her bladder is distended and she is unable to void.
   5. Conduct the delivery when it is a single, vertex, normal, and spontaneous vaginal delivery.
   6. Participate in twin, breech, and premature deliveries with appropriate physician collaboration.
   7. Perform an episiotomy, if needed.
   8. Perform the immediate appraisal of the newborn, assign Apgar scores, and consult with a physician or neonatal nurse practitioner, as indicated.
C. Third stage of labor
   1. Deliver and inspect the placenta, cord, and membranes.
   2. Collect cord blood to determine the type, Rh factor, and VDRL and HIV data, as required.
   3. Collect cord blood for gases if fetus had a nonreassuring fetal heart rate pattern, terminal bradycardia, or difficult delivery. Send data to the lab if the 1-minute Apgar score is 5 or below.
   4. Control postpartum bleeding by massage of the fundus and use of oxytocin if needed.
   5. Culture the placenta if prolonged rupture of membranes or fever occurred.
   6. Perform perineal, vaginal, and cervical inspection.
   7. Perform local infiltration or pudendal block anesthesia if needed.
   8. Repair perineal, vaginal, and cervical lacerations or episiotomy.
   9. Promote early infant-parent contact and breast-feeding.
D. Medication: The nurse-midwife may order the following:
   1. Phenergan 25 to 50 mg IM or IV every 3 to 4 hours as necessary for relief of anxiety or nausea
   2. Vistaril 50 to 100 mg IM only, every 3 to 4 hours as necessary for relief of anxiety or nausea
   3. Stadol 1 to 2 mg every 2 to 4 hours as necessary for pain
   4. Nubain 10mg IV push every 3 to 4 hours as necessary for pain
   5. Morphine sulfate, 10 to 15 mg administered subcutaneously (SQ), to stop latent labor and permit rest
   6. A hypnotic such as Ambien 5–10 mg orally to take home for sedation in latent labor
E. Postpartum care
   1. In hospital
      a. Manage patient's hospital course.
         (1) Fourth stage of labor
            (a) Vital signs
            (b) Estimated blood loss and current lochia flow

       (c) Fundus for consistency and location

       (d) Bladder status

       (e) Condition of genital area

       (f) Status of hydration and nutrition

       (g) Psychosocial status

       (h) Maternal-infant bonding

    (2) Order appropriate lab work.

       (a) Hemoglobin and hematocrit 12 to 24 hours after delivery as indicated

       (b) Cultures as indicated (see Puerperal Infection in Part V)

         (i) Endocervical

         (ii) Urine

         (iii) Blood

       (c) Other lab work, as indicated

    (3) Visit patient daily while hospitalized.

       (a) Review history and progress to date.

       (b) Perform daily physical exam, to include:

         (i) Breasts and nipples.

         (ii) Abdomen and uterus.

         (iii) Lochia.

         (iv) Vulva and perineum.

         (v) Costovertebral angle tenderness.

         (vi) Extremities (Homans' sign).

       (c) Provide postpartum instruction.

b. Foster family bonding and adjustment to the newborn.

c. Identify deviations from the normal puerperium.

    (1) Manage frequently encountered problems according to approved guidelines.

    (2) Consult or refer patient when indicated.

d. Identify patient's informational needs and instruct her regarding

    (1) Normal anatomic and physiologic changes.

    (2) Nutrition and weight loss.

    (3) Exercise and activities.

    (4) Hygiene.

    (5) Danger signs and when to seek help.

    (6) Community resources for newborn care.

    (7) Breast-feeding or lactation suppression.

    (8) Sexuality and contraception.

    (9) Referral to appropriate community resources.

e. Obtain relevant laboratory tests.

    f. Assist in planning home care.

    g. Keep adequate hospital records according to standard chart forms. Chart progress notes on any events out of the ordinary.

    h. Discharge patients from the hospital under the following circumstances:

      (1) The patient has no medical problems requiring close supervision (e.g., high blood pressure, diabetes).

      (2) The patient has no antepartum or intrapartum OB complications requiring close postpartum observation (e.g., hemorrhage, infection).

      (3) The patient is asymptomatic with hemoglobin and hematocrit equal to or above 9.0 and 27%, respectively.

      (4) The baby has been released by the pediatrician or family practice physician.

2. In office (4 to 8 weeks postpartum): Evaluate the physical and emotional condition of the mother.

    a. History

      (1) Antepartum and intrapartum course review

      (2) General health of the mother: weight loss or gain, rest, and fatigue

      (3) Family's and mother's adjustment to newborn

      (4) Breast-feeding

      (5) Amount and type of lochia

      (6) Resumption of sexual relations and any problems

      (7) Emotional state

    b. Physical exam

      (1) Record blood pressure, pulse, and weight

      (2) Auscultate the heart and lungs.

      (3) Examine the breasts for nipple integrity, masses, inflammation, and engorgement.

      (4) Palpate the abdomen for tenderness, masses, involution of the uterus, and diastis recti.

      (5) Examine the legs for indications of thrombophlebitis.

      (6) Examine the external genitalia for lesions, healing of the episiotomy or lacerations, and abnormalities of the Bartholin's and Skene's glands.

      (7) Perform speculum exam. Note lacerations of cervix, discharge, and lesions. Obtain a specimen for a Pap smear.

      (8) Perform a bimanual exam. Check for any abnormalities of the cervix, uterus, adnexa, state of involution, presence of cystocele or rectocele, and vaginal muscle tone.

    c. Provide the mother with the opportunity to discuss any problems concerning her baby, family, or self.

    d. Observe the mother-infant interaction if the baby is present.

      e. Initiate a contraceptive method if desired.

      f. Encourage regular aerobic, abdominal, and Kegel exercises.

III. Consultation or Collaborative Management

  A. Consultation or collaborative management with a physician is appropriate for the following situations:

     1. Vaginal birth after cesarean section

     2. Premature or prolonged rupture of membranes

     3. Abnormal presentation

     4. Abnormal vaginal bleeding

     5. Twin pregnancy

     6. Polyhydramnios or oligohydramnios

     7. Hypertension

     8. Diabetes mellitus

     9. Prolonged active labor: no progress for 3 hours with a questionable contraction pattern or no progress for 2 hours with an adequate contraction pattern

    10. Prolonged second stage: no progress for 1 hour or a second stage lasting longer than 2 hours

    11. Preterm labor: 36 weeks or less

    12. Cord prolapse

    13. Fetal distress

      a. Extended bradycardia or tachycardia

      b. Multiple late or variable decelerations

      c. Nonreassuring fetal heart rate pattern

    14. Postterm: Over 42 weeks

    15. Other maternal or fetal distress

    16. Inappropriate gestational size

    17. Signs of genital herpes

    18. Moderately or heavily meconium-stained amniotic fluid

    19. Abnormalities immediately after delivery

      a. Retained placenta

      b. Postpartum hemorrhage that does not respond to the following measures:

        (1) Oxytocic drugs

        (2) An oral dose of 200 μg of misoprostol

        (3) Fundal massage, bimanual compression, or both

        (4) Supine position

        (5) Rapid administration of IV fluids

        (6) Oxygen per mask

  B. Referral to physician care is required in the following situations:

     1. Multiple pregnancy of more than two fetuses

     2. Severe preeclampsia or eclampsia

     3. Diabetes mellitus greater than class I insulin-dependent diabetics

  4. Cesarean section (maternal or fetal indication) with a documented classical uterine incision

IV. Oxytocin Induction or Augmentation

A. Admission procedures

1. Be sure the prenatal record and indication for procedure are in hospital chart.
2. Take a brief history, including onset of labor, status of membranes, and presence of bleeding.
3. Conduct a brief physical exam according to the standard form in the hospital chart.
4. Indicate selection of standing orders and sign them.
5. Lab work
   a. CBC, if necessary
   b. Clot tube to be held, if necessary
   c. Blood type and screen only if high likelihood of hemorrhage and surgery

B. Induction

1. Indications
   a. Postdates
   b. Premature rupture of membranes
   c. Polyhydramnios or oligohydramnios
   d. Fetal indications
      (1) Nonreactive nonstress test
      (2) Biophysical profile below 8
      (3) Large for gestational age
      (4) Suspected intrauterine fetal growth retardation
   e. Maternal indications
      (1) Diabetes
      (2) Hemolysis, elevated liver function, and low platelets (HELLP) syndrome
      (3) PIH
      (4) Multiple gestation
      (5) History of genital herpes or GBS in past or current pregnancy
      (6) Social indications
2. Criteria
   a. Patient must be at greater than 37 weeks' EGA.
   b. Prior consultation must have occurred with a collaborative physician.
3. Method
   a. Amniotomy
   b. Prostaglandin gel or Prepidil administration, according to hospital protocol
      (1) Unripe cervix

   (2) Bishop's score of 4 or below, with or without ruptured membranes (see Table 5-2, Bishop's Score, in Part V)

  c. Misoprostol administration, according to hospital protocol[13]

  d. Pitocin administration, according to hospital protocol

C. Augmentation

 1. Indications

  a. Rupture of membranes without active labor

  b. Poor uterine contractions

  c. Failure to progress with active labor; cervix unchanged in 3 hours in primipara or 2 hours in the multiparous patient

 2. Criteria

  a. Vertex presentation

  b. Reassuring fetal heart rate pattern

  c. Physician consultation

D. Management: See Ongoing Management earlier in this section.

 MENOPAUSE AND PERIMENOPAUSE

I. Definitions

 A. Menopause is the permanent cessation of menses resulting from ovarian failure.

 B. Perimenopause is the term used to describe the years that surround the actual experience of menopause. This transition usually takes 4 to 5 years and is characterized by menstrual irregularity. Conception is unlikely but can still occur.

II. Etiology

 A. Six percent of women enter menopause by 35 years of age, 25% by 44 years of age, 75% by 50 years of age, and 94% by 55 years of age.

 B. Estrogen and progesterone levels begin to fluctuate unpredictably.

 C. The cells lining the follicles in the ovary no longer respond as predictably to follicle-stimulating hormone (FSH) or luteinizing hormone (LH), resulting in anovulatory menstrual cycles.

 D. Surgical menopause: Removal of the ovaries and uterus will cause immediate symptoms of change. Removal of only the uterus will allow the ovaries to continue producing estrogen, and the signs of change will be more gradual.

III. Clinical Features

 A. Change in menstruation

  1. Menstrual cycles

   a. Menstrual cycles are often anovulatory.

   b. Breakthrough bleeding with spotting during days 19 to 25 may occur, followed by menses at the regular time.

---

[13]Physician's Desk Reference, 2001, p. 2576

      c. More than 60% of women experience less frequent periods and skipping of cycles.

  2. Amount

      a. The majority of women experience short, scant bleeding.

      b. Heavier periods with clots and cramps can occur.

B. Increased signs and symptoms of PMS

  1. Bloating

  2. Pelvic discomfort

  3. Headaches

  4. Irritability

  5. Mood swings

C. Vasomotor disturbances (hot flashes, night sweats)

  1. Vasomotor disturbances occur in 45% of women.

  2. Twenty-five percent of women have hot flashes for more than 5 years; two percent experience them for life.

  3. Hot flashes occurring during sleep cause profuse perspiration.

D. Urogenital atrophy

  1. Urinary frequency and urgency caused by thinner urethral epithelium and less urethral tone

  2. Susceptibility to UTIs

  3. Loss of support for pelvic viscera

  4. Loss of rugae in vagina and paleness of mucosa

E. Osteopenia and osteoporosis

  1. Bone is lost at an annual rate of 0.5% after age 40.

  2. Many women do not experience any associated symptoms until a fracture occurs.

      a. The most common fractures are vertebral, forearm, and hip.

      b. Hip fractures and sequelae are lethal in 12% to 20% of women.

  3. Symptoms include pain radiating along the back, backache, curvature of the spine, and height loss.

  4. The Osteopenia and Osteoporosis section in Part IV provides further information.

F. Cardiovascular disease

  1. When women reach age 55, the incidence of cardiovascular disease overtakes that of cancer and becomes the leading cause of death.

  2. The cause is multifactorial.

      a. Throughout the reproductive cycle, serum levels of low-density lipoprotein (LDL) cholesterol in women are lower than they are in men. Levels of LDL cholesterol rise at menopause and become equal to those of men. There are no significant changes in high-density lipoprotein (HDL) cholesterol. Therefore, after menopause, women's risk of cardiovascular disease equals that of men.

        b. Age, sex, and genetic predisposition are nonmodifiable. Fortunately their effects can be influenced by diet, exercise, stress reduction measures, weight loss, avoidance of toxic substances (e.g., nicotine, alcohol, cocaine, and amphetamines), and use of hormone replacement therapy (HRT).

  G. Skin changes

     1. Thinning and loss of subcutaneous fat

     2. Dryness

     3. Loss of hair

     4. Minor hirsutism of face

  H. Psychological, social, and sexual issues

     1. Depression and mood changes caused by hormone changes and insomnia are common during the perimenopause.

     2. The attitudes of society, cultural background, family, and the patient's own feelings are all reflected in her response to menopause.

     3. Sexual desire and coital enjoyment decrease in many women.

IV. Management

  A. History

     1. Menstrual history

        a. Menstrual cycles can be either longer or shorter than what they consider normal.

        b. Some women may skip cycles entirely.

        c. There may be incidences of breakthrough bleeding.

        d. The color, amount, and consistency of menses may change.

     2. Signs and symptoms

        a. Hot flashes

        b. Anxiety

        c. Depression

        d. Mood swings

        e. Insomnia

        f. Fatigue

        g. Increase in PMS symptoms

        h. Decreased vaginal lubrication

        i. Increased number of vaginal infections

        j. Increased number of bladder infections

        k. Changes in fatty deposits in the body

     3. Stress incontinence

     4. Symptoms and risks for cardiovascular disease

     5. Gynecologic surgery

  B. Physical exam: This should include

     1. A thorough breast exam.

     2. Inspection of vaginal mucosa for paleness and loss of rugae.

3. A careful bimanual exam.

   a. In menopause, the ovaries should be very small or not palpable.

   b. The uterus should be small with normal consistency. A firm, irregular, or enlarged uterus may indicate a fibroid or other problems.

4. Inspection for cystocele, rectocele, and uterine prolapse.

5. A rectal exam, noting hemorrhoids.

C. Lab work

   1. Pap smear

      a. A yearly Pap smear is the standard.

      b. Some are recommending that practitioners should not perform routine Pap smears on postmenopausal women within 2 to 4 years of a normal Pap result. "These cause needless concern and are unnecessary."[14]

      c. In hysterectomy patients, some cervical cells may be left during the operation. It is recommended that the vaginal area be checked and a Pap smear be taken from the cuff area every 2 to 3 years.

   2. Mammogram—The American Cancer Society recommends the following practices:[15]

      a. Have one mammogram done every 2 years beginning at 40 years of age.

      b. Have one mammogram done every year beginning at 50 years of age.

      c. If a close family member on either side of the family has had breast cancer before the age of 50, get a yearly mammogram, beginning 10 years before the age of onset in the youngest family member.

   3. Blood workup

      a. Human chorionic gonadotropin levels will determine if the patient is pregnant.

      b. FSH should be measured on day 6 or 7 of a BCP-free week. If FSH is above 40 mIU/mL, the patient is in menopause and may be switched to, or started on, HRT.

      c. LH changes little throughout adulthood: female not midcycle, less than 30 IU/L; midcycle, 30 to 150 IU/L; and postmenopausal, 30 to 120 IU/mL. Note that an FSH:LH ratio of more than 1 is diagnostic of menopause.

      d. Estradiol below 3 ng/dL indicates a postmenopausal female.

      e. Progesterone (serum) should be measured on days 20 to 24 before menses. Patient is anovulatory if below 300 ng.

      f. A thyroid profile may be done to rule out problems in this area.

      g. Prolactin should be measured if nipple discharge is present.

---

[14]Swaya, Grady, and Kerlikoske, 2000, p. 942
[15]American Cancer Society, 2000, p. 9

    h. A cardiac risk assessment of HDLs, LDLs, and triglycerides should be performed.

    i. Stool should be examined for occult blood every year past 40 years of age.

D. Special considerations

    1. Consider an endometrial biopsy in the following situations:

        a. When any abnormal uterine bleeding occurs and the patient is older than 35

        b. Before the initiation of HRT (optional)

        c. If a postmenopausal patient presents with vaginal bleeding (biopsy is a necessity)

    2. If adnexa are found to be young-adult size or enlarged in a menopausal woman, consider ultrasound plus a cancer antigen (CA) 125 test.

    3. If uterus is firm, enlarged, and has an irregular contour, do an ultrasound and refer the patient as appropriate.

    4. If the patient has urinary incontinence or cystocele, take the following measures:

        a. Advise the patient to do Kegel exercises—see instructions for these exercises at end of this section.

        b. If the patient is not a good surgical candidate, try a pessary or Introl system.

        c. Refer the patient for a workup and probable surgery.

    5. If the patient has a family history of osteoporosis or is at high risk because of lifestyle or physical characteristics, consider bone density studies.

E. Perimenopausal medications

    1. Irregular bleeding of recent onset, *without* other signs and symptoms

        a. In a nonsmoker over 35 years of age, start low-dose BCPs.

            (1) If irregular bleeding continues past 2 to 3 months, the patient needs further evaluation. See Dysfunctional Uterine Bleeding in Part IV.

            (2) Contraception is an added benefit. Women over 40 have the second-highest proportion of unintended pregnancies.[16]

        b. In either smoker or nonsmoker, try the following:

No estrogen		No estrogen
Progestin* 5–10 mg, first 10 days of the month	OR	Progestin* 5–10 mg, day 14 or 16 to day 25

*Common progestins: Provera, Cycrin, Aygestin, and Amen

---

[16]Hatcher, Robert A. et al. Contraceptive Technology. Seventeenth Edition. 1998 p 78

2. Irregular bleeding *with* other signs and symptoms
   a. In a nonsmoker over 35 years of age, give low-dose BCPs. If she gets signs of estrogen withdrawal (e.g., hot flashes, headaches) during the inactive pills, two to three cycles of active BCPs may be given before allowing a period. The patient may also be given a low dose of estrogen or an OTC soy product, such as
      (1) Premarin 0.3 or 0.625 mg.
      (2) Estrace 0.5 or 1 mg.
      (3) OTC products, such as Estroven, Remifemin, Healthy Women.
   b. In a smoker over 35 years of age, give Premphase or OTC products. Be sure to counsel the patient that these products do not protect against pregnancy.

Premphase	
Premarin 0.625 daily	Provera 5–10 mg, day 14 or 16 to day 25

F. HRT medications
   1. Advantages
      a. Relief of menopausal symptoms
      b. Prevention and treatment of osteoporosis
      c. Prevention of cardiovascular disease
   2. Risks
      a. Endometrial cancer: Two to 6 times greater in women with a uterus, using unopposed estrogen
      b. Breast cancer: Slight increased risk of breast cancer with prolonged use of HRT
   3. Contraindications
      a. Known breast cancer
      b. Known or suspected endometrial cancer
      c. Known or suspected pregnancy
      d. Undiagnosed genital bleeding
      e. Active thrombophlebitis and thrombotic disorders
      f. Acute liver disease or chronic impaired liver function
G. Menopausal medications: A continuous-dose regimen leads to further atrophy and thinning of the endometrium. If there is still occasional spotting, the combination of medication in the following chart will ultimately eliminate it. If periods have stopped for more than 1 year, they are unlikely to restart.

Estrogen daily	Progestin 2.5 mg daily, increasing up to 10 mg daily, as needed

H. Hysterectomy: Daily estrogen is indicated for women without a uterus. There is no need for progestin administration.

Estrogen daily	No progestin

I. HRT options: See Table 1-5 at the end of this chapter.

J. Special problems

1. The following medications help relieve symptoms for patients unable to take estrogen:

   a. Bellergal-S 0.2 mg orally twice a day for hot flashes

   b. Clonidine 0.1 mg orally or transdermally for hot flashes

   c. Megestrol acetate 20 mg orally twice a day for hot flashes

   d. Effexor XR—75 mg orally once a day for hot flashes in breast cancer survivors

   e. Evista (raloxifene) for osteoporosis prevention; does not help hot flashes or vaginal dryness

2. The following medications help decreased libido: Estratest 1.25 mg/2.5 mg or Estratest H.S. 0.625 mg/1.25 mg taken daily.

3. Atrophic vaginitis sometimes appears as abnormal squamous cells of undetermined significance (ASCUS) on a Pap smear. Some treatments are as follows:

   a. Vaginal creams, such as Ortho Dienestrol, Estrace, Ogen, and Premarin. When starting an estrogen cream, it should be given every day for 1 to 2 weeks, every other day for a week, and then two times a week. Some patients can remain symptom-free using estrogen cream once a week.

   b. Vagifem tablets—One tablet vaginally per day for 2 weeks and then twice weekly for maintenance.

   c. Estring 2 mg may be placed in the vagina. It needs to be changed every 90 days.

4. If the patient is unable to take Provera because of increased PMS, bloating, gas, and cramps, she should try an HRT that has norethindrone or another progestin.

5. If increasing the estrogen dose does not relieve symptoms, an injectable estrogen every month with or without testosterone (Depo-Estradiol, Depo-Testadiol) might work better.

6. If osteopenia or osteoporosis is a problem, see Osteopenia and Osteoporosis in Part IV.

V. Teaching. Counsel the patient to

A. Learn the signs and symptoms of menopause.

B. Wear light clothes and dress in layers to deal with hot flashes.

C. Alleviate insomnia by napping during the day and decreasing caffeine and spicy foods, especially at night.

D. Improve mood swings, irritability, and depression with regular diet and exercise. Talking with friends helps. If depression is severe (having crying spells or suicidal thoughts), a complete physical and HRT may help. Referral to a counselor or psychologist may be indicated.

E. View exercise as a way of living and being healthier.

F. Eat a diet that is average in protein, low in fat, and high in fiber with calcium-rich foods.

G. Take 1000 mg of calcium per day (perimenopausal) and 1500 mg of calcium per day (menopausal) through diet plus supplements. Take adequate amounts of vitamin D and magnesium. Avoid nicotine and limit caffeine and alcohol.

H. Take all medication as prescribed. (In women with a uterus, estrogen, when taken without a progesterone product, may do more damage than not taking any medication.)

I. Remove the backing on the Estraderm, Climara, or other transdermal patch and wait 30 to 60 seconds to allow alcohol to evaporate before applying the patch, if there is local irritation at the application site.

J. Discuss individual problems, such as incontinence and pain with intercourse, with her health care provider. Many of these problems can be helped or eliminated.

 KEGEL EXERCISES

I. **Definition.** These exercises were originally developed by Dr. Arnold Kegel to help with problems controlling urination. They are designed to strengthen and give voluntary control of the pubococcygeus (PC) muscle. The PC muscle is part of the sling of muscle stretching from the pubic bone in front to the tailbone in back. Because the muscle encircles not only the urinary opening but also the outside of the vagina, the exercise may increase sexual awareness as well.

II. **Teaching.** Initiate Kegels on the second or third day after childbirth, at any time a woman is found to have lax vaginal muscles on exam, or if there is a complaint of stress incontinence.

A. Identification of the PC muscle: Sit on the toilet. Stop and start the flow of urine. The PC muscle is the one that turns the flow on and off. Once the muscle is identified, it is best not to practice this exercise while urinating, but after.

B. The exercises

1. Perform slow Kegels—Tighten the PC muscle. Hold it for a slow count of three and then relax it.

2. Perform quick Kegels—Tighten and relax the PC muscle as rapidly as possible.

3. At first, do 10 (one "set") of each exercise five times every day. Each week, increase the number of repetitions by five (e.g., 15, 20, 25). Keep doing five sets each day.

4. Suggest the patient complete a set of exercises each time she goes to the bathroom, just before she wipes.

5. These exercises can be done while driving, watching television, doing dishes, or lying in bed.

Table 1-5. Hormone Replacement Therapy Options

Brand Name	Generic Name	Dosing Information
Oral Estrogens (taken daily)		
Premarin	Conjugated estrogens	0.3, 0.625, 0.9, 1.25, or 2.5 mg conjugated estrogens
Estratab	Esterified estrogens	0.3, 0.625, or 2.5 mg estrogen
Menest	Esterified estrogens	0.3, 0.625, 1.25, or 2.5 mg estrogen
Estrace	Micronized estradiol	0.5, 1, or 2 mg micronized estradiol
Ortho-Est	Estropipate	0.75 or 1.5 mg estropipate (supplied as Ortho-Est 0.625 or 1.25)
Ogen	Estropipate	0.625, 1.25, 2.5, or 5 mg estropipate
Cenestin	Synthetic conjugated estrogen	0.625 and 0.9 mg estrogen, titrated to 1.25 mg
Oral Estrogen and Progestin Combinations		
Premphase	Conjugated estrogens and medroxyprogesterone acetate (MPA)	2-tablet regimen: conjugated estrogens 0.625 mg daily on days 1–14; conjugated estrogens 0.625 mg and 5 mg MPA on days 15–28
Prempro	Conjugated estrogens and MPA	1 tablet containing 0.625 mg conjugated estrogens and 2.5 or 5 mg MPA taken daily
Ortho-Prefest	17 beta-estradiol and norgestimate combination	1 mg estradiol for 3 days, followed by 1 mg estradiol and 0.09 mg norgestimate for 3 days, repeated continuously
Femhrt	Progestin–estrogen combination	1 tablet containing 5 μg ethinyl and 1 mg norethindrone taken daily
Activella	Estradiol and norethindrone	1 tablet containing 1 mg estradiol and 0.5 mg norethindrone taken daily
Transdermal Estrogens		
Estraderm	Estradiol	0.05 or 0.1 mg estradiol per day via 4- or 8-mg patch used 2 times per week
FemPatch	Estradiol	0.025 mg estradiol per day via 10.3-mg patch used once every 7 days

(continued)

Table 1-5. Hormone Replacement Therapy Options *(Continued)*

Brand Name	Generic Name	Dosing Information
Vivelle	Estradiol	0.0375, 0.05, 0.075, or 0.1 mg estradiol per day via 3.28-, 4.33-, 6.57- or 8.66-mg patch used 2 times per week
Climara	Estradiol	0.025, 0.05, 0.075, or 0.1 mg estradiol per day via 2-, 3.9-, 5.7-, or 7.6-mg patch used once every 7 days
CombiPatch	Estradiol and norethindrone acetate	0.05 mg estradiol and 0.14 or 0.25 mg norethindrone acetate per day; applied two times per week
Oral Estrogen and Testosterone		
Estratest, Estratest HS	Esterified estrogen and methyltestosterone	1.25 mg esterified estrogen and 2.5 mg methyltestosterone (Estratest); 0.625 mg esterified estrogen and 1.25 mg methyltestosterone (Estratest HS); both taken daily
Oral Progestins		
Provera	MPA	5 or 10 mg a day for 12–14 days per month along with conjugated estrogens; if menopausal, 2.5 or 5 mg daily
Cycrin	MPA	5 or 10 mg for 5–12 days beginning on day 14, 16, or 21 of the menstrual cycle; if menopausal, 2.5 or 5 mg taken daily
Prometrium	Progesterone	200 mg a day for 12 days per 28-day cycle along with conjugated estrogens
Aygestin	Norethindrone acetate	5 or 10 mg a day for 12–14 days per month along with conjugated estrogens; if menopausal, 2.5 or 5 mg daily

PART 2

Common Discomforts of Pregnancy

Anita Pendo, MSN, NP

Discomfort	Etiology	Differential Diagnosis	Relief Measures	Danger Signs
Back Pain, Lower	• Muscle strain caused by a shift in the center of gravity, caused by an enlarging uterus • A high blood level of progesterone, which softens cartilage and loosens stable pelvic joints, allowing movement • Lax abdominal muscle tone, especially in multiparas	• Uterine contractions • Genital infections • Urinary tract infections (UTIs) • Sciatica • Herniated disk • Vertebral tumor • Muscle sprain or strain • Kidney infection or disease	• Wear maternity support girdle. • Take warm tub baths. • Sleep on a supportive mattress and assume the lateral recumbent position with pillows supporting the back and legs. • Use local head and back rubs. • Use relaxation techniques. • Avoid excessive twisting, bending, stretching, excessive standing, or walking. • Use proper body mechanics, pelvic tilt, and other exercises to strengthen the back; refer the patient to a physical therapist for such instruction. • Start an exercise program that encourages general fitness.	History of back injury or other back problems, surgery, UTI symptoms, ruptured membranes, uterine contractions, neurologic deficit, costovertebral angle tenderness (CVAT) pain with straight-leg raises, abnormal deep tendon reflex (DTRs), and abnormal vaginal discharge

(continued)

Discomfort	Etiology	Differential Diagnosis	Relief Measures	Danger Signs
			• When standing for long periods, rest one foot on a low stool. When sitting for long periods, rest feet on a low stool, raise knees above the waist, and sit with the back firmly against the back of a chair.	
			• When driving, sit straight with knees slightly bent when using pedals.	
			• Maintain good posture and wear shoes with 2-inch heels.	
			• Take 1000 mg of acetaminophen every 4 hr or as needed for minor discomfort.	
Back Pain, Upper	• Muscle strain caused by a shift in the center of gravity, caused by an enlarging uterus	• Uterine contractions	• Wear a good, supportive bra.	History of back injury or other back problems, surgery, UTI symptoms, ruptured membranes, uterine contractions, neurologic deficit, CVAT, pain with straight-leg raises,
	• High blood levels of progesterone, which soften cartilage and	• Kidney infection or disease	• Take warm tub baths.	
		• UTIs	• Sleep on a firm supportive mattress and assume the lateral recumbent position with pillows supporting back and legs.	
		• Sciatica		
		• Herniated disk		
		• Vertebral tumor		

	Cause	Differential Diagnoses	Interventions	Warning Signs
	loosen stable pelvic joints • Increased breast size	• Muscle sprain or strain • Gallbladder disease	• Use local heat and back rubs. • Use relaxation techniques. • Avoid excessive twisting, bending, stretching, walking, or standing. • Use exercises to strengthen the back; refer the patient to a physical therapist for instruction. • Start an exercise program that encourages general fitness. • Maintain good posture. • Take 1000 mg of acetaminophen every 4 hr or as needed for minor discomfort.	abnormal DTRs, and abnormal vaginal discharge
Constipation	• Increased progesterone levels in pregnancy, which cause relaxation of smooth muscle in bowel, resulting in decreased motility, tone, and peristalsis of the gastrointestinal (GI) tract	• Preterm labor • Irritable bowel syndrome • Appendicitis • Intestinal obstruction • Fecal obstruction	• Increase roughage and fluids (fresh fruits and vegetables, dried fruits, bran, and whole grain foods). Drink 6 to 8 glasses of liquids daily, and a hot drink upon arising. • Increase exercise.	Changes in stool, diarrhea, abdominal pain, fever, anorexia, periumbilical pain, rectal bleeding, emotional distress, or excessive laxative use for weight control

(continued)

Discomfort	Etiology	Differential Diagnosis	Relief Measures	Danger Signs
	• Mechanical compression of the large bowel by an enlarging uterus • Changes in food and fluid intake or exercise level because of pregnancy changes • Prenatal vitamins with iron or calcium		• Maintain regular bowel habits. • If taking prenatal vitamins, use one with a stool softener. • If needed, take a nonsystemic bulk laxative stool softener or combination of softener and laxative. • If constipation is acute, try Dulcolax, Milk of Magnesia, or a glycerin suppository. • If all else fails, try a Fleets enema. Do not use acute measures regularly.	

Dependent Edema	• High estrogen levels, which make blood vessels more fragile and "leaky" • Impaired venous circulation and increased pressure in lower extremities from the pressure of an enlarging uterus on the veins • Expanding blood volume of pregnancy	• Pregnancy-induced hypertension—usually more severe than physiologic hypertension, with a sudden onset and more generalized symptoms • High sodium intake—sodium restriction not necessary during pregnancy, but an excessive amount may result in edema • Hemolysis, elevated liver function and low platelets (HELLP) syndrome, renal disease, varicosities, local trauma to extremities, carpal tunnel syndrome, and congestive heart failure	• Avoid constrictive clothing. • Take rest periods lying down on left side with legs elevated periodically throughout day to aid venous return. • Wear elastic stockings to aid venous return. • Avoid excessive sodium. • Call office if edema suddenly becomes more severe or general.	Sudden onset of generalized edema (facial or upper extremity)—may be a sign of PIH. Numbness or loss of sensation in fingers of either or both hands. Confusion, headache, flashing lights, fatigue, nausea and vomiting, dyspnea, upper abdominal pain, decreased fetal movement, decreased urine output, rapid weight gain (more than 2 lb/wk), and increase in blood pressure (BP) of 30 mm Hg systolic or 15 mm Hg diastolic over baseline
Dyspareunia	• Pressure from enlarging uterus • Inflammation • Anatomic abnormalities	• Vulvovaginitis • Atrophic vulvovaginitis • Hymeneal strands • Scar tissue	• Try to alternate positions during intercourse. • Use a water-soluble lubricant.	Uterine contractions, vulvar or vaginal inflammation, lesions, discharge, pelvic masses (other than pregnancy), *(continued)*

Discomfort	Etiology	Differential Diagnosis	Relief Measures	Danger Signs
		• Episiotomy	• Refer patient to psychologic therapy if appropriate.	cervical motion tenderness, loss of pelvic support, and symptoms of UTI
	• Pelvic pathology	• Vaginismus		
	• Atrophy	• Pelvic relaxation	• Explore alternate methods to express intimacy and affection.	
	• Failure of lubrication	• PID		
	• History of sexually transmitted diseases (STDs)	• Pelvic masses	• Take medication for inflammation and infection, if appropriate.	
	• Recurrent infection	• Bartholin's cyst		
	• Psychologic conflicts	• Inappropriate sexual technique		
		• Psychologic factors, such as previous sexual trauma or stress		
Fatigue	• Which occurs primarily during the first and third trimesters	• Most pathologic problems—emotional, physical, or dietary	• Expect increased fatigue in the first and third trimester.	A history of depression or anxiety, difficulty with concentration, anorexia, anemia, exercise intolerance, chest pain or discomfort, change in bowel habits, flulike symptoms, sore throat, coughing or dyspnea, or other symptoms or signs indicating other conditions requiring medical or other
			• Verbalize psychosocial problems and seek apt interventions.	
	• First trimester—increased oxygen consumption, progesterone levels, and fetal demands, as well as psychosocial changes		• Accept offers of help.	
			• Avoid, if possible, major life stresses during pregnancy.	
	• Third trimester—sleep disturbances		• Take supplemental iron if anemic.	
			• Get adequate sleep, take	

	from increased weight, physical discomforts, and decreased exercise		rest periods, maintain good posture, wear low-heeled shoes, and perform pelvic-rock exercises. • Correct nutritional inadequacies. • Avoid caffeine and heavy meals at the end of the day.	follow-up. Abnormal vital signs or lab work, especially complete blood count (CBC)
Gas	• Increased progesterone levels in pregnancy, which cause relaxation of smooth muscle in the bowel, resulting in decreased motility, tone, and peristalsis of the GI tract	• Irritable bowel syndrome • Lactose intolerance • Medication side effects • Hyperventilation	• Learn measures to avoid constipation. • Learn symptoms of hyperventilation or air swallowing. • Avoid gum chewing, large meals, and smoking. • Limit gas-forming foods (e.g., carbonated beverages, cheese, beans, bananas, and calcium carbonate supplements). • Take Phazyme.	Changes in bowel habits; dark, tarry stools; grey, mucus-covered stools; or abdominal pain or tenderness
Headache	• Increased circulatory volume • Vasodilation from high levels of circulating progesterone	• Tension, migraine, cluster, sinus, or benign vascular headaches • PIH	• Keep a diary of activities, foods, and environmental stimuli that occur around time of the headaches. • Learn the symptoms of PIH.	A history of injury to the head, neck, or back; occupational exposure to chemicals; consumption of alcohol, chocolate, or

(continued)

Discomfort	Etiology	Differential Diagnosis	Relief Measures	Danger Signs
	• Tissue edema resulting from vascular congestion • Stress • Fatigue • Low blood sugar	• Upper respiratory infection (URI) or sinus infection • Fever • Cardiovascular disease • Cervical arthritis • Muscle tension headache • Cerebellar mass or hemorrhage • Central nervous system (CNS) infection • Hypoglycemia	• Take 325 to 650 mg of acetaminophen every 4 hrs or as needed for pain. • Avoid activities and situations that may trigger headaches. • Reduce stress as much as possible, get adequate sleep, and have neck and shoulders massaged with heat or coolness applied. • Practice relaxation techniques. • Eat a regular, balanced diet and avoid an intake of food that triggers headaches. • Refer the patient to a pain center if the pain is unrelieved by these measures or counseling.	aged cheese; an unbalanced intake of calories, or fatigue—these signs and symptoms may indicate conditions requiring follow-up. A history of facial edema; changes in level of consciousness; memory changes; motor, visual, or sensory changes; N & V; stiff neck; fever; ear or eye pain; rhinitis; flulike symptoms; or injury. Urine dipstick with more than a trace of protein or ketones, low-serum glucose, or an abnormal CBC
Heartburn	• An increase in levels of circulating progesterone that causes decreased peristalsis and reflux of gastric or duodenal contents into the lower esophagus	• Cardiac disease • Gallbladder disease • Epigastric or pancreatic disease	• Counsel patient that heartburn is related to pregnancy and should improve or disappear after pregnancy.	Chest pain; shortness of breath; exercise intolerance; palpitations; sweating; anxiety; upper abdominal pain

- Tissue edema resulting from vascular congestion
- Stress
- Fatigue
- Low blood sugar

- An increase in levels of circulating progesterone that causes decreased peristalsis and reflux of gastric or duodenal contents into the lower esophagus

- GERD or hiatal disease

- Do not lie down, bend, or stoop for 2 hr after eating.
- Elevate the head of the bed 6 in.
- Avoid clothing that constricts around the abdomen or waist.
- Stop smoking.
- Avoid hot, spicy, fatty, gas-forming foods; coffee; alcohol; and gum chewing.
- Eat small, frequent meals and chew food thoroughly.
- Avoid excessive weight gain.
- Take antacids (e.g., Maalox, Mylanta, and Pepcid AC) to relieve hyperacidity and gas; if they contain aluminum and magnesium hydroxide, iron absorption may be impaired; so take iron and vitamin supplements at least 2 hr before or after taking antacids.

(especially after heavy, fatty, or spicy meals); fatty, foul-smelling stools; N & V; fever; or flulike symptoms

(continued)

Discomfort	Etiology	Differential Diagnosis	Relief Measures	Danger Signs
Hemorrhoids	• Impaired venous circulation with resulting congestion in pelvic veins • Increased venous pressure on pelvic veins caused by pressure of enlarging uterus • Relaxing effects of progesterone on vein walls and valves • Constipation • Straining at stool • Family tendency	• Abscessed or thrombosed hemorrhoids • Cancerous lesions • Idiopathic pruritus ani • Condyloma acuminata • Rectal fissure	• Use calcium carbonate with caution; it may cause rebound hyperacidity. • Avoid sodium bicarbonate. • Ask the physician to examine the hemorrhoids for severity, trauma, and possible thrombosis. If the hemorrhoids are thrombosed, the physician will refer the patient to a surgeon for lancing. • Inform the patient that if there is no improvement after 1 wk, the physician will reexamine the patient for trauma or thrombosis. Comfort measures: • Review diet and modify it to keep stools soft. • Relieve constipation. • Recommend frequent sitz baths. • Recommend ice packs, witch hazel packs, and	Decreased hemoglobin caused by prolonged or extensive bleeding, severe pain, blue-black colored hemorrhoids, and thrombosis

			History of or present depression, anxiety, difficulty with concentration, anorexia, anemia,

Epsom salt compresses to reduce swelling.

- Provide patient with a rubber ring to sit on for reduction of pressure.
- Instruct patient to keep hemorrhoids reduced by gently pushing them inside the rectum and tightening the rectal sphincter to give them support and to contain them within rectum.
- Advise bed rest with the hips and lower extremities elevated.
- Order medical suppositories, Preparation H, a topical analgesic, anesthetic spray, or ointment if needed.
- If the patient is bleeding, consider suppositories medicated with cortisone.

General measures:

- Alleviate or reduce sources of anxiety.

- Depression
- Anxiety or worry
- Stress

Insomnia

- Anxiety
- Discomforts of late pregnancy

(continued)

Discomfort	Etiology	Differential Diagnosis	Relief Measures	Danger Signs
	• Normal changes in the sleep–wake cycle in late pregnancy • Early labor		• Avoid stimulation activity just before bedtime. • Read a dull book. • Take a hot bath. • Use massage techniques. • Use relaxation techniques. • Drink hot liquids such as herb teas. • Take 20 mg of Unisom before retiring. • Exercise regularly during the day. • Modify schedule to allow for naps during day. • Avoid regular use of alcohol and sleeping pills. • Deal with specific concerns; refer the patient, if necessary, to a mental health counselor. • Alleviate specific discomforts of pregnancy where possible. • Conserve energy at the beginning of labor. Comfort measures:	exercise intolerance, and chest pain or discomfort

Leg Cramps	The etiology of leg cramps is not clear. Theories include the following: • Inadequate or impaired calcium intake • Lack of balance in calcium/phosphorus ratio in the body • Inadequate or impaired potassium intake or excessive loss of K^+ • Pressure from the enlarging uterus on the nerves to the lower extremities, occur primarily in the second and third trimesters	• Varicosities • Thrombophlebitis • Excessive activity (especially prolonged standing or walking in high heels) • Dehydration • Nerve root compression	• Straighten the affected leg and point the heel. • Participate in general exercise and maintain a habit of good body mechanics to improve circulation. • Elevate the leg periodically throughout the day. • Review diet. Balance calcium and phosphorus intake. Calcium intake consists of dairy products, calcium gluconate or lactate, or Tums. Foods rich in protein are high in phosphorus. Watch for excess phosphorus (excessive protein or soda).	A history of deep-vein thromboembolic disease, positive Homans' sign, abnormal pulses in one or both lower extremities, redness, tenderness, heat, swelling, coldness, numbness, or whiteness in calf or leg
Leukorrhea	• High levels of estrogen, which cause increased vascularity and hypertrophy of cervical glands and vaginal cells	• Ruptured membranes • Vaginitis • Cervicitis • Condyloma acuminatum • Genital herpes	• Keep vulva clean and dry. • Avoid panty hose and tight or layered clothing. • Wear cotton underwear or a nightgown without underwear at night.	Green, watery, bloody, itchy, or irritating discharge that smells foul or fishy; fever; flulike symptoms; abdominal pain; bleeding after

(continued)

Discomfort	Etiology	Differential Diagnosis	Relief Measures	Danger Signs
		• STDs and cervical dysplasias or neoplasia	• If using panty liners, use unscented or nondeodorant ones and change frequently. • Avoid douching and tampon use. • Avoid large amounts of simple sugars. • Eat sugar-free yogurt with active *L. acidophilus* cultures • Maintain a high carbohydrate diet.	intercourse; dyspareunia; (and the presence of *Candida*, trichomonads; clue cells; and abnormal numbers of coccal, bacteria, or red and white blood cells)
Nausea	The etiology is unknown. Theories include the following: • Sudden rise in hormone levels, especially estrogen • An endocrine effect on the CNS center that controls N & V • Smooth muscle relaxation of the stomach and	• Severe emotional problems • Hyperemesis gravidarum • Hydatidiform mole • Hiatal hernia • Gastroenteritis • Multiple gestation • Cholecystitis • Hepatitis • Inner ear infection • Sinusitis	• Avoid spicy, greasy foods and those with strong or offensive odors. • Eat small, frequent meals. • Avoid large amounts of fluids at one time, with meals. • Keep crackers, popcorn, or dry toast at the bedside to eat before arising. • Eat or drink something sweet before going to bed and before getting up	Fever, lethargy, muscle aches, abdominal pain, cramping, diarrhea, jaundice, dark urine, changes in the shape or color of bowel movements, vaginal bleeding, head injury, headaches, projectile vomiting, vomiting of blood, neurologic signs, ataxia, chest pain, ear pain, dehydration, or psychosocial distress

(continued)

intestine, caused by increased progesterone levels

- A decrease in muscular peristalsis, muscle tone, and secretion of acid and pepsin
- Overeating
- Enlarging uterus in last half of pregnancy
- Emotional factors

- Diabetes
- Thyroid dysfunction
- Increased intracranial pressure
- Migraine headaches
- Pica
- Food poisoning

(e.g., peppermint tea, hot lemonade or lemon juice, and hard lemon candy).

- Do not permit stomach to get completely empty—eat every 2 to 3 hr; immediately upon awakening, before retiring, and in middle of night, if awake.
- Drink one-fourth to one-half cup of grapefruit juice with meals to increase stomach acidity.
- Take 50 to 100 mg of vitamin B_6 twice a day.
- Try 10 mg of Unisom in the morning and 1 tablet at night with vitamin B_6.
- Take 800 to 1000 mg of Gingerroot twice a day and as needed.
- Take antiemetic medication (e.g., Tigan, Phenergan, or Compazine) as prescribed

Discomfort	Etiology	Differential Diagnosis	Relief Measures	Danger Signs
Nocturia	• Enlargement of the uterus in the pelvis, causing pressure on the bladder during the first trimester The following etiology for nocturia occurs in the third trimester: • Pressure from the fetal presenting parts • Hyperplasia and hyperemia of pelvic organs • Increased kidney output	• UTI • Pyelonephritis • Gestational diabetes • Preexisting diabetes mellitus • Hypocalcemia • Spontaneous rupture of membranes	• Refer the patient to a dietitian. • Consider hospitalization if significant dehydration, weight loss, or persistent ketonuria occurs. • Rest and sleep in the lateral recumbent position to encourage kidney function. • Perform Kegel exercises. • Maintain adequate fluid intake (6 to 8 glasses of water). • Decrease water intake 2 to 3 hr before bedtime. • Discontinue drinking beverages that contain caffeine.	Back pain, fever, flulike symptoms, hematuria, dysuria, urgency, dribbling, suprapubic pain, positive nitrazene or fern test, and CVAT
Round Ligament Pain	• Growth in pregnancy, which causes the ligaments (supporting structures for the uterus) to stretch and	• PID • Appendicitis • Gallbladder disease • Peptic ulcer	• Reassure the patient that the physician can explain the reason for the pain. Comfort measures: • Avoid sudden movements.	Contractions; constipation; diarrhea; low-grade fever; anorexia; periumbilical or right lower

	Causes	Possible complications	Interventions	Call provider for
	often contract, resulting in sharp pain along the side of the abdomen and just above the groin area • Sudden movements, coughing, lifting, and similar activities, which accentuate the stretching and contracting of ligaments	• Pancreatitis • Other GI or abdominal disease • UTI • Placental abruption • Labor	• Apply heat. • Try a change of activity. • Use a maternity girdle. • Support the uterus with a pillow when sitting or lying down. • Take 650 mg of acetaminophen every 4 hr as needed. • If there is no relief, refer the patient to a physical therapist. • Call the office if the sharp abdominal pain does not subside within 30 min.	abdominal flank pain or tenderness; a tender lump in the groin that worsens with standing; a one-sided constant pain that increases (if pregnancy is at 14 to 16 wk); cervical dilation, effacement, or softening; rupture of membranes; adnexal or abdominal masses; hernias; and decreased bowel sounds
Shortness of Breath	• The enlarging uterus, pressed against the abdominal organs and diaphragm, which prevents full expansion of the lungs • An increased awareness of the need to breathe • The pressure of the gravid uterus against the vena cava, which reduces venous	• URI • Pulmonary or cardiac problems	• Avoid exercise that precipitates dyspnea, and rest after exercise. • Avoid restrictive clothing. • Sit up very straight, elevate the head with pillows, or lie in the lateral recumbent position.	Headaches; sore throat; coughing; flulike symptoms; chest pain; indigestion; exercise intolerance with vomiting, sweating, or anxiety; and history of smoking, respiratory, or cardiac problems

(continued)

Discomfort	Etiology	Differential Diagnosis	Relief Measures	Danger Signs
	return to heart and may aggravate the shortness of breath			
Supine Hypotensive Syndrome	Pooling of blood in the lower extremities, expansion of the vena cava, and compression of the vena cava and lungs by the uterus	• Orthostatic hypotension • Compression of the vena cava • Hyperventilation • Anemia • Substance abuse • Exposure to a toxic agent • Psychosocial stress • CNS, cardiac, respiratory, endocrine, eye, ear, or sinus pathology	• Rest in lateral recumbent position. • Change position gradually, holding onto something when rising; lower the head below the level of the heart if feeling faint. • Apply compression stockings before getting out of bed, and perform leg-pumping exercises.	History of exposure to toxic agents; report of substance abuse, sinus, or ear problems; numbness or tingling in digits or around mouth; N & V; melena; heart palpitations; shortness of breath; double vision; loss of strength or sensation; incoordination; anxiety; depression; and anemia
Tingling and Numbness of Fingers	• Increased lordosis and pressure on the lower back with a thrust of the shoulders forward (most common at night and early in the morning)	• Carpal tunnel syndrome • Brachialgia • Herniated intervertebral (cervical) disk • Hyperventilation	• Practice good posture. • Elevate affected hand. • Sleep with hand(s) elevated on pillows. • Perform stretching and relaxation exercises for the shoulders. • Perform exercises to	Paresthesia over the thumb, index, or middle fingers and the medial portion of the ring finger; pain in the lateral aspect of the hand and forearm; blanching of the fingers; pain; loss of

Discomfort	Causes	Complications	Preventive and Treatment Measures	Danger Signs
	• Possible progression to partial anesthesia and impairment of manual proprioception		• strengthen the shoulder muscles. • Use splinting. • When hyperventilating, breathe into a paper bag or cupped hands.	sensation; or numbness in the hand, wrist, or arm
Varicosities	• Familial tendency • Impaired venous circulation and increased venous pressure in the extremities because of the pressure of the enlarging uterus • Increased levels of progesterone, which causes relaxation of the vein walls and valves and surrounding smooth muscle • Constrictive clothing or prolonged periods of standing, which impairs venous return from the extremities	• Venous thrombosis • Thrombophlebitis • Edema from PIH • Physiologic edema of pregnancy	Preventive measures: • Avoid constrictive clothing, long periods of standing and sitting, and crossing legs when sitting. • Whenever possible, sit (with legs elevated) rather than stand. • Maintain good posture and good body mechanics. Treatment measures: • Wear support hose. • Take rest periods throughout the day. • Lie on back with legs straight and at a 45° angle for 20 min several times daily. • For vulvar varicosities, lie on the shoulders, with body and legs straight	History of, or present, clotting, swelling, redness, or tenderness; cold, white, and numb leg; inflammation over varicosities; dependent cyanosis; positive Homans' sign; deep pain on palpation; distention of veins on the dorsal side of the foot after elevation

(continued)

Discomfort	Etiology	Differential Diagnosis	Relief Measures	Danger Signs
			from the waist and at 45° angle to waist (resting against wall) for 15 to 20 min several times a day; support the vulva with a foam rubber pad or perineal pad, held in place with sanitary belt; lie on the side or the back with the hips elevated for 15 to 20 min several times daily.	

PART 3

Abuse, Domestic Violence, and Sexual Coercion or Assault

Geri Morgan, CNM, ND

I. **Definition.** Abuse or violence in a relationship occurs when one person physically, verbally, emotionally, or sexually hurts another person or destroys his or her property. Experiencing fear for one's self in a relationship is characteristic of an abusive situation, regardless of whether there is physical violence. Another hallmark of abuse is one person's desire to exert power and control over another.

II. **Incidence.** Because of underreporting, accurate statistics are hard to come by. Domestic violence has been reported to occur to as many as 1 in 4 to 1 in 10 women. One in 2 to 1 in 4 women may have experienced sexual coercion, and 1 in 10 to 1 in 20 women may have been raped.

III. **Features**

   A. The patient may
   1. On rare occasions, come forward and state to you that she is being abused, was forced to have sex, was forced to do things she was uncomfortable with, or was sexually assaulted.
   2. Seem fearful, embarrassed, or evasive while giving a history.
   3. Have numerous psychosomatic complaints without physical evidence.

   B. The abusive partner may
   1. Insist on being present for the interview and exam.
   2. Give a history of the problem and state what is needed.
   3. Answer questions, even when they are directed to the patient.

   C. Consider sexual abuse as a possibility until proven otherwise when a prepubertal female presents with vaginitis or repeated bladder infections.

   D. During a physical examination, consider abuse or domestic violence if
   1. The patient presents with unexplained bruises, whiplike injuries, lacerations, burn marks, and similar evidence—especially if the injured areas are usually hidden by clothing.
   2. The patient has injuries inconsistent with common accidents.
   3. The explanation of the "accident(s)" does not fit the findings.
   4. The patient exhibits a high anxiety state during physical examination.

IV. **Management**

   A. Provide a quiet, private, safe place to discuss this problem before or after the physical examination.

   B. Phrase all questions in a nonthreatening empathetic way, especially if the patient has not come forward and stated that she is in an abusive relationship or that she was sexually coerced or assaulted. For example, you might ask, "I noted some bruises on your arm. How did that happen? Did someone grab or pinch you?"

   C. Assure the patient of confidentiality.

   D. Provide support that conveys that she is an important person and that no one deserves abuse.

E. Teach the patient about patterns of violence (e.g., the perpetrator may be very contrite after the abuse, followed by a "honeymoon" phase, and then a return to power and control).

F. Offer emergency numbers for police, domestic violence shelters, and counseling. If the abused person is willing, assist her with appointments, referrals, or police notification.

G. Whenever possible, plan a return visit with the patient. Another contact means another opportunity.

V. **Special Considerations.** Know the laws in your state. How can they help the woman or child (<14 years old)? Know when confidentiality is expected and when you are required to make a report to child protective services or the police.

A. Child abuse: A report is usually required for actual or suspected child abuse, whether it is physical, emotional, or sexual.

B. Sexually active children: A report may be required for all sexually active children under the age of 14. It may also be required if the female is younger than 17 or if the partner is 5 or more years older than her.

C. Domestic violence

1. A suicidal woman needs appropriate referral and good follow-up.

2. A woman who expresses homicidal thoughts needs counseling. Serious threats may need to be reported to the police.

D. Sexual assault and rape victims need to be seen in facilities equipped to handle rape cases. The victim needs to be told to

1. Call the police.

2. Go directly to a rape crisis facility. Do not wash or change clothing. (Although the woman needs understanding and support, evidence will be lost if strict protocols are not followed during the interview and subsequent physical examination.)

NOTES

PART 4

Management of Common Problems and Procedures in Pregnant and Nonpregnant Women

Geri Morgan, CNM, ND
Carole Hamilton, CNM, OGNP

AMENORRHEA

I. Definition

    A. Primary

        1. No period by age 14 in the presence of normal growth and development of secondary sexual characteristics. Menses usually begins within 12 months after the appearance of pubic hair.

        2. No period by age 16, regardless of the presence of normal growth and development and the appearance of secondary sexual characteristics

    B. Secondary: Absence of periods for more than 6 months in a woman who has established her menstrual cycle

II. Etiology

    A. Primary amenorrhea

        1. Abnormal chromosomes

        2. Anatomic defects

            a. Imperforate hymen

            b. Vaginal agenesis

        3. Emotional stress

        4. Excessive exercise

        5. Bulimia or anorexia

    B. Secondary amenorrhea

        1. Pregnancy

        2. Menopause

        3. Pituitary disorder

        4. Obesity

        5. Eating disorder

        6. Excessive exercise

        7. Rapid weight loss

        8. Use of oral contraception or Depo-Provera

        9. Stress

      10. Thyroid disease

      11. Polycystic ovary disease

      12. Some medications, including Depo-Provera

III. Clinical Features

    A. History

        1. Menstrual history

        2. Contraceptive history

        3. Sexual history

        4. Symptoms of galactorrhea

        5. Family history of sexual development

        6. Medications

7. Sources of emotional stress
8. Symptoms of climacteric
9. History of chronic illness
10. Present weight and weight 1 year ago
B. Physical exam
   1. Check thyroid gland for enlargements.
   2. Check heart rhythm and rate for palpitations.
   3. Check breasts for
      a. Development.
      b. Discharge (milky or clear, dark or light, thick or thin).
   4. Perform a vaginal exam to check for
      a. An imperforate hymen.
      b. Atrophic vagina.
      c. Absence of cervical mucus.
   5. Perform a bimanual exam to check for
      a. An enlarged uterus.
      b. Enlarged, cystic ovaries.

IV. **Lab Tests**
A. Primary: chromosomal karyotyping
B. Human chorionic gonadotropin (hCG)
C. Sensitive pregnancy test
D. Prolactin level
E. Thyroid-stimulating hormone (TSH)
F. Follicle-stimulating hormone (FSH)
G. Luteinizing hormone (LH)
H. Dehydroepiandrosterone (DHEA) sulfate
I. Complete blood count (CBC) with a comprehensive metabolic profile for a suspected eating disorder
J. Serum testosterone if patient is hirsute
K. Papanicolaou (Pap) smear

V. **Management**
A. Lab results
   1. If a urine pregnancy test or blood hCG is positive, advise the patient that she is pregnant.
   2. If TSH levels are elevated, order a thyroid panel and refer the patient as necessary for primary hypothyroidism.
   3. If the prolactin level is above 20 mg/mL and all other tests are negative, give 2.5 mg of Parlodel every day; if it is above 80 mg/mL, request a magnetic resonance imaging (MRI) or a coned-down view of the sella turcica. The patient may have a pituitary tumor.
      a. If either image is abnormal, refer the patient for further studies.

    b. If the sella turcica looks normal, give Parlodel to reduce prolactin to normal level. If the prolactin level remains above 30 mg/mL after 2 months, obtain consultation.

  4. If the patient is 40 or older with elevated FSH or an elevated FSH:LH ratio, advise the patient that she is menopausal.

  5. If the patient is younger than 40 with an elevated FSH level, consider ovarian failure and rule out endocrine disorders.

  6. If DHEAS levels are elevated or the LH:FSH ratio is 3:1 or greater, evaluate the patient for polycystic ovary syndrome.

  7. If the blood hCG test is negative,

    a. Give 5 to 10 mg of medroxyprogesterone acetate (Provera) orally for 5 to 10 days, 400 mg of Prometrium (four 100-mg tablets), or 100 to 200 mg of progesterone in oil intramuscularly (IM).

    b. If the patient is sexually active, give the patient a pregnancy test prior to the administration of Provera or Prometrium.

      (1) If withdrawal bleeding occurs with Provera, instruct the patient to call if there are no menses within 90 days; she is anovulatory. (To protect against unopposed estrogen effects, a period is necessary every 3 to 4 months.) Consider treatment with birth control pills (BCPs). If desired, the patient may cycle with progestin 10 to 12 days every 1, 2, or 3 months.

      (2) If no withdrawal bleeding occurs,

        (a) Give BCPs with high endometrial activity for two to three cycles.

        (b) Give 1 to 2 mg of Estrace or 0.625 to 2.5 mg of Premarin orally for 25 days. Give 5 to 10 mg of Provera orally during days 16 to 25 of the cycle. If no bleeding occurs, repeat this procedure one time.

B. Physical exam

  1. If breast discharge is present (usually bilateral) see Galactorrhea later in Part IV.

  2. Conduct a normal physical examination on a patient who has not had her period by age 16, regardless of the presence or absence of secondary sex characteristics. Also refer the patient for further workup.

 ANEMIA

I.   **Definition.** Anemia is indicated when hemoglobin (Hgb) is less than 12 in nonpregnant women or less than 10 in pregnant women.

II.   **Etiology**

  A. Acquired

    1. Iron deficiency anemia

    2. Anemia from blood loss

    3. Megaloblastic anemia

    4. Acquired hemolytic anemia

    5. Pernicious anemia

  B. Hereditary

    1. Thalassemia

    2. Sickle cell anemia

    3. Hereditary hemolytic anemia

III. Clinical Features

  A. History

    1. Heavy menses

    2. Chronic blood loss

    3. Family history

    4. Poor diet

    5. Closely spaced pregnancies

    6. Anemia with previous pregnancies

    7. Pica

  B. Signs and symptoms

    1. Fatigue, malaise, or drowsiness

    2. Dizziness or weakness

    3. Headaches

    4. Sore tongue and mouth

    5. Anorexia, nausea, or vomiting

    6. Skin pallor

    7. Pale mucous membranes or conjunctiva

    8. Pale fingernail beds

    9. Tachycardia

IV. Management

  A. At the initial visit, obtain patient history information.

    1. Discover any history of anemia, blood-clotting problems, sickle cell disease, glucose-6-phosphate dehydrogenase (G6PD) anemia, or other hereditary hemolytic diseases.

    2. Obtain a family history.

  B. Order a CBC at the initial visit.

    1. Morphology

      a. Normal morphology indicates mature healthy red blood cells (RBCs).

      b. Microcytic, hypochromic RBCs indicate iron deficiency anemia.

      c. Macrocytic, hypochromic RBCs indicate pernicious anemia.

    2. Hemoglobin and hematocrit (Hct) in pregnancy

      a. An Hgb greater than 13 with an Hct greater than 40% may indicate hypovolemia. Be alert for dehydration and preeclampsia.

    b. An Hgb of 11.5 to 13 with an Hct of 34% to 40% is normal and healthy.

    c. An Hgb of 10.5 to 11.5 with an Hct of 31% to 32% is low but normal.

    d. An Hgb of 10 with an Hct of 30% indicates anemia.

        (1) Refer the patient to a dietitian, diet counseling, or both.

        (2) Supplement with iron tablets once or twice a day or one time-release capsule, such as Slow-Fe, every day.

    e. An Hgb of 9 to 10 with an Hct of 27% to 30% may indicate megaloblastic anemia.

        (1) Refer the patient to a dietitian or diet counseling.

        (2) Recommend ferrous sulfate 325 mg by mouth two or three times a day.

    f. An Hgb of <9 with an Hct of <27%, or anemia that does not respond to above treatment measures, requires the following measures:

        (1) Look for occult bleeding or an infection.

        (2) Consider ordering the following lab work:

            (a) Hemoglobin and hematocrit (to rule out lab error)

            (b) Serum iron concentration level

            (c) Iron-binding capacity

            (d) Cell indices (white blood cell [WBC] and RBC counts)

            (e) Reticulocyte count (measures the production of erythrocytes)

            (f) Platelet count

            (g) Stool guaiac for occult bleeding

            (h) Stool culture for ova and parasites

            (i) G6PD screen (see guidelines for Anemia: Acquired Hemolytic) if client is African American

        (3) Consult with a physician.

        (4) Refer the patient to a dietitian or diet counseling.

C. If the patient is pregnant, check her hematocrit at the initial visit, at 28 weeks, and 4 weeks after initiating therapy.

    1. Manage signs of anemia (according to the previous information under section IV—Management, B2).

    2. Consult with a physician if

        a. There is a steadily downward trend in hematocrit despite treatment.

        b. There is a significant drop in hematocrit compared to previous readings (rule out lab error first).

        c. There is no response to treatment after 4 to 6 weeks.

        d. The Hgb is below 9.0 or Hct is equal to or below 27%.

ANEMIA: ACQUIRED HEMOLYTIC

I. Definition. An inherited, X-linked, enzymatic defect in which the body does not produce the G6PD enzyme, which acts as a catalyst for aerobic use of glucose by RBCs. Acquired hemolytic anemia is seen in African Americans, Asians, and persons of Mediterranean descent.

II. Incidence. Two percent of all African American women have the disease.

III. Etiology. Infections and several oxidic drugs in the presence of G6PD deficiency will precipitate RBC hemolysis, with resultant mild-to-severe hemolytic anemia.

IV. Management

   A. Screening: Patients who are African American who have anemia or frequent urinary tract infections (UTIs) should have a G6PD screen.

   B. Treatment

   1. Prescribe 1 mg of folic acid every day.
   2. Give the patient a list of medicines to avoid.
   3. If the patient is pregnant, obtain a urine culture and sensitivity (C&S) monthly.
   4. Consult with a physician when the patient is in crisis or has severe anemia.

   C. Medications: Patients should avoid the following:

   1. Aldomet
   2. Antimalarial drugs
   3. Aspirin
   4. Ascorbic acid (massive doses)
   5. Chloramphenicol
   6. Diaphenylsulfone
   7. Isoniazid
   8. Methylene blue
   9. N^1-Acetylsufanilamide
   10. Nalidixic acid
   11. Naphthalene (mothballs)
   12. Nitrofurantoin
   13. Nitrofurazone
   14. Orinase
   15. Para-aminosalicylic acid
   16. Pentaquine
   17. Phenacetin
   18. Primaquine
   19. Probenecid
   20. Quinacrine (atabrine)

21. Quinidine
22. Quinine
23. Quinocide
24. Sulfa
25. Sulfacetamide
26. Sulfamethoxypyridazine (Kynex)
27. Sulfanilamide
28. Sulfapyridine
29. Sulfasalazine (Azulfidine)
30. Sulfisoxazole (Gantrisin)
31. Sulfoxone
32. Trimethoprim/sulfamethoxazole (Bactrim, Septra)

 ANEMIA: IRON DEFICIENCY

I. **Definition and Etiology**
   A. Iron deficiency anemia is the most common anemia of pregnancy; it constitutes about 95% of pregnancy-related anemias.
   B. The morphology consists of microcytic, hypochromic RBCs.
   C. Serum iron is decreased, and iron-binding capacity is increased.

II. **Clinical Features**
   A. Suspect iron deficiency anemia if
      1. One or more of the predisposing factors for anemia exist.
      2. The Hct is <30%.
   B. Confirm the diagnosis as iron deficiency anemia if
      1. The morphology indicates microcytic, hypochromic RBCs.
      2. The serum iron saturation is <15% after the patient is off iron therapy for 1 week.

III. **Management**
   A. Routine screening
      1. At the initial visit, ask about any past history of anemia or blood-clotting problems.
      2. Order a CBC at the initial visit.
      3. Discuss the importance of taking prenatal vitamins (with iron).
      4. Recheck the hematocrit at 28 weeks of pregnancy.
   B. Treatment of anemia
      1. If the Hgb is <10 and the Hct is <30%, perform the following functions:
         a. Offer diet counseling.
            (1) Review the patient's diet.
            (2) Discuss dietary sources of iron.

(3) Give the patient a handout on foods high in iron.

(4) Offer the patient a referral to a dietitian.

b. Advise supplemental iron in addition to prenatal vitamins. The iron requirement in pregnancy is 60 mg of elemental iron.

(1) Time-release iron tablets are best but much more expensive. Any standard iron salt preparation is adequate.

(2) Take one to three tablets daily in divided doses.

(3) Iron is better absorbed on an empty stomach. Take it 1 hour before meals or 2 hours after meals.

(4) Vitamin C aids iron absorption. Take iron with a juice high in vitamin C or a vitamin C tablet.

(5) Antacids and dairy products can hinder absorption.

(6) It is preferable to take iron with antacids or food than not to take it at all.

2. If the Hgb is <9 and the Hct is <27%, consider megaloblastic anemia. Manage this patient according to the following anemia guidelines.

3. If the Hgb is <9 and the Hct is less than or equal to 27% at the start of labor, consider administering an intravenous (IV) line or heparin lock in labor.

 ## ANEMIA: MEGALOBLASTIC

I. Definition and Etiology

A. Megaloblastic anemia is a disease in which the RBCs are reduced in number and are macrocytic and hypochromic.

B. It is commonly associated with iron deficiency anemia. It's rare to see megaloblastic anemia alone.

C. Megaloblastic anemia is associated with a diet lacking in fresh vegetables or animal protein.

II. Clinical Features

A. Symptoms

1. Nausea and vomiting

2. Anorexia

B. Morphology

1. Hypochromic, macrocytic RBCs

2. Low hemoglobin and hematocrit levels that do not respond to iron therapy

C. A diet history indicating a low intake of fresh vegetables, animal protein, or both

III. Management

A. Supplements

1. Prenatal vitamin containing folic acid and iron

2. Folic acid, 1 to 2 mg per day, to correct folic acid deficiency
3. Supplemental iron, considering megaloblastic anemia rarely exists in the absence of iron deficiency anemia

B. Diet counseling
1. Review the patient's diet.
2. Recommend dietary sources of folic acid.
3. Offer referral to a dietitian.

C. CBC
1. Repeat a CBC in 1 month.
2. Look for an increase in the reticulocyte count of 3% to 4% in 2 to 3 weeks and a slight increase in the hemoglobin and hematocrit count.

 ## ANEMIA: PERNICIOUS

I. Definition and Etiology

A. Pernicious anemia is caused by lack of intrinsic factor in the gastric juices, which is necessary for the absorption of vitamin B_{12} from food. Because B_{12} is not absorbed, the RBCs do not mature normally.

B. It is rarely seen in persons under age 35.

II. Clinical Features

A. Pernicious anemia is characterized by macrocytic RBCs, which may also be normochromic or hyperchromic.

B. RBCs may easily be mistaken for those seen in folic acid deficiency.

C. Treatment with folic acid may mask pernicious anemia, because the RBCs may become normocytic, even though the disease still exists.

III. Diagnosis

A. Suspect pernicious anemia if, after treatment with folic acid, the RBCs become normal in morphology but the hematocrit does not increase.

B. A diagnosis may be made if improvement occurs after a trial treatment with 1000 ng of parenteral B_{12} for 3 months.

IV. Management

A. Review the patient's diet for animal products. If her diet is lacking in sources of vitamin B_{12}, give diet counseling.

B. Give 1 cc (1000 ng) of parenteral B_{12} IM every month.

C. Offer a referral to a dietitian.

D. Repeat the CBC in 1 month.
1. The condition is alleviated if
   a. The morphology is normal.
   b. The hematocrit has increased.
2. If there is no change, consult with a physician.

ANEMIA: SICKLE CELL

I. **Definition and Etiology**

    A. Types

        1. In sickle cell trait, there is one normal gene and one Hgb-S gene. Symptoms do not appear except in severe oxygen deprivation.

        2. In sickle cell disease, both genes are Hbg S. The disease is chronic and debilitating. Morbidity and mortality are high.

    B. Incidence

        1. One in 12 African Americans has sickle cell trait.

        2. One in 500 African Americans has the disease.

II. **Management**

    A. Order a sickle cell screen on all African American patients.

        1. If the test is negative, both genes are normal and no problem exists.

        2. If the test is positive, order a hemoglobin electrophoresis.

            a. If the gene is homozygous, the patient is considered high risk and should be referred to physician.

            b. If the gene is heterozygous, the patient is considered low risk and can be managed normally throughout pregnancy and labor.

    B. Consider a monthly urine C&S because of the increased risk of UTIs during pregnancy.

    C. Counsel the patient.

        1. Inform the patient of her sickle cell trait.

        2. Advise testing of the father of the baby. If he is also heterozygous, there is a chance that the baby could have the disease.

        3. Refer the patient for genetic counseling, as necessary.

 ## BACTERIAL VAGINOSIS

I. **Definition.** Bacterial vaginosis is a vaginal inflammation caused by the Gardnerella bacteria, which is normally found in the vagina and causes symptoms when it overgrows.

II. **Etiology and Characteristics**

    A. Bacterial vaginosis is the most frequent cause of vaginitis.

    B. The bacteria do not invade the vaginal mucosa; the tissue underlying the discharge is healthy.

    C. A significant percentage of women are asymptomatic.

    D. The bacteria may be found in the gastrointestinal (GI) tract and bladder.

    E. Although males are not usually symptomatic, they can harbor the bacteria in their urethras and transmit the bacteria to women.

F. Bacterial vaginosis is implicated in chorioamnionitis, preterm labor, premature rupture of membranes, spontaneous abortion, and second-trimester loss.

III. **Clinical Features**

A. Signs and symptoms

1. The patient may be asymptomatic.
2. A major presenting symptom is yellow or creamy-gray vaginal discharge and a fishy odor.
3. The vaginal mucosa may look normal.
4. Bacterial vaginosis is usually not associated with pain, burning, or itching.
5. If bacterial vaginosis is present, look for a concomitant infection.

B. Laboratory findings

1. The following findings are positive for bacterial vaginosis:
   a. A positive whiff (sniff) test when vaginal discharge is mixed with potassium hydroxide
   b. Microscopic findings on a wet mount of clue cells (epithelial cells that appear "sandy" because they are studded with the *Gardnerella* bacteria)
2. Cultures are not reliable, because *Gardnerella* bacteria are found in 60% of normal vaginal cultures.
3. Pap smears are 90% accurate in diagnosing bacterial vaginosis.

IV. **Management**

A. Make a diagnosis. (See vaginal discharge guidelines for a differential diagnosis.)

B. Consider the following options regarding treatment:

1. Flagyl (metronidazole) orally or vaginally is the drug of choice. If the patient is unable to take Flagyl, 2% Cleocin vaginal cream every night vaginally for 7 days; or Cleocin Vaginal Ovules for 3 days.
2. Treatment of the male partner is controversial. It seems prudent to evaluate or treat steady partners. Condoms should be used until 1 week after treatment is completed.

C. Treat the patient with the following medications in first trimester of pregnancy:

1. Flagyl has been used without any known ill effects.[1] However, it does not carry a recommendation for use during the first trimester.
2. If the patient is symptomatic, the following medications may be tried:
   a. Metrogel vaginal cream, one application vaginally at bedtime for 5 to 7 days.

---

[1]Caro-Paton et al., 1997

   b. Acid-gel, Tri-Sulfa, or other vaginal creams or suppositories

D. If bacterial vaginosis is present in the second or third trimester, strive for effective treatment because of the association between *Gardnerella*, premature rupture of membranes, and postpartum endometritis. Use one of the following:

   1. Metronidazole, 250 to 500 mg orally, twice to three times a day for 5 to 7 days

   2. MetroGel-Vaginal cream, one applicator vaginally at bedtime for 5 to 7 days

E. With treatment by either metronidazole or penicillin, warn patient that monilia vaginitis may develop secondary to antibiotic therapy. The patient should be alert for signs and symptoms and may want to use prophylactic acidophilus tablets.

 ## CARDIOVASCULAR ASSESSMENT

I. **Definition.** Cardiovascular assessment is evaluation of the patient for physiologic changes and problems relating to the heart and blood vessels.

II. **Clinical Features.** Normal cardiovascular changes in pregnancy include the following:

A. Stroke volume increases by one third in the first 8 to 10 weeks.

   1. Increased estrogen levels cause the heart rate to increase 10 to 15 beats per minute in some women.

   2. Total blood volume increases by 20% to 30%.

      a. Plasma increases 40% to 50%.

      b. RBCs increase 20%.

B. A reduction in exercise tolerance occurs because of

   1. Greater body weight to move.

   2. Cardiac output that has already increased, leaving less reserve for an increase with exercise.

C. Progesterone causes blood vessel tone to decrease, so peripheral vascular resistance falls, leading to

   1. A greater incidence of varicosities and aneurysms.

   2. A drop in blood pressure (BP) at the end of the first trimester, returning to normal or slightly above normal in the final weeks of pregnancy.

D. The diaphragm elevates, and the transverse diameter of the thorax increases, pushing the heart upward and to the left; it lies almost horizontally.

E. Cardiac volume increases by about 75 mL.

F. A systolic murmur may occur because of

   1. Increased cardiac output.

   2. Acceleration of blood flow (heart rate).

   3. Changes in the position of the heart.

    4. Decreased blood viscosity—a smaller ratio of RBCs to plasma.

  G. Blood flow increases to most areas of the body from early pregnancy.

III. Management of Cardiovascular Abnormalities

  A. At the first visit, take a good history of the cardiovascular system.

    1. Any history of the following indicates consultation and a workup by a cardiologist:

      a. Palpitations or abnormalities in the heart rate or rhythm

      b. Anything more than a nonproblematic (grade I or VI) murmur (which does not need a cardiac workup)

      c. Any of the following conditions, if they are chronic or if the cause is unknown:

        (1) Chest pain

        (2) Cyanosis

        (3) Dependent edema (differentiated from normal pregnancy edema)

    2. Any history of the following indicates referral to an obstetrician for care:

      a. Rheumatic fever with resultant damage

      b. Heart disease or coronary artery disease

      c. Persistent hypertension

      d. Heart surgery

      e. Signs and symptoms of congestive heart failure

        (1) Persistent rales at the base of the lungs

        (2) An increased inability to carry out her usual physical activity

        (3) Increased dyspnea with exertion

        (4) Hemoptysis

        (5) Cyanosis

        (6) Edema in the lower extremities (differentiated from normal pregnancy edema)

  B. Physical exam

    1. Do a routine assessment, which includes

      a. Taking the BP.

      b. Auscultating the heart for the following:

        (1) The rate, rhythm, and quality of heart sounds at the four valvular areas

        (2) Extra sounds, murmurs, splitting, rubs, and thrills

      c. Observation of the limbs for cyanosis or edema

    2. If the history or routine exam indicates possible abnormal cardiac function, perform a more extended exam.

      a. Observe the anterior chest wall for bulging, heaving, or pulsation.

b. Palpate the anterior chest wall for the point of maximum intensity (PMI), thrills, and rubs.

c. Percuss the anterior chest wall for heart size.

3. If the following conditions are present, consult with or refer the patient to a cardiologist:

    a. An irregular heartbeat or tachycardia (more than 100 beats per minute) in the absence of other findings indicative of heart disease or hyperthyroidism

    b. Any systolic murmurs with a classification of grade II or greater.

 ## CERVICAL ABNORMALITIES

I. Etiology

    A. Congenital abnormalities or exposure to diethylstilbestrol (DES) in utero

    B. Atrophy or stenosis

    C. Cervicitis

    D. Endometriosis

    E. Erosion or ulcerations

    F. Human papilloma virus (HPV) or condylomata

    G. Polyps

    H. Trauma or surgery

II. Clinical Features

    A. Congenital abnormalities: A double cervix and other structural anomalies

    B. Atrophy or stenosis

        1. Menopausal women often have a pale cervix and a small canal due to decreased estrogen.

        2. Cryosurgery, cone biopsy, or radiation can cause atrophy or stenosis.

    C. Cervicitis

        1. The mucous membrane of the cervix will be red, inflamed, and friable.

        2. The mucous membrane of the cervix will bleed with intercourse.

        3. Chlamydia, gonorrhea, bacterial vaginosis, trichomoniasis, vaginitis, moniliasis, and herpes must be ruled out before cervicitis can be confirmed.

    D. Endometriosis

        1. Patients may have a history suspicious of endometriosis; a diagnosis may be made after a laparoscopic exam.

        2. A blue or black bump may be seen on the cervix.

    E. Erosion or ulcerations

        1. Herpes must be ruled out before erosion or ulcerations can be confirmed.

2. The patient may have a history of using tampons or a cervical cap.

F. HPV

1. Patients with HPV may have visible warts on the cervix.

2. Fifty to sixty percent of patients with external condylomata test positive for HPV on the cervix.

3. Herpes and nabothian cysts need to be ruled out before HPV can be confirmed.

G. Polyps

1. A history of spotting with intercourse may indicate polyps.

2. Growth on the stalk is sometimes visible.

H. Trauma or surgery

1. Trauma resulting in cervical abnormalities may be caused by delivery, elective abortion, or instruments inserted into the vagina.

2. Surgery causing cervical abnormalities may include a loop electrosurgical excision procedure (LEEP) or a cone biopsy.

3. The cervix may fail to dilate or tear during labor.

III. Management

A. Congenital abnormalities or exposure to DES in utero

1. Congenital abnormalities may present problems in labor and delivery and need to be managed collaboratively with a physician.

2. Exposure to DES in utero (used prior to 1971) changes the location of the squamocolumnar junction, which is often located in the vagina rather than the ectocervix, predisposing the patient to more frequent cervical infections and cervical cancer. A Pap smear every year, even when everything looks and has been normal, is a must.

B. Atrophy or stenosis

1. No treatment is necessary.

2. Nothing further is needed unless the patient complains of vaginal dryness. See Part I-Menopause and Perimenopause, HRT guidelines.

3. Dilation of the cervical os may be necessary if no endocervical cells appear on two Pap smears.

C. Cervicitis: See guidelines on Vaginal Discharge in Part IV.

D. Endometriosis: No management is needed for a cervical manifestation.

E. Erosion or ulceration

1. The cause should be treated.

2. Amino-Cerv Crème may be used at bedtime for 10 to 14 days.

F. HPV: See guidelines on Human Papilloma Virus (HPV) later in Part IV.

G. Polyps

1. Polyps may be removed if the stalk can be seen.

2. They should be sent to pathology.

H. Trauma or surgery: Monitor an antepartal patient for an incompetent cervix.

 CHLAMYDIA

I. Definition. Chlamydia trachomatis is a Gram-negative intracellular parasite that is smaller than bacteria and larger than viruses. It is the chief agent of bacterial sexually transmitted diseases (STDs) in the United States today.

II. Incidence

A. Infection by *Chlamydia trachomatis* has been identified in half of men with nonspecific urethritis and 20% to 60% of women with gonorrhea.

B. Chlamydial diseases are the most prevalent STDs in the United States today—several times more prevalent than gonorrhea.

C. Five percent of babies born in the United States have a chlamydia infection; fifty percent of these develop conjunctivitis, and 20% develop pneumonia.

III. Etiology

A. Chlamydia is often found in conjunction with other STDs.

B. The genus *Chlamydia* has two species.

1. *Chlamydia psittaci* does not cause an STD and is not relevant in obstetrics and gynecology (OB/GYN) care. It causes a mild flu-like disease, contracted following exposure to bird droppings containing the parasite.

2. *C. trachomatis* is the STD species referred to in the remainder of this section and is responsible for the following diseases:

a. Pelvic inflammatory disease

b. Nongonococcal (and postgonococcal) urethritis

c. Chronic conjunctivitis

(1) Chronic conjunctivitis may be associated with an infected sibling, in which case reinfection is generally more severe than the initial episode.

(2) It has been cited as a major cause of blindness.

(3) Adult infection generally occurs by exposure to genital discharges containing chlamydia.

d. Chlamydiae blennorrhea

(1) The fetus generally contracts this disease by passing through an infected birth canal.

(2) There are many clinical manifestations of this disease including

(a) Benign to severe conjunctivitis.

(b) Pneumonitis, which can become quite severe to fatal.

     e. Lymphogranuloma venereum

       (1) Lymphogranuloma venereum is a strain of *C. trachomatis* characterized by a transient minor genital ulcer and inguinal adenopathy (and possibly urethritis).

       (2) It can be cultured in the same specific medium as the other genital chlamydia and is differentiated as the lymphogranuloma venereum strain on culture.

IV. Clinical Features

A. Although patients with a chlamydial infection may be asymptomatic, they may have the following signs and symptoms:

    1. General

      a. Mucopurulent, foul-smelling vaginal discharge draining from the cervical os

      b. Erythema, edema, and congestion of the cervix and vagina

    2. Cervicitis

      a. Cobblestone ectopy

      b. Increased friability and bleeding

      c. Mucopurulent discharge from the os

    3. Urethritis

      a. Mild dysuria or lower abdominal pain

      b. Sterile pyuria

      c. Gradual onset

      d. Mucopurulent discharge from the urethra

B. Chlamydia can mimic the following conditions:

    1. Cervicitis of chlamydia may look like cervicitis of herpes simplex. Chlamydia causes inflammation and ulceration of both the ectocervix and the endocervix, while herpes simplex affects the ectocervix alone.

    2. Chlamydia may result in a pelvic inflammatory disease (PID) similar to that caused by gonorrhea.

C. Patients with chlamydia may experience a latency period of many decades, similar to syphilis, after the initial infection.

D. Chlamydia is a major cause of

    1. Mucopurulent cervicitis.

    2. Urethral infection.

    3. PID and acute perihepatitis.

    4. Neonatal conjunctivitis and pneumonia.

E. Chlamydiosis is associated with

    1. Infertility (secondary to PID).

    2. Cervical dysplasia.

    3. Fetal wastage and stillbirth.

    4. Neonatal infections.

    5. Postpartum endometritis and salpingitis.

V. Management

A. Suspect chlamydia in the following situations:

1. WBCs are too numerous to count on a wet prep slide without large amounts of bacteria or yeast present.

2. Other STDs have been ruled out or treated unsuccessfully (especially in the presence of mucopurulent, foul-smelling vaginal discharge, which is indicative of either gonorrhea or chlamydia).

3. Dysuria and urinary frequency are present, and a UTI and urethritis have been ruled out.

4. Cervicitis is present.

5. The Pap smear report is suggestive of chlamydia.

6. There is a recent history of chlamydia, especially with symptoms.

7. The patient's partner has nongonococcal urethritis.

B. Test all new OB patients and those suspected of, or exposed to, chlamydia.

1. Specific tissue culture

   a. Obtain chlamydia culture kit.

   b. Swab transitional zone of cervix.

   c. Swab area vigorously; it is essential that enough epithelial cells be collected.

   d. Use the Dacron swabs provided in the kit; cotton swabs are toxic to chlamydia.

   e. Obtain results in 72 hours.

2. Rapid detection test for chlamydia antigen

   a. The positive predictive value is 100%; the negative predictive value is 94% to 98%.

   b. The test may be done in the office. A cervical swab needs to be taken with the swabs provided in the kit.

   c. Test results are ready within ½ hour.

C. Before beginning treatment, obtain a Venereal Disease Research Laboratory (VDRL) test for syphilis and a gonorrhea culture if either disease has not been ruled out.

D. Treat chlamydia as follows:

1. Nonpregnant women not breast-feeding

   a. Zithromax (azythromycin), 1g orally in a single dose

   b. Doxycycline, 100 mg, one tablet orally twice a day for 7 days

   c. Ofloxacin, 400 mg twice a day for 7 days

2. Pregnant or breast-feeding women

   a. Zithromax (azithromycin), 1 g orally in a single dose

   b. Erythromycin, 500 mg, one tablet orally four times a day for 7 to 10 days

E. Refer the patient's partner(s) for treatment. Caution the patient and her partner(s) not to have intercourse while being treated to avoid reinfection. If they are unable to wait for the test of cure (TOC), counsel them to use a condom.

F. Repeat a cervical culture for a TOC 6 weeks after the treatment is recommended.

1. If the patient is pregnant, reexamine her cervix and repeat the culture at 34 to 36 weeks of estimated gestational age (EGA).

2. If culture is still positive, check the following:

    a. Compliance with medications

    b. Treatment of partner

3. Repeat treatment with a different medication.

 ## COLDS, FLU, AND UPPER RESPIRATORY INFECTIONS

I. **Etiology.** Colds, flu, and upper respiratory infections (URIs) are usually viral, characterized by general malaise.

II. **Clinical Features.** Each of the following symptoms are frequently associated with colds, flu, and URIs and are discussed separately:

    A. Sore throat

    B. Cough

    C. Nasal congestion

    D. Sinusitis

    E. Allergies including hay fever

    F. Diarrhea

    G. Nausea and vomiting

III. **Management**

    A. Increase rest.

    B. Increase fluids.

    C. Use a humidifier or vaporizer.

    D. For general aches and pains, take one or two acetaminophen tablets every 4 hours, as needed, not to exceed 4 g per day.

    E. Consider that over-the-counter (OTC) medications such as Actifed and Sudafed contain multiple ingredients. Discourage the use of NyQuil during pregnancy, because it contains alcohol. Recommend gargling with NaCl and taking Robitussin for a cough while pregnant.

    F. Consider the following treatments, which are optional:

        1. Vitamin C, 2 to 5 g a day, divided into equal dosages every 3 to 4 hours. If toxicity symptoms occur (e.g., slight burning during urination, loose bowels, gas retention, or skin rashes), reduce dosage.

        2. Oscillococcinum, a homeopathic remedy. One tube can be placed under the tongue every 6 hours.

        3. Echinacea, which comes in many forms, from tablets to tincture; patients should follow the dosage on the label.

COUGHS

I. **Clinical Features**
   A. History
      1. Onset, duration, course, and any self-treatment measures
      2. History of smoking
      3. Previous history of coughs
      4. Presence of sputum, color of sputum, and blood in sputum
      5. Associated signs and symptoms
         a. Nasal congestion
         b. Fever or myalgias
         c. Nausea or vomiting
         d. Headache
         e. Lung involvement
         f. Sore throat
   B. Physical exam
      1. Inspect throat for infection, edema, or an abscess. Differentiate between infection and irritation from coughing.
      2. Palpate the submental, submaxillar, tonsillar, and cervical lymph nodes. If they are swollen and tender, suspect an infection.
      3. Percuss and auscultate the lungs for decreased breath sounds, wheezes, rales, rhonchi, and areas of consolidation. If any of these are present, suspect lung involvement.
      4. Take the patient's temperature. If it is elevated, suspect infection.
   C. Lab work
      1. If the patient's throat is infected, obtain a throat culture.
      2. Obtain a CBC and other lab work, as necessary.
II. **Management**
   A. Mild symptoms
      1. Mix lemon and honey together and use it as a cough syrup.
      2. Try OTC cough syrups.
         a. Robitussin plain or DM
         b. Phenergan expectorant
      3. Gargle with saline or mouthwash.
      4. Use throat lozenges (or hard candy).
   B. Severe symptoms
      1. Take Robitussin AC.
      2. Take Nucofed.
      3. Recommend a medication for the patient.
   C. Cough that persists more than 7 days
      1. Reassess the patient and consider a chest radiograph.
      2. Rule out pneumonia, tuberculosis (TB), allergies, and asthma.

3. For treatment of an uncomplicated productive cough, prescribe an antibiotic.

D. Physician consultation

1. Consult with a physician when the cough is chronic or does not respond to the previously described measures.

2. Consult with a physician when the clinical picture suggests pneumonia.

 ## "CRABS" (PEDICULOSIS PUBIS)

I. Definition and Etiology. "Crabs" is the common term for pediculosis pubis, an infestation of the vulva caused by crab louse, Pthirus pubis, or its nits. It is contracted by contact with an infested person or object, such as clothing, bed linens, and upholstered furniture.

II. Clinical Features

A. The patient may have no symptoms or may notice lice or nits on body hair.

B. Diagnosis is made by finding the lice or nits attached to body hair.

1. The usual location for lice or nits is pubic hair.

2. Occasionally the following body hair may be involved:

   a. Hair on the thighs or the trunk

   b. Eyelashes or eyebrows

   c. Hair in the axilla

   d. Hair on the scalp

III. Management

A. If the patient is pregnant or breast-feeding, follow these recommendations:

1. Use a medication such as Stop-X, RID, or another OTC choice. These are contraindicated in patients with ragweed sensitivities.

   a. Apply sufficient liquid to completely wet the hair and skin of any infected areas. Avoid contact with eyes and mucous membranes.

   b. Leave the medication on for 10 minutes.

   c. Wash and rinse the affected areas with plenty of warm water.

   d. Use a clean, fine-tooth comb to remove nits and dead lice.

   e. If head hair is treated, shampoo the hair after treatment.

   f. If retreatment is necessary, do not exceed two applications within 24 hours.

2. During the first trimester, limit treatment to one, if possible. Treat as many times as necessary in the second and third trimesters.

B. If the patient is not pregnant or breast-feeding, use 1% Kwell cream or lotion (4 oz).

1. Bathe or shower before beginning treatment and dry with a clean towel.

2. Apply lotion or cream over the entire body from the neck down.

3. Leave on lotion or cream for 24 hours.

4. Wear clean clothes and sleep in clean bed linen during the 24-hour treatment.

5. Reapply lotion or cream to hands after each washing during 24-hour treatment.

6. Take a cleansing bath 24 hours after application (*no sooner*)**.**

7. If the scalp is involved, follow these steps:

   a. Use Kwell shampoo.

   b. Leave it on for 5 minutes before rinsing.

   c. Then shampoo with regular shampoo.

   d. Use a clean, fine-tooth comb to remove nits and dead lice.

8. Comb pubic, underarm, and other infested body hair to remove nits and dead lice.

C. Consider the following factors when dealing with crabs:

1. Crabs can live more than a month on inanimate objects.

   a. All combs, hairbrushes, curlers, and other hair-grooming objects should be cleaned with Kwell.

   b. All clothing and bed linens should be washed in hot water with detergent and dried in an electric dryer. A commercial washer is better because the water is hotter.

   c. Clothing and bed linens that cannot be washed should be dry-cleaned.

   d. Upholstered furniture, beds, and pillows should be cleaned.

2. If eyelashes are involved, occlusive ophthalmic ointment should be applied before treatment.

3. Retreatment may be necessary in 1 week because eggs will hatch that were not killed during treatment.

4. Sexual partner(s) within the preceding month also need treatment.

 DIARRHEA

I. Etiology

A. Viruses, bacteria, or protozoa

1. Flu (see the previous entry, Colds, Flu, and Upper Respiratory Infections)

2. Gastroenteritis

B. Diet

C. Lactose intolerance, especially in dark-skinned races

D. Antibiotic therapy

E. Contaminated water or exposure to a new puppy (*Giardia*)

II. Management

A. With an acute onset of diarrhea, take a patient history.

1. Elicit information on the onset, severity, occurrence in other family members, relief measures, and any other symptoms.
2. Gather a diet history.
   a. Any recent change in eating habits
   b. Seasonal food choices, for example, access to fresh fruits or vegetables
   c. Food choices that include bran, whole grains, beans, or other legumes
   d. Potentially contaminated dairy products, eggs, meat, or other foods
   e. A recent increase in dairy products because of pregnancy or a history of lactose intolerance in the family
   f. Large doses of vitamin C

B. Manage an acute onset of diarrhea in the following ways:
   1. Avoid dairy products for 24 hours.
   2. Try acidophilus-cultured milk or adding lactase to dairy products if there is a history of lactose intolerance in the family.
   3. Reduce the dose of vitamin C if the patient is taking large doses.
   4. Maintain a clear liquid diet for 24 hours.
   5. Take Kaopectate, Imodium A-D, or Pepto-Bismol, as needed. The patient may need Lomotil if the diarrhea is severe.
   6. If abdominal cramping occurs with the diarrhea, take one Phazyme before each meal and one at bedtime.
   7. Check for ketonuria. Advise the patient to check her urine 2 hours after eating. Advise the patient to call the office if more than a trace of ketonuria is discovered for more than 48 hours.
   8. If the diarrhea is unrelieved in 48 hours, get a stool specimen to check for ova and parasites.
   9. If *Giardia* is present, treat it with 250 mg of Flagyl, orally, three times a day for 5 to 7 days or 375 mg, orally, twice a day for 7 days.
   10. Consult with a physician if:
       a. Diarrhea persists despite treatment.
       b. Significant dehydration is present.
       c. Ketonuria is unrelieved in 24 hours.

C. Manage chronic diarrhea in the following ways:
   1. Ascertain whether prenatal vitamins contain a stool softener. If so, try a vitamin without a stool softener.
   2. Consult with a physician; chronic diarrhea may indicate colitis or another condition.

 ## DYSFUNCTIONAL UTERINE BLEEDING

I. **Definition.** Dysfunctional uterine bleeding is abnormal uterine bleeding with no demonstrable or organic cause. It is a diagnosis of exclusion.

II. **Incidence**
   A. Fifty percent of sufferers are 40 to 50 years old.
   B. Twenty percent are adolescents.

III. **Etiology**
   A. Anovulation—the most common cause
   B. Coagulation defects
   C. Perimenopause
      1. Shortening of the proliferative phase
      2. Corpus luteum dysfunction

IV. **Lab tests**
   A. Pap smear, endometrial biopsy, quantitative beta human chorionic gonadotropin (QBHCG), CBC, coagulation studies, TSH, FSH, and DHEAS if masculinization is present
   B. Ultrasound

V. **Differential diagnosis**
   A. Pathology of pregnancy
      1. Ectopic pregnancy
         a. Positive hCG test
         b. Unilateral pain
         c. Bleeding
      2. Abortion
         a. Threatened
         b. Incomplete
         c. Missed
      3. Trophoblastic disease—very high QBHCG
      4. Postpartum condition
         a. Subinvolution
         b. Retained products of conception
         c. Infection
   B. Malignancy
      1. Cervical cancer
      2. Uterine cancer
      3. Fallopian tube cancer
   C. Chronic endometritis
      1. Episodic intermenstrual spotting
      2. TB endometritis
   D. Uterine defects
      1. Fibroids
      2. Endometrial polyps
   E. Pathology of cervix, vagina, and ovaries
      1. Cervical polyps
      2. Severe infections

      3. Corpus luteum dysfunction

      4. Ovarian tumors, especially hormone-secreting tumors

  F. Systemic diseases

      1. Coagulation defects

        a. von Willebrand's disease

        b. Leukemias

        c. Severe sepsis

      2. Hypothyroidism—elevated TSH

      3. Adrenal insufficiency

        a. Usual cause of oligomenorrhea or amenorrhea

        b. Rare cause of irregular vaginal bleeding

      4. Cirrhosis

        a. Reduced capacity of liver to metabolize estrogens

        b. Possible accompanying hypoprothrombinemia

      5. Iatrogenic causes

        a. Birth control pills

        b. Depo-Provera

        c. Hormone replacement therapy (HRT)

        d. Danazol

        e. Gonadotropin-releasing hormone (GnRH) agonist

          (1) Synarel

          (2) Lupron

        f. Tranquilizers

        g. Intrauterine devices (IUDs)

VI. Management

  A. Evaluation

      1. History and physical

        a. Last menstrual period (LMP)

        b. Previous menstrual period (PMP)

        c. Dysmenorrhea

        d. Menorrhagia

      2. Pregnancy

      3. Contraception

      4. Trauma

  B. Possible therapies

      1. BCPs

      2. Provera

      3. Premarin and Provera

      4. Clomid, if pregnancy is desired

      5. Mirena or Progestasert IUD, which will decrease bleeding and cramping over time

  C. Referral, as appropriate

1. Hysteroscopy
2. Dilation and curettage (D&C)
3. Uterine ablation
4. Hysterectomy with or without bilateral salpingostomies

 DYSMENORRHEA

I. **Definition**

   A. Primary dysmenorrhea: Painful menstruation unrelated to an obvious physical cause

   B. Secondary dysmenorrhea: Painful menstruation related to a demonstrable pelvic disease

II. **Incidence**

   A. Occurs to some degree in 40% to 80% of all women

   B. Is so severe that it is incapacitating in 5% to 10%

III. **Etiology**

   A. Primary dysmenorrhea is believed to be caused by high endometrial levels of prostaglandins.

      1. Under the influence of progesterone during the luteal phase of the menstrual cycle, the endometrial content of prostaglandins is increased, reaching a maximum at the onset of menstruation.

      2. Prostaglandins cause strong myometrial contractions that constrict the blood vessels, resulting in ischemia, endometrial disintegration, bleeding, and pain.

   B. Secondary dysmenorrhea may be caused by any of the following:

      1. Endometriosis
      2. Uterine polyps or fibroids
      3. PID
      4. Dysfunctional uterine bleeding
      5. Uterine prolapse
      6. Maladaptation to an IUD
      7. Retained products of conception following a spontaneous abortion, therapeutic abortion, or childbirth
      8. Uterine or ovarian cancer

IV. **Clinical Features**

   A. Primary dysmenorrhea

      1. Description of course

         a. Primary dysmenorrhea presents as low, midline cramping, spasmodic in nature that may radiate to the back or inner thighs.

         b. Discomfort commonly begins 1 or 2 days before the onset of flow, but pain is characteristically most severe during the first 24 hours of flow and subsides by the second day.

         c. It is frequently accompanied by side effects such as

            (1) Vomiting.

      (2) Diarrhea.

      (3) Headache.

      (4) Syncope.

      (5) Leg pains.

  2. Characteristics and associated factors

    a. Primary dysmenorrhea characteristically begins 1 to 3 years after menarche.

    b. It increases in severity over several years to ages 23 to 27 and then begins to decline.

    c. It is more common in nulliparous women; it frequently decreases significantly after the birth of a child.

    d. It is more common in obese women.

    e. It is associated with a prolonged menstrual flow.

    f. It is less common in athletes.

    g. It is less common in women who have irregular cycles.

B. Secondary dysmenorrhea

  1. Indications

    a. Dysmenorrhea begins after the age of 20.

    b. The pain is unilateral.

  2. Associated factors according to cause

    a. PID

      (1) Acute onset

      (2) Dyspareunia

      (3) Tenderness to palpation and with movement

      (4) Possible palpable adnexal mass

    b. Endometriosis

      (1) Cyclic dyspareunia

      (2) Pain that increases in intensity throughout the period (does not precede the flow and does not end within a few hours, as in primary)

      (3) Pain that is steady rather than crampy and may be specific to the lesion site

      (4) Occasional nodules, which may be palpated upon exam

    c. Uterine fibroids and polyps

      (1) Later onset of dysmenorrhea in the reproductive years than primary dysmenorrhea

      (2) Accompanying changes in the menstrual flow

      (3) Cramping pain

      (4) Palpable fibroids

      (5) Polyps that may or may not protrude from the cervix

    d. Uterine prolapse

      (1) Later onset of dysmenorrhea in the reproductive years than primary dysmenorrhea

      (2) More common in multipara patients

  (3) Initial backache, beginning premenstrually and persisting through the period

  (4) Accompanying dyspareunia and pelvic pain, which are more severe premenstrually and may be relieved by a recumbent or knee-chest position

  (5) Concurrent cystocele and urinary stress incontinence

C. Differentiation of primary and secondary dysmenorrhea according to history and physical exam

1. History

  a. Menstrual history

  (1) Onset of menarche

  (2) Onset of dysmenorrhea in relation to menarche

  (3) Frequency and regularity of cycles

  (4) Duration and amount of flow

  (5) Relationship of dysmenorrhea to cycle and flow

  b. Description of pain

  (1) Onset in relation to menstrual period

  (2) Cramping—spasmodic or steady

  (3) Generalized or in a specific location

  (4) Unilateral or all over lower abdomen

  (5) Location in lower abdomen, back, or thighs

  (6) Worse upon palpation or movement

  c. Associated symptoms

  (1) Extragenital symptoms—see Part IV-Clinical Features, A1c

  (2) Dyspareunia—constant or cyclical relationship to menstrual cycle

  d. Obstetric history—parity

  e. An IUD in place

  f. Any history of conditions that may result in secondary dysmenorrhea

2. Physical exam

  a. Age and weight notation

  b. Speculum exam

  (1) Observe the os for polyps.

  (2) Note any unusual color or odor of the vaginal discharge; do a wet prep.

  (3) Prepare a cervical culture, STD cultures, and blood work, as necessary according to the patient's history.

  c. Bimanual exam

  (1) Note cervical motion tenderness.

  (2) Note the size, shape, and consistency of the uterus; feel for fibroids.

  (3) Note any adnexal masses or nodules.

  (4) Note uterine or adnexal tenderness, especially unilateral.

(5) Note a cystocele or uterine prolapse.

V. Management

A. Primary dysmenorrhea

1. Exercise

   a. Moderate exercise, such as a walk or swim

   b. Pelvic-rocking exercises

   c. Exercises with knees to chest, lying on the back or side

2. Heat

   a. Heating pad or hot-water bottle applied to lower back or lower abdomen

   b. Hot bath, shower, or sauna

3. Orgasm, which relieves pelvic congestion. Warning: Intercourse without orgasm may increase pelvic congestion.

4. Avoidance of caffeine, which can increase the release of prostaglandins

5. Massage of back, leg, or calf

6. Rest

7. Drugs

   a. Oral contraceptives inhibit ovulation and thus relieve the symptoms.

   b. The Mirena or Progestasert IUD may prevent cramping.

   c. The drug of choice is ibuprofen, 200 to 250 mg, taken orally every 4 to 12 hours, depending on the dosage not to exceed 600 mg in 24 hours.

   d. Aleve (naproxen sodium), 200 mg, may also be taken orally every 6 hours.

8. Complementary therapies

   a. Biofeedback

   b. Acupuncture

   c. Meditation

   d. Black cohosh

B. Secondary dysmenorrhea

1. PID

   a. PID may include endometritis, salpingitis, tubo-ovarian abscess, or pelvic peritonitis.

   b. Causative organisms often include *Neisseria gonorrhoeae* and *C. trachomatis*, as well as Gram-negatives, anaerobes, group B streptococci, and genital mycoplasmata. Take appropriate cultures.

   c. Treatment with broad-spectrum antibiotics should begin as soon as the diagnosis is made to prevent permanent damage (e.g., adhesions, sterility). Recommendations by the Centers for Disease Control and Prevention (CDC) are as follows[2]:

---

[2]CDC, 1998, p. 79

      (1) Take 400 mg of ofloxacin orally twice a day for 14 days, plus 500 mg of Flagyl twice a day for 14 days.

      (2) Take either 250 mg of ceftriaxone IM or 2 g of cefoxitin IM, and 1 g of probenecid orally plus 100 mg of doxycycline orally, twice daily for 14 days.

      (3) For serious cases, consult a specialist about hospitalizing the patient for a course of IV antibiotics.

    d. Although the effect of an IUD removal on the patient's response to treatment is unknown, removal is recommended.

  2. Endometriosis

    a. Confirmatory diagnosis needs to be made by laparoscope.

    b. The patient may be treated with BCPs, Lupron, or other medications, as directed by a physician.

  3. Uterine fibroids and polyps

    a. Cervical polyps need to be removed.

    b. A patient with symptomatic uterine fibroids needs to be referred to a physician.

  4. Uterine prolapse

    a. Definitive treatment involves a hysterectomy.

    b. Concurrent cystocele and urinary stress incontinence can be relieved to some degree with the following:

      (1) Kegel exercises

      (2) Pessary and Introl devices to reposition and raise the bladder

ENDOMETRIAL BIOPSY

I.   **Definition.** An endometrial biopsy involves obtaining a sample of the endometrial lining to screen for endometrial cancer or hyperplasia.

II.   **Indications**

  A. Irregular uterine bleeding of unknown etiology in a woman of 35 years or older

  B. Presence of any vaginal bleeding in a postmenopausal woman

  C. A screening precaution before initiating HRT. Routine screening is controversial.

  D. Staging of the endometrium of the infertile patient or of the patient with recurrent fetal wastage to diagnose luteal phase defect

III.   **Contraindications**

  A. Pregnancy

  B. PID

IV.   **Technique**

  A. Give 600 to 800 mg of ibuprofen orally or some other antiprostaglandin 20 to 30 minutes before the procedure. If desired, give an antibiotic prophylactically before and 6 to 8 hours after the procedure.

B. Select one of several instruments designed for endometrial sampling. The Pipelle endometrial suction curette is described here. It is a disposable, flexible curette, 23.5-cm long, with color markings 4, 7, 8, and 10 cm from the end.

C. Perform a bimanual exam to determine the size, shape, and position of the uterus.

D. Visualize the cervix and clean it with an antiseptic. If desired or necessary, the cervix may be straightened by grasping it with a tenaculum. A sound may be introduced to determine the length of the uterus. Gently introduce the Pipelle up into the uterine fundus. Pull back the piston of the Pipelle, creating a negative pressure while rotating it 360°, as the Pipelle is moved from the fundus toward the os. Tissue being collected should be seen within the sheath.

V. Complications. These are rare and reported in less than 1 per 1000.

A. Infection, which may be prevented by premedication and postmedication with a broad-spectrum antibiotic

B. Bleeding

C. Potential perforation of the uterus (there are no reported cases using the Pipelle)

VI. Management

A. Benign: proliferative or secretory

1. Prescribe BCPs.

2. Cycle with Provera or another progestational agent.

B. Cystic or adenomatous hyperplasia

1. If the patient desires pregnancy:

a. Induce ovulation.

b. Repeat an endometrial biopsy if she is not pregnant within 6 months.

2. If the patient does not desire pregnancy or is postmenopausal:

a. Remove unopposed estrogen source by cycling with BCPs or 10 mg of Provera taken orally, starting on days 14 to 16 of the patient's period for 10 to 12 days each menstrual cycle. Megace or another progestational agent may be used.

b. Repeat an endometrial biopsy in 6 months.

(1) If it is normal, continue to follow up.

(2) If it indicates hyperplasia, refer the patient for a D&C or a possible hysterectomy.

C. Atypical adenomatous hyperplasia: Refer the patient to a physician.

 GALACTORRHEA

I. Definition. Galactorrhea is lactation in women who have not breast-fed within the past 6 months.

II. Etiology

A. Physiologic

1. Nipple stimulation

    2. Pregnancy

    3. Postpartum changes

  B. Pathologic

    1. Chiari-Frommel syndrome

    2. Hypothalamic disorders, hypothyroid, or tumors

    3. Prolactin-secreting pituitary tumors

    4. Trauma or chronic irritation from intraductal papillomas and infected milk ducts, or sexual activity

  C. Pharmacologic

    1. Psychotropic drugs

    2. Antihypertensives

    3. Oral contraceptives

III. Management

  A. Take a good history and perform a breast exam. If the discharge is unilateral, consider infection, intraductal papilloma, or local tumor instead of lactation, pregnancy, pituitary problems, and drugs.

  B. Rule out pregnancy.

  C. Perform a smear of breast discharge using Pap smear slide and fixative.

  D. Order lab tests.

    1. TSH: If elevated, refer the patient for hypothyroidism.

    2. Prolactin level: This level needs to be taken before the breasts are stimulated with a breast exam.

      a. If the patient is not pregnant, prolactin levels should be less than 20 mg/mL.

      b. If the patient is lactating, prolactin levels should be less than 40 mg/mL.

      c. If prolactin levels are greater than 40 to 80 mg/mL

        (1) Recommend 2.5 to 7.5 mg of bromocriptine (Parlodel) every day. Monitor blood pressure for elevation.

        (2) Consult a specialist regarding the need for computed tomography (CT) or an MRI of the sella turcica.

        (3) Following treatment, measure prolactin levels every 1 to 3 months.

      d. If prolactin levels are greater than 80 mg/mL

        (1) Order a CT or an MRI of the sella turcica.

        (2) Refer the patient to a physician.

  E. Recommend a mammogram; if it is abnormal, refer the patient appropriately.

 GENETIC SCREENING

I. **Genetic Disorders in the Fetus**

  A. **Definition.** Genetic screening is the process of determining, from parental history, the risk of genetic disorders in the fetus and recommending appropriate testing.

B. Etiology

1. Single-gene defect

   a. Autosomal dominant disorders

      (1) Characteristics

         (a) An abnormal gene dominates, while a normal gene is recessive.

         (b) The likelihood in the fetus is 50% if a parent has the condition.

         (c) Unaffected children of affected parents are not carriers.

      (2) Examples

         (a) Achondroplasia (a form of dwarfism)

         (b) Huntington's disease

         (c) Neurofibromatosis

   b. Autosomal recessive disorders

      (1) Characteristics

         (a) The abnormal gene is recessive, so a gene must be contributed by each parent for offspring to be affected. Offspring who inherit one normal and one abnormal gene are carriers. All affected persons are homozygous.

         (b) If both parents are carriers, there is a 25% chance of producing either an affected child or a normal child and a 50% chance of producing a carrier.

      (2) Examples

         (a) Cystic fibrosis

         (b) Sickle cell anemia

         (c) Tay-Sachs disease

         (d) Phenylketonuria

         (e) Galactosemia

   c. Sex-linked disorders

      (1) An abnormal gene is carried on an X chromosome. Men are always affected. Women are affected only if both X chromosomes are abnormal, and they are carriers if one X chromosome is abnormal.

      (2) Examples

         (a) Duchenne's muscular dystrophy

         (b) Hemophilia

         (c) Red-green color blindness

2. Chromosomal aberrations

   a. Aberrations in chromosome structure: Rearrangement of genes between two paired chromosomes

   b. Aberrations in chromosomal number

      (1) Monosome: Cells contain one less chromosome than the basic number or are aneuploid, for example, Turner's syndrome (XO).

      (2) Trisomy: Cells contain three chromosomes instead of a normal pair (e.g., trisomy 21 or Down syndrome).

      (3) Mosaic: Only a portion of the body's cells contains the variation in chromosome number.

C. Management: Screening should be done at the initial visit.

  1. High-risk factors

    a. Maternal age older than 35-The incidence of Down syndrome is as follows:

      (1) Under age 25: 1 in 2000

      (2) At age 30: 1 in 885

      (3) At age 35: 1 in 250

      (4) At age 40: 1 in 109

      (5) At age 45: 1 in 12

    b. Paternal age older than 55, which has shown a slight increase in genetic problems

    c. A family history of hereditary abnormality

    d. Ethnic or racial groups at high risk for specific genetic diseases

      (1) African Americans may inherit sickle cell disease or trait. All African American patients should be screened for sickle cell trait.

      (2) African Americans, Asians, and those of Mediterranean descent may inherit G6PD anemia. People with this heritage should be screened only if they experience severe or persistent anemia or UTIs.

      (3) People of English descent are at risk for an increased incidence of spinal cord defects.

      (4) People of Jewish descent are at risk for Tay-Sachs disease.

      (5) Asians and those of Mediterranean descent should be screened for thalassemia.

    e. Parents who have already had one child with a birth defect

    f. Patients who have had two or more first-trimester spontaneous abortions

    g. Those with known or suspected exposure to teratogens—Ask patients about the following:

      (1) Exposure to high temperatures (over 102°F) during the first trimester, for example, a fever, hot tub, sauna: If exposed to heat during neural tube formation, embryos may suffer spinal cord defects.

      (2) A fever in the first trimester: If caused by a viral infection, a fever could also result in a viral-type syndrome in the fetus, such as that seen in cytomegalovirus.

      (3) Primary herpes: Ask the patient about any history of herpes; if positive, ascertain whether the primary episode was in first trimester.

(4) An intake of drugs since becoming pregnant, including OTC, prescription, or street drugs

(5) Exposure to cat litter or ingestion of raw meat

(6) Smoking, which increases the chance of low-birth-weight babies

(7) Ingestion of alcohol: If positive, ask about fetal alcohol syndrome in present children.

(8) Caffeine intake: If excessive, recommend cutting down on caffeine.

(9) Syphilis: Screen the patient if there is a previous history.

2. Chorionic villi sampling (9–11 weeks) or amniocentesis (16–18 weeks)

  a. These tests should be offered to

    (1) Patients age 35 or older

    (2) A parent with a chromosome abnormality

    (3) A patient with previous offspring with a chromosome abnormality

    (4) A parent with a carrier state for metabolic disorders

    (5) A parent with a previous child with a neural tube defect or a patient with elevated serum alpha-fetoprotein (AFP)

  b. Such clients should be encouraged to make an appointment with a geneticist before deciding for or against amniocentesis. Factors in the decision include

    (1) Chances of a defect occurring.

    (2) The patient's feelings about abortions. If she would not abort the fetus regardless of a defect, she may decide against amniocentesis. Even if she would not abort, knowing the diagnosis may prevent months of needless anxiety or help her prepare for parenting an affected child.

    (3) Patient's feelings about the defects in question. Some are more severe or possibly more unacceptable than others.

3. Serum AFP when the EGA is 15–18 weeks. The AFP will detect between 85% to 90% of neural tube defects and 20% of Down syndrome babies. The AFP test has a false-positive rate of 30% when taken and calculated with the correct EGA.

  a. The AFP or AFP-Plus test should be offered to all patients who qualify.

  b. If AFP levels are elevated, an ultrasound should be done to confirm the dates; the AFP test should be repeated as indicated. If the results are abnormal, the patient should be referred for genetic counseling.

  c. If the AFP is decreased, an ultrasound should be done to confirm the dates, and an AFP-Plus should be done to reconfirm a possible problem. The patient should be referred for genetic counseling and possible amniocentesis, as necessary.

4. AFP-Plus testing

   a. The AFP-Plus test can detect 3 times as many cases of Down syndrome as AFP testing alone.

   b. It will detect 85% to 90% of open neural tube defects and 60% to 70% of Down syndrome babies.

   c. AFP-Plus measures AFP, unconjugated estriol, and hCG.

   d. It should be done between 15 and 18 weeks of pregnancy.

      (1) Encourage all patients who do not want an amniocentesis to have this test.

      (2) Offer AFP-Plus to patients who have a family history of anacephaly, neural tube defects, or Down syndrome.

D. **Preventive Measures:** Encourage patients to

   1. Maintain a healthy lifestyle, eat well-balanced meals, and avoid substances harmful to a baby when planning a pregnancy.

   2. Avoid excess vitamins; vitamin A, in particular, is teratogenic in high doses.

   3. Consider taking 2 to 4 mg of folic acid every day before conception to prevent neural tube defects.

   4. Avoid hot tubs, saunas, and tanning beds if there is a possibility of pregnancy.

II. **Genetic Predisposition to Breast and Ovarian Cancer**

A. **Definition.** Between 5% and 10 % of breast and ovarian cancers are hereditary. BRCA1 and BRCA2 are tumor suppressor genes that protect and preserve DNA. Mutations in BRCA1 are responsible for up to 40% of inherited breast cancer and confer a lifetime risk of 50% to 85% for breast cancer in the person who inherits the mutation and 15% to 45% for ovarian cancer. Mutations in BRCA2 are responsible for 30% of inherited female breast cancers and 40% of inherited male breast cancers. Such mutations confer a lifetime risk of 50% to 80% for breast cancer and 20% for ovarian cancer.[3] TP53, phosphate and tensin homolog (PTEN), and ataxia telangiectasia (ATM) mutations account for less than 2.5% of all breast and ovarian cancers; the remaining gene mutations have yet to be discovered.

B. **Etiology**

   1. Germline mutations, in which a mutation occurs in an egg or sperm, affect all cells of the person who inherits them.

   2. Of persons who have the altered gene who go on to develop cancer, the cancer appears to be age related. As a person ages, he or she is exposed to more environmental carcinogens, hormones, and DNA damage.

   3. Tumor development requires a combination of mutations, genetic defects, and failed immune surveillance.

   4. Breast and ovarian cancer heredity syndrome is autosomal dominant.

      a. An abnormal gene dominates, while a normal gene is recessive.

---

[3]Olopade & Cummings, 2000, p. 1809

      b. The likelihood of transmission is 50% from *either* parent if they have the mutation.

      c. Unaffected children of unaffected parents are not carriers.

  5. Some ethnic or racial groups have a higher frequency of mutations.

      a. Ashkenazi Jews have two specific mutations in BRCA1 and one in BRCA2.

      b. Some subpopulations of French Canadians, Icelanders, and African Americans have BRCA1 mutations.

C. Management

  1. Take a detailed family history that includes any incidence of cancer in the family, the type, which family member, the relationship of this relative to the patient, and the age of onset. Be sure to include paternal as well as maternal family.

  2. Teach and encourage all women to do a breast self-exam monthly. It is mandatory for those at risk by history.

  3. Thoroughly screen the patient for abdominal female problems every year; include a pelvic examination for those at high risk.

  4. Initiate a mammogram screening for those at risk 10 years prior to the onset of cancer in the youngest family member, according to American Cancer Society recommendations.[4]

  5. Consider BRCA analysis[5] those at high risk for breast and ovarian cancer by family history and race.

      a. Screen the patient for BRCA1 and BRCA2 genes.

      b. Ensure counseling is provided prior to testing. Positive, negative, or uncertain results will have implications for the individual, as well as her entire family.

      c. Inform the patient that BRCA analysis currently remains a costly option.

 GONORRHEA

I.   **Definition.** Gonorrhea is an STD caused by the anaerobic Gram-negative intracellular diplococcus *Neisseria gonorrhoeae*.

II.   **Etiology**

  A. The gonococcus (GC) organism is a kidney bean–shaped diplococcus, which is a pathogen for epithelium. Common sites of infection include the following:

    1. Oropharynx

    2. Conjunctiva of eyes

    3. Male urethra

---

[4]American Cancer Society, 2000
[5]For more more information on genetic testing, research, and development, access www.myriad.com on the Internet.

4. Female reproductive tract. The GC stay in the vagina until menses, when the cervical canal is open, and then ascend to the uterus and fallopian tubes.

5. Rectum

B. Prior infection confers antibodies but no immunity. Both the virulence of the bacteria and individual resistance vary.

III. Clinical Features

A. Course of the disease: The onset is 3 to 7 days after first menstrual period following exposure. Symptoms begin to subside 7 to 10 days later and are usually gone after 21 days without treatment (sooner with treatment).

B. Signs and symptoms

1. Often asymptomatic: Gonorrhea is detected only on routine cervical screening or following possible exposure. About 40% to 60% of women with gonorrhea develop some symptoms.

2. Urethra: Urinary frequency or a slight burning during urination may occur.

3. Paraurethral (Skene's) glands: Pus can be expressed from the urethral meatus.

4. Bartholin's glands: Gonorrhea may cause an abscess (redness, edema, pain), which may require an incision and drainage or heal with resulting cysts.

5. Cervix: Leukorrhea, which may be green or yellow-green, is discharged and irritates the vulvar tissues.

6. Endometrium: Infection is transitory, heals spontaneously, and is asymptomatic.

7. Endosalpinx: Pus forms in the fallopian tubes and can spill out onto the ovaries, peritoneum, muscle of the tubes, and broad ligament. Endosalpingitis is the predominant feature of GC infection. Symptoms include the following:

   a. Fever—up to 103°F

   b. Nausea and vomiting

   c. Pain, moderate or severe, in both lower abdominal quadrants. It may be more severe on the onset side.

   d. Tenderness and rigidity in both lower abdominal quadrants upon exam—involuntary guarding upon abdominal palpation

   e. Cervical motion tenderness and pain in lateral fornices during bimanual exam

   f. Adnexal or uterine tenderness during bimanual exam

   g. Adnexal mass palpable during bimanual exam

   h. Tender inguinal adenopathy

8. Perihepatitis: Palpation elicits pain in the lower portion of the liver, caused by the spread of gonorrhea to the peritoneum and fibrotic bands that form between the liver and the peritoneum.

9. Local infection: Gonorrhea causes pharyngitis, proctitis, and conjunctivitis.

10. Disseminated infection (arthritis-dermatitis syndrome): GC spreads to the bloodstream.

   a. Disseminated infection occurs in 1% to 3% of women with gonorrhea, particularly during pregnancy or the menstrual period.

   b. It is a benign condition but mimics serious conditions, so it must be carefully differentiated. Meningitis and endocarditis are rare.

   c. It presents a classic triad of symptoms:

      (1) Chills and fever

      (2) Maculopapular rash on wrists and joints, which progresses to vesicles and hemorrhagic pustules

      (3) Arthritis of the joints

   d. Diagnosis is almost always made from a culture of the original infection site. Cultures of the blood, joint aspirate, and skin lesions are often negative.

C. Residual of GC PID

   1. Narrowing and thickening of the fallopian tubes—adnexa are palpable and fixed. This condition may lead to sterility or an increased incidence of ectopic pregnancy.

   2. Closure of the tubes, usually at the fimbriated ends, resulting in sterility

   3. Pelvic masses secondary to adhesions

   4. A fixed and nonmobile uterus secondary to adhesions

   5. Chronic pain, abnormal uterine bleeding, or dyspareunia

D. Effects in pregnancy

   1. GC PID during pregnancy can be of greater clinical severity than in nonpregnant women because of suppression of the immune response during pregnancy.

   2. There is a greater risk of disseminated GC in pregnant women than in nonpregnant women.

   3. Gonorrhea infection is associated with chorioamnionitis, premature rupture of membranes, and premature delivery.

   4. After delivery, the gonococci that were present in the vagina can ascend and cause postpartum endometritis.

E. Effects on the fetus and neonate

   1. Gonorrhea causes increased fetal loss and low birth weight if the mother is infected during pregnancy.

   2. GC infects the infant's conjunctivae as the fetus passes through the vagina during birth, and it can cause blindness.

   3. The infant can contract disseminated GC.

IV. **Differential Diagnosis.** Diagnoses should be considered and ruled out, depending on the site of the GC infection.

   A. Urethra: Rule out a UTI or chlamydia.

   B. Cervix, vagina, and Bartholin's glands: Rule out nongonococcal infection, particularly chlamydia.

    C. Endometrium or endosalpinx: Rule out the following conditions:

      1. Round ligament pain

      2. Diverticulitis

      3. Appendicitis

      4. Ectopic pregnancy

      5. Septic abortion

      6. Pelvic endometriosis

      7. Kidney stone

V. Management

    A. Diagnose the disease by examining a GC culture of the cervix or urethra, if signs and symptoms of urethritis exist.

    B. Do a GC culture of the cervix under the following circumstances:

      1. When there are signs and symptoms of gonorrhea

      2. When the patient is diagnosed with syphilis or chlamydia

      3. When the patient expresses a concern that she may have a sexually transmitted infection (STI)

    C. If the culture is positive, perform the following procedure:

      1. Obtain a VDRL result to rule out syphilis before treatment.

      2. Consider treating the patient in the office. Notify the health department of the infection and treatment.

    D. Follow the standard treatment recommended by the CDC.[6]

      1. Nonpregnant patient

        a. Recommend 125 mg of Rocephin (ceftriaxone) IM in a single dose or 400 mg of ofloxacin, orally, in a single dose, followed by either 1 g of Zithromax (azithromycin), orally, in a single dose or 100 mg of doxycycline, orally, twice a day for 7 days.

        b. Alternate regimens

          (1) Recommend 2 g of spectinomycin IM in a single dose, followed by either 1 g of Zithromax, orally, in a single dose or 100 mg of doxycycline, orally, twice a day for 7 days.

          (2) If the infection was acquired from a source not proven to be penicillin resistant, give 3 g of amoxicillin orally with 1g of probenecid, followed by 100 mg of doxycycline, orally, twice a day for 7 days.

      2. Pregnant patient: Give 125 mg of Rocephin IM in a single dose or 2 g of spectinomycin IM in a single dose, followed by either 1 g of Zithromax, orally, in a single dose or 500 mg of amoxicillin, orally, 3 times a day for 7 days.

    E. After treatment, follow up with these practices:

      1. Reculture the cervix after treatment at the following times:

        a. One week after treatment is completed

        b. Gonorrhea diagnosis during pregnancy

---

[6]CDC, 1998, pp. 61–63

       (1) Reculture the cervix within 1 month of the estimated date of confinement (EDC) to verify cure or rule out reinfection before delivery.

       (2) Reculture the cervix at the 6-week postpartum visit.

    2. If results are positive at any time, retreat the patient. Tell the patient her diagnosis, educate her about GC, and emphasize the necessity of completing the treatment and follow-up practices.

    3. Contact the patient's sexual partner(s) (every effort must be made) and confirm his or her treatment through the health department.

  F. If gonorrhea was diagnosed during pregnancy,

    1. Be sure the pediatrician or neonatal nurse practitioner is notified of the diagnosis after delivery.

    2. Be alert for signs of GC PID in the postpartum patient and consult with physician if it develops.

 HEADACHE

  I. **Definition.** A headache is a diffuse pain in various parts of the head, which varies in intensity, site, and duration. Headaches are classified as chronic, acute, or episodic.

  II. **Etiology.** Symptoms vary depending upon the type of headache; the most common types are as follows:

  A. Migraine: Usually provoked by the menstrual cycle, odors, food, and stress. Migraine headaches occur more often in females than males. They may be unilateral and throbbing, with visual disturbances.

  B. Cluster: Often triggered by alcohol or tobacco. Cluster headaches frequently occur in sleep and occur 5 to 6 times more frequently in men than women. They are associated with constant or excruciating pain.

  C. Tension: Often triggered by emotional stress, fatigue, or worry. Tension headaches frequently involve the posterior head and neck.

  D. Sinusitis: Caused by pressure built up in the sinuses, causing a deep, dull ache around the nose, cheeks, and teeth. They worsen when the patient bends over.

  E. Hormone-related headaches

    1. Pregnancy: Occur early in pregnancy through the second trimester. Headaches during pregnancy result from hormonal changes and increased capillary permeability, causing increases in cerebral edema.

    2. Pill-related: Often occur during the pill-free week of BCPs because of hormonal withdrawal. They may occur at any time during the cycle.

    3. Menopausal: Migraine headaches decrease by up to 70% during menopause. Other types of headaches are triggered by hormonal and serotonin imbalances, insomnia, or stress.

    F. Less-common types of headaches

        1. Hypoglycemia—Severe headache in the absence of regular meals, caused by a drop in glucose levels

        2. Eye strain—Caused by squinting to compensate for difficulty reading and watching television

        3. Preeclampsia—Occurs late in pregnancy. Is associated with elevated blood pressure and edema.

        4. Anemia—Usually occurs in the afternoon because of fatigue

        5. Cerebral tumor—Caused by increased pressure

III. Management

    A. Migraines

        1. Severe and frequent migraines with focal and neurologic symptoms need to be referred to a neurologist for a complete workup.

        2. Those with a prior history or known cause may be managed as follows:

            a. In pregnancy

                (1) Suggest lifestyle modifications, such as regular sleep, exercise, decreased stress, meditation, or biofeedback.

                (2) Order medications, such as Tylenol with Codeine No. 3, Fioricet, and transnasal butorphanol (Stadol).

                (3) Do not use ergot-based medications. The oxytocic properties of these medications are dangerous in pregnancy, as they cause uterine contractions.

            b. In lactation

                (1) Use triptans, which have a very short half-life. After use, pump the breasts and discard the milk after two feedings.

                (2) Use beta-blockers and divalproex sodium (Depakote) prophylactically.

            c. With oral contraceptives

                (1) Do not prescribe BCPs to patients who have frequent, severe, or uncontrolled migraines with focal and neurologic signs and symptoms. Consider Depo-Provera, an IUD, or other forms of birth control. Progestin-only pills are another option.

                (2) Because estrogen and frequent hormonal changes have been implicated in headaches, try a monophasic, low-dose estrogen BCP, such as Loestrin 1/20 or Lo/Ovral.

                (3) Give two or three cycles of active BCPs prior to having a pill-free week and having a period.

                (4) Discuss lifestyle changes such as stopping smoking, trying biofeedback, decreasing stress, and finding and eliminating triggers that start a migraine.

            d. Menstrual migraines

                (1) Give three cycles of active BCPs prior to having a pill-free week and having a period. This will decrease headaches to four or five per year.

(2) Start 400 to 600 mg of nonsteroidal anti-inflammatory drugs (NSAIDs) orally every 6 to 8 hours, 3 days prior to the expected onset of menses.

(3) Give triptans 24 hours prior to the expected onset of a headache or as rescue therapy for a breakthrough headache.

(4) Review the patient's diet. Certain foods are associated with migraines (e.g., ripened cheese, chocolate, MSG, vinegar, fermented foods, and alcohol).[7]

e. In menopause

    (1) Recommend continuous low-dose oral or transdermal HRT.

    (2) Initiate prophylactic therapy such as beta-blockers, calcium channel blockers, selective serotonin reuptake inhibitors, and tricyclic antidepressants, which may prevent attacks.

    (3) Avoid triptans in the elderly, because they constrict arteries.

B. Cluster headaches

    1. A sumatriptan injection or nasal spray may be given.

    2. Oxygen inhalation has been shown to benefit patients who suffer from cluster headaches. Give 6 liters for 15 to 20 minutes.

    3. The following medications can be used prophylactically: verapamil (Calan), lithium, divalproex sodium (Depakote), and cyproheptadine (Periactin).

C. Tension headaches

    1. Find and avoid provocative factors.

    2. Recommend OTC NSAIDs, aspirin, or acetaminophen.

    3. Take antidepressants to reduce frequency.

    4. Refer the patient for counseling, biofeedback, yoga, and other stress-reduction and relaxation techniques.

D. Sinusitis

    1. Give the patient antibiotics if the infection is severe or present for more than a week.

    2. Try relief measures such as hot compresses and humidifier use.

    3. Use nasal sprays with caution. If used too frequently or too long, they may have a rebound effect when stopped and cause the very problem they were taken initially to prevent.

E. Hormone-related headaches

    1. If pregnant

        a. Eat frequent, small meals, rest, drink plenty of fluids, and use stress-reduction techniques.

        b. Modify lifestyle patterns to incorporate regular sleep, exercise, decreased stress, meditation, or biofeedback.

---

[7]Diamond, 2001, p. 1131

    c. Consider taking the following medications: Tylenol with Codeine No. 3, Fioricet, and transnasal butorphanol (Stadol).

    d. Consult with a neurologist if these methods fail.

  2. If not pregnant

    a. Have the patient document on her menstrual chart the day the headaches began, severity, type of medication taken, time taken, dose, and degree of relief.

    b. See the previously described treatment for menstrual migraines.

F. Less common types of headaches

  1. Hypoglycemia

    a. Eat small, frequent meals.

    b. Have some proteins at each meal or snack.

    c. Avoid concentrated sugars and refined foods.

    d. Avoid long periods without eating.

    e. Consider a referral to a dietitian.

  2. Eyestrain

    a. Recommend an eye exam.

    b. Instruct the patient in the use of proper lighting.

    c. Ascertain if the patient is working on a computer or is using her eyes for prolonged fine eye work. Suggest taking breaks.

  3. Preeclampsia

    a. Rest, drink plenty of fluids, and carefully check blood pressure.

    b. See management under prenatal care regarding magnesium sulfate.

  4. Anemia

    a. Because headaches often occur in the afternoon, recommend a rest break during that time.

    b. See Anemia at the beginning of Part IV for treatment options.

  5. Confirmed or suspected cerebral tumor—Refer the patient as soon as possible.

 ## HEMORRHOIDS

I. **Definition.** Hemorrhoids are anal varicosities.

II. **Etiology**

A. Genetic predisposition

B. Pregnancy

  1. Increased venous pressure on the pelvic veins caused by the pressure of the enlarging uterus

  2. The relaxing effect of progesterone on the vein walls and valves, surrounding muscle tissue, and large bowel

  3. Trauma from pushing during the second stage of labor and the pressure of the baby and distention at birth

C. Anal intercourse

III. Management

    A. Examine the hemorrhoids for severity, trauma, and possible thrombosis.

    B. If the hemorrhoid is thrombosed, refer the patient to a surgeon or GI specialist for lancing.

    C. If bleeding continues over 1 month, refer the patient to a GI specialist.

    D. Begin the following comfort measures and medications. If no improvement occurs after 1 week, reexamine the hemorrhoids. Rule out rectal fissures.

    E. Comfort measures

       1. Review the patient's diet and modify it to keep the stools soft.

       2. Relieve constipation.

       3. Recommend frequent sitz baths. The heat of the water not only gives comfort, but it also increases circulation.

       4. Apply ice packs for reduction of swelling.

       5. Provide a rubber ring to sit on to reduce pressure on the hemorrhoids without interfering with circulation. Ensure the rubber ring is

          a. Not fully inflated, but inflated only enough to relieve pressure.

          b. Large enough to avoid a small area of concentrated pressure.

          c. Positioned so that there are no pressure points in the pelvic area.

       6. Keep hemorrhoids reduced by gently pushing them inside the rectum with a lubricated finger cot or glove and then tightening the rectal sphincter to give them support and to contain them within the rectum.

       7. Rest in bed, with the hips and lower extremities elevated.

    F. Medications

       1. Take 50 mg of Colace orally every day or twice a day.

       2. Apply Preparation H.

       3. Use suppositories, as needed, such as Anusol, one twice a day and after bowel movements.

       4. Use Tucks (witch hazel packs) to reduce swelling and ease pain.

       5. Apply epsom salt compresses for reduction of swelling.

       6. Apply a topical analgesic/anesthetic spray or ointment, such as Americaine Spray and Dibucaine ointment.

       7. If the hemorrhoids are bleeding, consider suppositories with cortisone (e.g., Anusol HC cream or suppositories).

 HEPATITIS

I. **Definition.** Hepatitis is an inflammation of the liver in which diffuse patchy necrosis affects all liver acini and destroys liver architecture.

II. **Etiology**

    A. See Table 4-1, Comparisons of Viral Hepatitis A, B, C, D, E, and G.

    B. Consider the other causes of acute hepatitis.

Table 4-1. Comparisons of Viral Hepatitis A, B, C, D, E, and G

Virus Type:	A RNA	B DNA	C RNA (6 genotypes)	D RNA (delta agent)	E RNA	G RNA
Mode of Transmission	Enteric Food/water	Blood, all bodily fluids	Blood	Blood	Enteric Food/water	Blood
Risk Factors	• Travel outside the United States to areas endemic for disease • Contaminated food and water • Institutionalization • Children in day care • Military personnel	• IV drug user • Anal intercourse • Intercourse with an infected person • Occupational exposure • Blood transfusion recipients • Dialysis patients • Close contact with an infected person (spouse, children)	• IV drug user • Intercourse with an infected person • Occupational exposure • Blood transfusion recipient (less than 1%)	• HBV—HDV is a defective RNA virus that requires HBV to replicate. • IV drug user • Occupational exposure	• Travel outside the United States to areas endemic for disease	• Blood transfusions—major source • HCV, which is present 10% of the time and related to HGV
Incubation Clinical Course	15–50 days • Has a rapid onset • Lasts 1 to 4 weeks • Does not become chronic	1–6 months • Is acute in 90% • Becomes chronic in 5% to 10% • Is associated with hepatocellular carcinoma	2–26 weeks • Is acute in 20% • Becomes chronic in 80%; may progress to cirrhosis or hepatocellular carcinoma • Is a leading cause of liver transplants	2–8 weeks • Is acute • When combined with HBV, increases the likelihood of fulminating hepatitis • Becomes chronically progressive in 15% • Mortality 2%–20%	2–9 weeks • Is acute • Is often self-limiting • During pregnancy, causes maternal mortality in up to 20%	

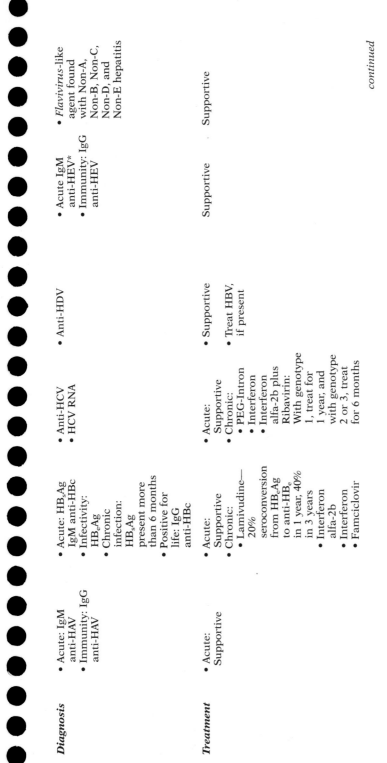

	HAV	HBV	HCV	HDV	HEV
Diagnosis	• Acute: IgM anti-HAV • Immunity: IgG anti-HAV	• Acute: HB$_s$Ag IgM anti-HBc • Infectivity: HB$_e$Ag • Chronic infection: HB$_s$Ag present more than 6 months • Positive for life: IgG anti-HBc	• Anti-HCV • HCV RNA	• Anti-HDV	• Acute IgM anti-HEV* • Immunity: IgG anti-HEV • *Flavivirus*-like agent found with Non-A, Non-B, Non-C, Non-D, and Non-E hepatitis
Treatment	• Acute: Supportive	• Acute: Supportive • Chronic: • Lamivudine—20% seroconversion from HB$_e$Ag to anti-HB$_e$ in 1 year; 40% in 3 years • Interferon alfa-2b • Interferon • Famciclovir	• Acute: Supportive • Chronic: • PEG-Intron • Interferon • Interferon alfa-2b plus Ribavirin: With genotype 1, treat for 1 year, and with genotype 2 or 3, treat for 6 months	• Supportive • Treat HBV, if present	Supportive

continued

Table 4-1. Comparisons of Viral Hepatitis A, B, C, D, E, and G

Virus Type	A RNA	B DNA	C RNA (6 genotypes)	D RNA (delta agent)	E RNA	G RNA
Vaccines	Inactivated HAV vaccine: >18 yr old—Havrix, 1440 EL. U. IM; second dose 6 months later	HBVac: >18 yr old—1.0 mL of Recombivax IM or 1.0 mL Engerix-B IM; second dose 1 month later; third dose 5 months after second dose	None	HBVac	None	None

HAV=hepatitis A virus, HBV=hepatitis B virus, HCV=hepatitis C virus, HDV=hepatitis D virus, HEV=hepatitis E virus.

1. Mononucleosis and cytomegalovirus
2. Syphilis
3. Cholangitis, especially gallstone obstruction
4. Drug-induced hepatitis: Many medications can cause acute liver injury. Most of the common ones are
   a. Aspirin in high doses.
   b. Acetaminophen in high doses.
   c. Nitrofurantoin.
   d. Sulfonamide.
5. Chronic alcohol intake

III. **Clinical Features**
   A. The disease is extremely variable.
      1. Mild, transient, or asymptomatic
      2. Severe, prolonged, and ultimately fatal
      3. Anywhere in between mild and severe
   B. Hepatitis is separated into four phases:
      1. Incubation phase
      2. Pre-icteric phase
      3. Icteric phase
      4. Convalescence
   C. Symptoms according to phase
      1. Incubation period: None
      2. Pre-icteric phase (2-15 days)
         a. Malaise: the most frequent complaint and the first symptom to appear and the last to resolve
         b. Anorexia: Possible intolerance for strong odors and tastes
         c. Weight loss of 2 to 10 pounds
         d. Intermittent nausea and vomiting, which may be provoked by eating or smelling food
         e. Distaste for cigarette smoking
         f. Right upper quadrant pain: Dull and mild to moderate in severity
         g. Less common symptoms
            (1) Low-grade fever
            (2) Headaches
            (3) Diarrhea
      3. Icteric phase
         a. Jaundice, which is maximal in 1 to 2 weeks and lasts for 6 to 8 weeks
         b. Pruritus secondary to jaundice
         c. Darkening of urine color
         d. Lightening of stool color
      4. Convalescent phase

        a. This phase begins with the disappearance of jaundice and major symptoms and lasts 2 to 6 weeks.

        b. Malaise may persist for weeks or months.

  D. Signs

    1. Mild to moderate hepatic tenderness to percussion

    2. Firm liver edge palpable slightly below the right costal margin

    3. Enlarged spleen, which may be palpable

    4. Skin manifestation

        a. Rash in 10% to 15% in pre-icteric phase

        b. Excoriations secondary to pruritus

    5. Signs of portal hypertension, cirrhosis, and hepatic failure

IV. Management

  A. At the initial visit, ask the patient the following questions:

    1. Have you ever had a blood transfusion? If so, did you have any unusual or abnormal reactions?

    2. Have you or anyone in your family ever had hepatitis?

  B. Order a hepatitis B screen on all OB patients.

  C. Order a total hepatitis screen, including antigens and antibodies, for the following patients:

    1. Those with a positive history of

        a. Blood transfusion, hepatitis, or hepatitis of a family member

        b. Rejection as a blood donor because they were found to be hepatitis B or C positive

        c. Identification as a hepatitis carrier

    2. Those with high exposure to hepatitis

        a. Who work or reside in institutions for the mentally retarded, military, or day care

        b. Who are exposed to blood and needles

        c. Who have family members who have hepatitis or are carriers

    3. Those who have traveled to or are from high-risk areas, such as Asia (except Japan), Africa, the Middle East, Central America, and South America

  D. Order a hepatitis screen for any patient who presents with a clinical picture of hepatitis.

  E. If the hepatitis screen is abnormal at any time, order liver function tests. Refer the patient to a physician if the liver function is impaired or active infection is indicated.

  F. Report any diagnosis of hepatitis to the health department for epidemiologic follow-up.

  G. Offer hepatitis A and B vaccines to those at risk, such as travelers from the United States, military and medical personnel, and those living with an infected person. Havrix and hepatitis B vaccine (HBVac) can be given separately or Twinrix (hepatitis A inactivated and hepatitis B [recombinant] vaccine) can be given at the office visit at 1 month and at 6 months.

H. Treat patients who have been exposed to hepatitis A as follows:

    1. For adults older than 18, give Havrix in 1440 enzyme-linked immunosorbent assay (ELISA) units (EL.U.) IM concurrently with immune globulin (Ig) at 0.02 to 0.06 mL/kg IM.

        a. With Havrix, the patient has 80% to 98% seroconversion by day 15 and 100% by 1 month.

        b. With the Ig, the patient has passive immunity in 24 hours, which dissipates in 4 to 6 months.

    2. For long-term immunity, give a second dose of 1440 EL.U. of Havrix 6 months after the first dose.

I. Treat patients who are exposed to hepatitis B as follows:

    1. For adults older than 18, give 1.0 mL of Recombivax HB or 1.0 mL of Engerix-B IM concurrently with 0.6 mL/kg of hepatitis immune globulin (HBIG) IM.

        a. HBIG provides short-term passive immunity within 24 hours and dissipates in 6 to 9 months.

        b. HBVac provides long-term immunity; use the following preexposure schedule.

    2. Follow the HBVac preexposure schedule for long-term immunity.

        a. First dose at time of the visit

        b. Second dose, 1 month after the first dose

        c. Third dose, 5 months after the second dose

J. For immunocompromised patients or those on dialysis, give 2.0 mL of Engerix-B IM or 1.0 mL of the special Recombivax for the immunocompromised.

K. Manage uncompromised, nonacute patients collaboratively.

V. Maternal, Fetal, and Neonatal Considerations

    A. Maternal considerations

        1. Maternal disease may cause an increase in spontaneous abortion and prematurity.

        2. Maternal disease may possibly increase in severity in the third trimester because of the added load on the liver from the pregnancy.

        3. Maternal hepatitis may be prevented with the following:

            a. Hepatitis B vaccine (Heptavax B) may be given to those who are at high risk for contracting hepatitis B. It consists of killed virus. It can be given in pregnancy when clearly indicated.

            b. Hepatitis A vaccine (Havrix) can be given during pregnancy when clearly indicated. It is an inactivated virus.

            c. Ig and HBIG confer passive immunity within 24 hours.

    B. Fetal considerations

        1. Maternal disease may cause an increase in spontaneous abortion and prematurity.

        2. There may be congenital effects from maternal type-B infection, irrespective of time of gestation, but it is rare.

3. The major effects on the fetus are secondary to the mother's condition, which may be compromised by the disease (e.g., poor nutrition, weight loss). The prognosis is good if the mother has good supportive care.

C. Neonatal considerations

1. The infant may contract the infection in utero or from the mother after birth. The following medications can be given to the infant prophylactically:

   a. Type A: Infants born to mothers who are incubating the virus or are acutely ill should receive one 0.5 mL dose of Ig as soon as possible after birth.

   b. Type B: Infants less than 1 year old born to HBsAg-positive mothers should receive 0.5 mL HBIG within 12 hours of birth concurrently with 0.5 mL of Recombivax HB or Engerix-B IM. Follow the regular dosing schedule for the second and third doses of HBVac injections.

2. The virus is shed in the breast milk, so breast-feeding is contraindicated if the mother is infected.

 HERPES SIMPLEX

I. Definition. Herpes simplex is a vesicular eruption of the skin and mucous membranes caused by the herpes virus.

II. Etiology

A. There are two types of herpes virus, which have cross-reacting antibodies.

1. Type 1 is almost always nongenital. The primary infection usually occurs in infancy through prepuberty.

2. Type 2 almost always involves the genitals. The primary infection usually occurs after puberty in the sexually active years.

3. There is some crossover. About 15% of type 1 herpes is genital, and 15% of type 2 herpes is oral.

B. Unlike most viruses, the herpes virus does not undergo elimination by the immune system. Despite the presence of specific antibodies, it persists as a latent virus in humans. Recurrences of herpes virus can be triggered by the following conditions:

1. Illness

2. Emotional stress

3. Intense sunlight

4. Genital irritation (e.g., intercourse or chafing)

5. Menstruation

6. Poor nutrition

III. Clinical Features

A. Course of illness

1. The incubation period is 2 to 20 days and averages 6 days.

2. Each outbreak consists of three stages:

a. Prodromal stage: The affected person feels a vague sensation at the site of viral entry. Sensations include the following:

(1) Feeling of pressure

(2) Dull, pulselike throbbing

(3) Intermittent prickly pain

(4) Tingly sensation

(5) Ache or soreness at site of viral entry

b. Vesicle stage: Red, painful vesicular lesions appear that are 1 to 5 mm in diameter, are in close proximity to each other, and become confluent.

(1) In primary episodes, lesions tend to be larger and cover a larger area. In recurrent episodes, lesions are fewer in number, are smaller, and usually appear only at the viral entry site.

(2) In primary episodes, lack of immediate cell-mediated immunity commonly causes systemic signs and symptoms.

(a) Chills and fever

(b) Headache

(c) Myalgia

(d) Immune adenopathy

c. Crusting-over stage: After 2 or 3 days, the vesicles rupture, leaving painful shallow ulcers with a pale yellow center and bright red border, which persist about a week and then heal without scarring.

B. Clinical features of oral herpes

1. Oral herpes is characterized by a vesicular eruption of gingival and buccal mucosa, tongue, and soft palate.

2. A yellow-gray membrane forms and sloughs, leaving an ulcer.

3. Submandibular lymph nodes are usually enlarged and tender.

4. This process may last 1 to 3 weeks.

C. Comparison of signs and symptoms of primary versus recurrent herpes: See Table 4-2, Signs and Symptoms of Herpes.

D. Diagnosis of herpes

1. Culture

a. The most accurate test takes 3 to 7 days before the results are known.

b. A culture can be obtained by following these steps:

(1) If the vesicle is roofed

(a) Unroof it with a sterile needle.

(b) Absorb the fluid with a sterile cotton applicator.

(c) Inoculate the medium.

(2) If the vesicle is ulcerated, swab it with a cotton applicator presoaked in a transport medium.

(3) If there are no lesions, but testing is desired for virus shedding, do the following:

Table 4-2. Signs and Symptoms of Herpes

Signs/Symptoms	Primary	Recurrent
Ulcerated lesions	Multiple	Scattered, 1–3
Location of lesions	Anywhere in genital region, multiple locations	Confined to one specific area
Size of lesions	Variable, some large	Tend to be smaller than ones in primary herpes
Duration of lesions	14–28 days	5–10 days
Inguinal adenopathy	Present	Absent
Viremia	Present	Absent
Systemic signs: Malaise, myalgia, headache, fever	Occur if no antibodies to other type of herpes	Absent
Local signs: Pain, vaginal discharge, dysuria, itching, dyspareunia	Present	Present Also possible prodromal feeling before lesions appear
Specific antibody titer	Fourfold	No significant change
	Between appearance of initial lesion and 1–2 wk later	

(a) Swab the cervical canal and the site of a previous lesion.

(b) Inoculate the medium.

(4) All swabs obtained at a single collecting session may go into a single vial, unless it is necessary to localize the site of viral shedding.

2. Blood antibody titers

a. Caution: False positives can occur. There may be a crossover effect if the person tested has ever had a cold sore, shingles, or chickenpox.

b. Titers should be obtained at the time of the initial lesion and repeated in 7 to 10 days, if necessary.

c. Results of blood antibody titers should be interpreted as follows:

(1) If the patient has a primary infection

(a) No antibodies should be in the blood when it is tested at the time of the initial lesion appearance, unless the affected person has had herpes elsewhere and has cross-reacting antibodies.

(b) Antibodies appear 7 to 14 days after the first sign of infection and reach a maximum increase of fourfold or greater within several weeks.

(c) Thereafter, titers fall to the baseline level and stay there for life.

(2) If the patient has a recurrent infection

(a) Antibodies are present in the blood when it is drawn, at the time of the lesion appearance.

(b) The blood titer does not increase fourfold as in a primary infection.

IV. Management

A. At the initial visit, ask the patient about any history of herpes.

1. Patients at risk in pregnancy include those who have

a. A history of diagnosed genital herpes

b. A history of recurrent vascular or painful genital lesions

c. A partner with herpes. If the partner has herpes and the patient does not, suggest the use of condoms during pregnancy and avoid intercourse from the time of the partner's prodromal feeling until all lesions are gone.

2. If the patient has a definite or probable history of herpes,

a. Educate her about the risks during pregnancy and at time of delivery.

b. Instruct her to call if any outbreaks occur.

c. Educate her about palliative measures.

3. Note the history of herpes in the patient's chart.

B. Perform a physical exam.

1. If lesions suggestive of herpes are seen

      a. Perform a herpes culture.

      b. Ascertain whether it is a primary or secondary infection.

        (1) Previous history of genital lesions

        (2) Recent exposure

        (3) Clinical symptoms, such as malaise, fever, or headache

      c. If it is a primary outbreak, consider antibody titers.

      d. Educate the patient regarding palliative measures.

    2. If a Pap smear suggestive of herpes is obtained, do a herpes culture of any lesions present. If no lesions are present, do a herpes culture of the cervix.

C. If lesions suggestive of herpes appear at any time during the pregnancy, instruct the patient to come in for a culture as soon as possible after the lesions appear.

D. Manage pregnant patients known to have had genital herpes according to these guidelines:

    1. Check the patient every week after 36 weeks' EGA for lesions.

    2. If a lesion is present

      a. Culture it and follow the patient closely for signs and symptoms of labor.

      b. Schedule a cesarean section if the sore has not been healed for approximately 7 days.

E. Medications

    1. Acyclovir is a drug that reduces the severity, duration, and length of viral shedding. It is not recommended for pregnant or lactating patients. It may be prescribed for patients as follows:

      a. Apply 5% Zovirax (acyclovir) ointment to all lesions every 3 to 4 hours until the lesions are gone.

      b. Take 200 mg of Zovirax orally, every 4 hours while awake (maximum of five per day) for 10 days if it is an initial outbreak or 5 days if it is a recurrent outbreak.

      c. Take 400 mg of Zovirax twice a day for 5 to 7 days at the first sign of a recurrent outbreak.

      d. For frequent outbreaks with lesions every 4 to 6 weeks, consider suppressive management, such as 400 or 800 mg of Zovirax, orally, once a day for a minimum of a year. Then reassess the patient.

    2. Valtrex (valacyclovir), in a 500-mg oral dose, may be taken twice a day for 10 days if it is an initial outbreak and for 5 to 7 days for a recurrent outbreak.

    3. Famvir (famciclovir), in a 125-mg oral dose, may be taken twice a day for 5 days for recurrent outbreaks.

    4. For cold sores, OTC Abreva Cream may be applied to the affected area 5 times daily; it has been FDA approved.

F. Comfort measures

    1. Urinate in a sitz bath or while pouring warm water over the vulva, which may reduce pain from urine passing over lesions.

2. Take a sitz bath for 15 to 20 minutes, three times a day, in warm or cool water, which reduces discharge, odor, and discomfort. Add Burow's solution (aluminum acetate) to the water to help dry out the infected area.

3. Dry the vulva and perineum after a sitz bath with a blow-dryer on lowest setting.

4. Do not use creams, ointments, or salves on lesions. They cut off lesions from the drying effect of air and light and could spread the virus to a larger area. An exception is Zovirax (Acyclovir) ointment, which may help control the lesions.

5. Apply warm damp tea bags (of black tea), which are soothing and drying, to active lesions.

6. Wear cotton underwear to aid drying; change underwear frequently.

7. Avoid the use of restrictive, chafing clothing and panty hose.

8. Take 2 g of L-Lysine supplements daily, which may help heal and prevent future outbreaks.

9. Use OTC pain medications.

G. For support measures, refer the patient to a herpes support group.

V. **Fetal and Neonatal Considerations**

A. Congenital problems

1. First trimester

a. Spontaneous abortion increases when the mother has a primary infection.

b. If the fetus survives, it may have congenital anomalies similar to those caused by cytomegalovirus.

2. Second and third trimesters

a. There is an increased rate of premature birth if the mother has a primary infection after 20 weeks' gestation.

b. Infections are associated with low birth weight.

B. Neonatal infection

1. Etiology

a. Usually caused by passing through an infected birth canal

b. Can be contracted from being handled by infected people

2. Incidence: If the mother had a primary case of genital herpes at term and the birth is vaginal, there is a 50% chance that the infant will have a clinically apparent infection. The incidence drops to less than 3% if the mother has a recurrent case of active herpes at delivery.

3. Signs and symptoms: These will appear 4 to 10 days after delivery. Some infected neonates have cutaneous lesions. Other signs and symptoms may include lethargy, high or low temperature, anorexia, nausea and vomiting, cough or respiratory distress, and irritability or convulsions.

HUMAN IMMUNODEFICIENCY VIRUS/ACQUIRED IMMUNODEFICIENCY SYNDROME (HIV/AIDS)

I. **Definition.** HIV is a retrovirus that compromises the competency of the immune system. Once acquired, HIV produces a spectrum of disease that will progress in most cases from a clinically latent or asymptomatic state to AIDS, characterized by a CD4 cell count <200 or any opportunistic infection, regardless of the CD4 cell count.

II. **Etiology.** HIV/AIDS is caused by two related retroviruses termed HIV-1 and HIV-2. HIV-1 is isolated most frequently in Central and Eastern Africa, the Americas, Europe, and Asia. HIV-2 is isolated most frequently in Western Africa (Angola, Mozambique), France, and Portugal. The presence of HIV-2 in the United States is extremely low. The retroviruses are transmitted by exchange of body fluids (e.g., semen, blood, or saliva) or by transfused blood products. The infected person will test negative for HIV for several weeks and possibly as long as a year. The pace of disease progression is variable. The median time for development of AIDS is 10 years. Ninety percent of infected persons will have developed AIDS within 17 to 20 years of infection.[8]

III. **Classification of Disease.** The CDC defines three categories of HIV/AIDS.

    A. Category A: Asymptomatic HIV infection

        1. Acute primary HIV infection characterized by fever, malaise, lymphadenopathy, and skin rash

        2. Asymptomatic persistent generalized lymphadenopathy

    B. Category B: Symptomatic conditions not included in Category A or C

        1. Candidiasis vulvovaginal—persistent beyond a month, poor response to treatment

        2. Candidiasis oropharyngeal

        3. Bacillary angiomatosis

        4. Cervical dysplasia—rapid progression to carcinoma in situ

        5. Constitutional symptoms such as fever or diarrhea—longer than a month

    C. Category C: AIDS

        1. CD4 cell count <200

        2. Any opportunistic infection

            a. Cytomegalovirus, which causes retinitis and cardiomyopathy

            b. Kaposi's sarcoma

            c. *Pneumocystis carinii* pneumonia

            d. Non-Hodgkin's lymphoma

            e. Toxoplasmic encephalitis

            f. Disseminated mycobacterium avium complex (MAC)

            g. TB

        3. Severe malnutrition, weight loss, and wasting

---

[8]For more information, access the following web site: www.cdc.gov/hiv/stats/internet.html.

IV. Counseling and Testing

   A. Pretest counseling

   1. Obtain confidential information, with special attention to the following:

   a. Current or most recent sexual activity

   b. Type of sexual activity

   c. Use of contraception

   d. Patient's knowledge of HIV and its routes of transmission

   (1) Unprotected oral, vaginal, and anal sex

   (2) IV drug use—sharing needles

   (3) Tattooing

   (4) Body piercing

   e. Knowledge of preventive measures

   (1) Condoms

   (2) Clean needles

   (3) Abstinence

   f. History of sexual or physical abuse

   g. Support system of resources

   (1) Financial

   (2) Emotional

   (3) Social

   (4) Religious

   2. Assure the patient that test results are confidential and protected by each individual state's discrimination laws.

   B. Testing

   1. Screen the patient for HIV-1 with a sensitive screening test such as enzyme immunoassay (EIA). Reactive tests *must* be confirmed with a supplemental test such as a Western blot analysis or immunofluorescence assay (IFA).

   2. Consider testing for HIV-2 in the following circumstances:

   a. When there is clinical evidence or suggestion of HIV disease with a negative HIV-1 test

   b. If the person is from a high-risk country such as West Africa, France, or Portugal

   C. Counseling of HIV-infected patients

   1. Counseling should be done by a person(s) who can discuss the behavioral, psychologic, and medical implications of HIV infection.

   2. Referrals should be made, as appropriate, to counselors, psychologists, social and financial services, support groups, substance abuse groups, and similar agencies.

V. Management. Management of HIV is a specialty area requiring a complexity of services and will not be covered in this guideline book except for a brief overview of testing and management during pregnancy.

A. Encourage all antepartal patients to take an HIV test.
  1. Medications that can slow disease progression are available.
  2. Zidovudine (ZDV) therapy can reduce the risk of mother-to-infant transmission from 15% to 25% to just 8%.
  3. Breast-feeding is contraindicated, because the retrovirus may be transmitted in the milk to the baby.

B. Collaboratively manage patients who test positive for AIDS but do not have an acute disease. When managing these patients consider doing the following:
  1. Perform a complete exam for HIV progression every trimester.
  2. Repeat labs every trimester.
     a. CD4
     b. CBC
     c. Hepatitis A, B, and C
     d. Syphilis screening
     e. Gonorrhea culture
     f. Chlamydia testing
     g. Toxoplasmosis
     h. Cytomegalovirus
     i. Chemistry panel
  3. Perform a routine OB fetal assessment, including
     a. An ultrasound at 16, 28, and 36 weeks' EGA.
     b. A nonstress test starting weekly at 32 weeks' EGA.
  4. Recommend organizations for social support: A peer group, buddy system, or appropriate social service, as necessary.
  5. Recommend psychologic services.
  6. Suggest substance abuse intervention support, as necessary.
  7. Refer the patient to a nutritionist.
  8. Consult with the managing physician on drug therapy.

C. During the intrapartum period,
  1. Use universal precautions.
  2. Avoid interrupting fetal scalp integrity with a scalp electrode.
  3. Consider a cesarean section according to standard indications.
  4. Deliver the baby over an intact perineum whenever possible.
  5. Drain the umbilical cord for cord blood. Do not use a needle to draw cord blood.
  6. Use wall rather than mouth suction for DeLee traps.
  7. Collect requested and patient-consented study samples.

D. During the postpartum period,
  1. Refer the patient for ongoing medical care.
  2. Refer the baby to a neonatologist.
  3. Discuss contraception with the patient.
  4. Counsel her on safe sex.

5. Give the patient a hepatitis A and B vaccine, if not given prenatally.

6. Give the patient a pneumococcal vaccine, if not given prenatally.

7. Give the patient a rubella vaccine, if indicated.

8. Follow up on social service, psychologic, psychiatric, and substance abuse counseling, as needed.

E. Refer an infant younger than 18 months old to a neonatologist for further testing and prophylactic medication. Because of transplacental passage of maternal HIV antibody, both infected and uninfected infants born to HIV-infected mothers will have positive HIV antibody test results.

HUMAN PAPILLOMA VIRUS (HPV)

I. Definition. HPV causes genital warts.

II. Etiology

A. Genital warts are most commonly caused by HPV types 6, 11, 16, 18, and 31, or by combinations of these.

B. HPV is sexually transmitted. However, if the disease is not active, the virus cannot be passed to others.

C. HPV carries a moderate infectivity.

D. HPV multiplies profusely when the immune response is lowered, for example, in cases of HIV, pregnancy, smoking, or malnutrition.

E. HPV cannot be cured. The infected person will always carry the virus.

III. Clinical Features

A. The incubation period is from 2 weeks to 9 months after exposure but could be longer.

B. Genital warts may appear on the vulva, vagina, anus, or cervix, as well as the penis and anal area in men.

C. The wartlike growths that are small, discrete structures that spread, enlarge, and coalesce to form narrow-based pedunculated cauliflower growths. They may appear in one small clump or in many clumps of varying size.

D. Lesions hypertrophy during pregnancy and may cover the vulva and perineum or extend over the vaginal mucosa and cervix. They regress after delivery.

E. Warts have been linked to the development of cervical cancer. Patients should be monitored carefully.

IV. Differential Diagnosis

A. Do not confuse genital warts with condylomata lata, which are highly infectious secondary syphilitic lesions caused by the spirochete *Treponema pallidum* (see Syphilis later in Part IV).

B. Genital warts caused by HPV can be differentiated from condylomata lata as follows:

1. Lata appear on the external genitalia only; HPV warts appear in the vagina and on the cervix.

    2. Lata look like a grouping of small, flat warts covered with a grayish exudate.

    3. Lata appear only as the primary lesion of syphilis; HPV may appear any time, but it proliferates greatly during pregnancy.

    4. *T. pallidum* can be cultured from lata; HPV can be cultured from genital warts.

V. Management

  A. General management, whether pregnant or not

    1. Perform a Pap smear if there are any cervical, atypical, or persistent warts.

    2. Encourage patients with external genital warts to get a yearly Pap smear for 3 to 5 years. Fifty to sixty percent of patients with external warts will test positive for HPV on the cervix.

    3. Identify and treat any accompanying vaginitis. Secondary infections are common.

    4. The warts may be treated with bichloracetic or trichloracetic acid therapy.

      a. Protect the surrounding tissue with petroleum jelly.

      b. Apply bichloracetic acid or trichloracetic acid to the affected area every week to 10 days. Continue this treatment as long as the warts are regressing.

      c. Consider alternative chemical methods in self-treatment kits.

        (1) Podophilox (Condylox) is a 0.5% topical solution applied twice a day for 3 days then stopped for 4 days. This can be repeated for up to 4 weeks.

        (2) Imiquimod (Aldara) 5% topical cream available in 0.25-g sachets, 12 sachets to a box, is applied at night twice a week to the infected area for up to 4 months.

        (3) If the warts are not gone by the end of the prescribed treatment period, the patient should return to her physician for alternate treatment.

    5. Consider other therapies, which include cryosurgery, laser surgery, or excision biopsy.

    6. Suggest the following practices and medications for pain relief:

      a. At the time of treatment

        (1) Dust baby powder onto the area.

        (2) Apply 2.5% topical Nupercainal ointment to the area.

      b. Later

        (1) Take warm or cool sitz baths for 10 to 20 minutes one to two times a day as needed.

        (2) Take 650–1000 mg acetaminophen every 4 hours, as needed.

    7. Advise the patient to keep the vulva as clean and dry as possible.

      a. Perform frequent perineal hygiene.

      b. Dry the vulva after washing or taking a sitz bath, using a blow-dryer set on the lowest setting.

c. Wear cotton underwear and change panties frequently.

d. Do not wear underpants around the house or to bed.

e. Do not use maxi or mini pads, which hold in heat and rub against the vulva, unless absolutely necessary.

8. Advise the couple to use condoms until all lesions are resolved.

9. Consider the possibility of coexisting STDs.

B. Additional management specific to the pregnant patient

1. Avoid an episiotomy or laceration through the lesions at the time of delivery, because they bleed profusely.

2. Consider cutting a right mediolateral or left mediolateral episiotomy instead of a midline episiotomy to avoid the lesions.

3. For extensive lesions, consult with a physician. A cesarean section may be indicated.

C. For management of cervical lesions, see the section on Cervical Abnormalities in Part IV.

 LUPUS

I. Definition

A. Lupus is a chronic inflammatory autoimmune disorder in which the body's immune system, instead of serving a normal protective function, forms antibodies that attack healthy tissues and organs.

B. Types

1. Discoid lupus erythematosus (DLE) affects the skin, causing a rash, lesions, or both.

2. Systemic lupus erythematosus (SLE) is usually more severe than DLE. It attacks body organs and systems, such as joints, kidneys, brain, heart, and lungs. It can be life threatening.

3. Drug-induced lupus symptoms usually disappear upon discontinuance of medication.

II. Etiology. The cause is unknown.

III. Clinical Features

A. Signs and symptoms

1. DLE

a. Exposure to sunlight often precedes the appearance of lesions. Half of patients have a history of photosensitivity.

b. Lesions are erythematous, round, scaling papules, 5 to 10 mm in diameter, often appearing in a butterfly shape over the bridge of the nose, with some appearing on the trunk, extremities, or both.

c. The disease is limited to the skin in 90% of DLE patients. Ten percent will also develop SLE.

2. SLE

a. Often nonspecific signs and symptoms that mimic other diseases

b. Rash, previously described

  c. Frequent UTIs to chronic renal problems

  d. Fever and malaise

  e. Joint pain (Jaccoud's fever) in 90% of patients

  f. Recurrent pleurisy

  g. Pericarditis

  h. Hypertension

  i. Splenomegaly

  j. Central nervous system problems: Chronic headaches, epilepsy, personality changes, or Chronic Brain Syndrome

  k. Depression of hemoglobin, WBCs, and platelets

  l. Infertility or increased fetal loss

B. Lab tests

 1. Skin biopsy studies will not differentiate DLE from SLE but will rule out other disorders.

 2. The SLE screening test is the fluorescent test for antinuclear antibodies (ANA). It is positive in 98% of cases. Drugs such as Procainamide, hydralazine, and isoniazid will also make this test positive.

IV. Management

A. After diagnosis, refer the patient to a specialist.

B. The patient may be collaboratively managed after the initial treatment and plan have been developed.

C. Consider the following in pregnancy:

 1. Lupus patients are considered to be high-risk patients.

 2. Twenty-five percent of patients have a problem getting pregnant.

 3. Pregnant lupus patients experience frequent miscarriages and stillbirths.

 4. Thirty-three percent of lupus patients have an antibody that is associated with early failure of the placenta (anticardiolipin), and about 10% have a related antibody, lupus anticoagulant, which allows early pregnancy, but at some point, causes the placenta to fail. The baby's growth slows as this occurs.

 5. Twenty-five percent of the remaining pregnant patients deliver prematurely.

 6. Sometimes pregnancy causes a flare-up of lupus.

  a. Thirty-three percent of patients will have a decreased platelet count.

  b. Twenty percent will have urine protein.

  c. Thirty-three percent will have a sudden increase in BP (PID) or eclampsia.

 7. Medications during pregnancy

  a. Safe: Prednisone, prednisolone, and methylprednisolone (Medrol). These do not go through the placenta.

  b. Probably safe: Azathioprine and hydroxychloroquine

  c. Not recommended unless the baby needs treatment as well: Dexamethasone and betamethasone

d. Harmful: Cyclophosphamide

8. Effect of lupus on the baby

    a. Prematurity is the greatest danger.

    b. There are no known congenital abnormalities peculiar to babies of lupus patients.

    c. Three percent of all lupus patients will have a baby with neonatal lupus. This is a syndrome *not* SLE, and it is transient. If heart problems occur (rare), they are treatable but permanent.

D. Discuss family planning with the patient.

    1. Barrier methods or IUDs are best and safest.

    2. BCPs might exacerbate lupus but are safer than an unwanted pregnancy.

 MAMMOGRAPHY

I. **Definition.** Mammography is the radiographic examination of the breast. It is a reliable means of detecting breast cancer before a mass can be palpated.

II. **Indications**

    A. Screening

    B. Evaluation of a questionable breast mass

    C. Follow-up after treatment

III. **Management**

    A. Normal mammogram: Recommend a mammogram according to American Cancer Society guidelines.

        1. A baseline mammogram should be done no later than 40 years old.

        2. A mammogram should be done every 2 years after age 40.

        3. A mammogram should be done every year after age 50.

        4. If there is a positive family history (on either side of family), it is recommended that a yearly mammogram be started 10 years before the age of onset of breast cancer in the youngest family member to have cancer.

        5. Mammograms should be done more frequently when there are fibrocystic breast changes or there is breast augmentation.

    B. Abnormal mammogram

        1. When findings suggest cysts on a mammogram, the patient should be sent for a breast ultrasound.

            a. If the ultrasound confirms a simple cyst, it may be drained or followed with mammograms every 6 months.

            b. If the ultrasound reveals a noncystic breast problem, refer for a needle-localization biopsy.

        2. When masses have a noncystic appearance on a mammogram, the patient should be referred to a surgeon.

3. Tiny specks of calcium in the breast, called microcalcifications, are often found in areas of rapidly dividing cells.

   a. **Benign appearance:** Repeat the mammogram in 3 to 6 months.

   b. **Clustered appearance or small grouping:** Refer the patient for a needle-localization biopsy or removal.

4. Macrocalcifications are calcium deposits frequently associated with degenerative changes in the breast caused by aging, old injuries, or inflammation.

   a. Reassure the patient that they are usually benign.

   b. **First appearance:** Repeat a mammogram in 6 months.

   c. **Stable:** Repeat a mammogram every year.

 MASTITIS

I. **Definition.** Mastitis is inflammation of the breast.

II. **Incidence.** Mastitis can occur in anyone but is almost exclusively a complication in the lactating woman.

III. **Etiology.** Mastitis develops as a result of invasion of breast tissue by bacteria in the presence of breast injury. The most common causative bacterium is *Staphylococcus aureus*.

A. Causes of injury are

   1. Bruising from rough manipulation or pumping.

   2. Breast overdistention.

   3. Milk stasis in a duct.

   4. Cracking or fissures of the nipple.

B. Sources from which bacteria may originate:

   1. The hands of the mother

   2. The hands of any person caring for the mother or baby

   3. The baby

IV. **Clinical Features**

A. Precursory signs and symptoms

   1. Severe engorgement

   2. Slight fever

   3. Mild pain in one segment of the breast, which is exaggerated when the baby nurses

   4. Slight redness over the affected area

B. Mastitis

   1. Signs and symptoms

      a. Rapid elevation in temperature from 100°F to 104°F

      b. Increased pulse rate

      c. Chills, general malaise, and headache

      d. Area of breast reddened, very tender, and painful, with a hard, sizable lump(s)

     2. Lab work: A C&S done on breast milk may identify the bacteria.

C. Untreated mastitis may progress to an abscess.

    1. Discharge of pus, especially if a high temperature continues for more than 48 hours

    2. Remittent fever with chills

    3. Breast swollen and extremely painful; a large, hard mass with an area of fluctuation, reddening, and bluish tinge to the skin, indicating the location of the pus-filled abscess

V. Management

  A. Advise the patient to take the prescribed antibiotic for the full course, even if her health improves sooner. Treatments of choice include 500 mg of Keflex or 500 mg of dicloxacillin, taken orally four times day for 7 to 10 days, or 250 to 500 mg of Augmentin, taken orally three times a day for 7 to 10 days. See the patient in 7 to 10 days; she may need retreatment.

  B. Warn the patient that monilia vaginitis may develop secondary to antibiotic therapy. The patient may want to use acidophilus tablets as a prophylactic while taking antibiotics.

  C. Obtain a milk C&S from the affected breast to confirm the diagnosis and treatment, as necessary.

  D. Advise the client to continue breast-feeding, unless an abscess is present. Try applying a hot compress to the site before breast-feeding. Continuation of breast-feeding in the presence of an abscess is not recommended. Suggest the following:

    1. Discontinue breast-feeding until the patient is afebrile for 24 hours, usually about 24 to 48 hours after starting antibiotics; then resume breast-feeding.

    2. During the time breast-feeding is discontinued, pump the breasts at least every 4 hours with an electric or manual pump after heat has been applied to the breasts. Avoid manipulation of the breast, which will exaggerate the already-existing breast injury.

    3. Discard any milk pumped during the time breast-feeding had been discontinued because it may contain pus.

  E. Provide firm, nonconstrictive support for the breasts.

  F. Prescribe pain medication. If acetaminophen is not effective, prescribe acetaminophen with codeine.

  G. If an abscess is present, consult with a physician. It may need an incision and drainage.

 MONILIA VAGINITIS

I. **Definition.** Monilia vaginitis is an infection of the vagina caused by the fungus *Candida albicans.*

II. **Etiology**

  A. Monilia is a normal inhabitant of the digestive tract. It is usually kept in check in the vagina by the inhospitable acidic environment, caused by lactic acid produced by lactobacilli in the epithelial cells. This keeps the pH of childbearing women between 4.0 and 4.5 and the pH of prepubertal girls and postmenopausal women at approximately 5.0.

B. Monilia thrives in a high glucose environment. Therefore, any situation that renders the vagina higher in glucose or increases the pH to 4.5 to 5.0 will encourage the growth of monilia. Situations that seem to predispose women to monilia growth include the following:

    1. Those related to high glucose

        a. Pregnancy

        b. Use of oral contraceptives containing progestin

        c. Diabetes mellitus

        d. High-glucose diet

        e. Obesity

    2. Those that increase vaginal pH

        a. Too-frequent douching

        b. Too-frequent use of oils, jellies, and creams, which upset the vaginal pH

        c. Use of broad-spectrum antibiotics (including Flagyl), which destroy the lactobacilli that make the vagina acidic

        d. Nylons, exercise, types of clothing, and heat from mini or maxi pads

        e. High-stress lifestyle

C. Monilia can grow on skin and mucous membranes, including the following:

    1. Vulva and vagina

    2. Penis and scrotum

    3. Mucous membranes of the oral cavity. This is called thrush and can be transmitted to the newborn while passing through the birth canal of an infected mother.

III. Clinical Features

A. Signs and symptoms

    1. Intense burning and itching of the vulva and vagina

    2. Red, patchy, excoriated appearance of the vulva

    3. Thick white or yellow discharge that resembles cottage cheese

    4. Curdy patches that stick to vaginal mucosa and the cervix

    5. Dyspareunia, dysuria, and urinary frequency

    6. Typical "yeasty" odor

    7. Symptoms that often develop premenstrually

B. Microscopic findings on a wet mount

    1. Filaments with budding spores

    2. Pseudohyphae; may be more apparent on a potassium hydroxide (KOH) slide

C. Identification from a Pap smear

IV. Management

A. Treat the active infection.

1. Take 150 mg of Diflucan orally; it takes 2 to 5 days to obtain complete relief. This may be refilled once if signs and symptoms still persist after 5 to 7 days.
2. Use Terazol vaginal cream or suppositories for 3 to 7 days.
3. Apply 5% Cleocin vaginal cream, vaginally, every night for 5 to 7 days. This may be used concurrently with Diflucan for dual infections.
4. Use OTC medications.
   a. Insert one full applicator or suppository of Monistat vaginal cream 3 or 7 at bedtime for 3 or 7days.
   b. Insert one full applicator or suppository of Gyne-Lotrimin cream 3 or 7 at bedtime for 3 or 7 days.
   c. Recommend the dual packs of Monistat and Gyne-Lotrimin. They contain a tube of cream as well as suppositories for a treatment period of 3 days. The combination allows for instant relief from symptoms.
5. To relieve itching and burning, follow these measures.
   a. Take sitz baths in cool or tepid water three times a day.
   b. Dry the vulva with a blow-dryer on a lower setting after the sitz bath.
   c. Apply extra vaginal cream or ointment to affected areas.

B. Educate the patient regarding prevention measures.
1. Avoid douching, oils, creams, and perfumed products, such as scented or deodorized tampons or pads and deodorized soaps.
2. Use white toilet paper, rather than colored paper.
3. Avoid refined sugar in the diet.
4. Avoid an excessively stressful lifestyle; get plenty of sleep and rest.
5. Wear panties with a cotton crotch. Avoid the use of nylon panties, panty hose, and tight slacks. Do not wear underwear to bed.
6. Avoid monilia infections by eating yogurt, which contains *L. acidophilus*. This promotes normal vaginal flora. OTC tablets can be purchased (e.g., Gyna.Tren, Probia). An alternative preventive treatment is to place boric acid capsules into the vagina nightly; this will restore the normal acid pH.
7. If the patient is put on a course of broad-spectrum antibiotics, advise her to do the following:
   a. Ask the medical provider for a Diflucan tablet, to be taken on the last day of the antibiotic.
   b. Start acidophilus tablets or boric acid the day the antibiotic is started and continue using them 3 days after completion of the antibiotic.

C. If the patient has frequent or chronic infections:
1. Examine the male partner; he may be harboring the fungus and infecting the woman, especially if he is uncircumcised. Apply antifungal cream to the penis and under the foreskin for 7 days. Take 150 mg of Diflucan, orally, as a second treatment option.

      2. Consider screening the patient for diabetes and HPV on the cervix.

D. Treat frequent or recurrent infections as follows:

      1. Diflucan, 150 mg orally, 3 to 5 days before the patient's period every month for 3 to 6 months.

      2. Nizoral, 200 mg orally, every day for a month. This may be repeated for 2 months; do a serum glutamic-oxaloacetic transaminase (SGOT) test before continuing past 3 months.

E. Pregnant patient with a history of frequent infections: Assess for an active infection near term according to her history and a wet prep. It is desirable to treat even a subclinical infection at term to avoid transmission of thrush to the neonate at the time of delivery.

OSTEOPENIA AND OSTEOPOROSIS

I. Definition

A. Osteopenia is defined by the World Health Organization (WHO) as a bone mineral density between 1 and 2.5 standard deviation (SD) below the young adult peak mean.

B. Osteoporosis is defined by WHO as a bone density 2.5 SD or more below the adult mean peak.

II. Incidence and Etiology

A. Osteopenia and osteoporosis can occur at any age.

B. One third of postmenopausal women have osteoporosis.

C. Osteoporosis-related fractures will occur in more than 40% of women over 50. Hip fractures account for 15% of the total fractures.

      1. Twelve to twenty percent of victims will die within the year.

      2. Fifty percent of patients will experience a loss of mobility.

      3. Twenty-five percent of survivors will be confined to long-term care facilities.[9]

D. Risk factors for osteopenia and osteoporosis are as follows:

      1. Women, especially after menopause

      2. Caucasian or Asian

      3. Small frame or underweight

      4. Irregular periods or amenorrhea

      5. Hyperthyroid or hyperparathyroid

      6. Steroid use

      7. High-risk behavior

          a. Eating disorders

          b. Chronic low-calcium intake—dieting, junk foods

          c. Heavy use of caffeine, alcohol, or cola drinks

          d. Smoking

          e. Inactivity—lack of weight-bearing exercise

          f. Endurance athletics

---

[9]American College of Obstetricians and Gynecologists 1998, p. 1

III. **Clinical Features**

A. Bone can be divided into two major types. Cortical bone forms the outer shell of all bone and 75% of bone mass. Trabecular bone accounts for 25% of bone mass and is the spongy, interchanging network that supports the cortical bone. Until age 30, reabsorption and formation of new bone are equal. After that, reabsorption exceeds formation by 0.4% per year. High bone loss occurs during the first 5 to 8 years after menopause, with an additional 2% cortical and 5% trabecular loss per year caused mainly by decreased estrogen and progesterone.

1. Estrogen inhibits bone reabsorption and helps control the rate of secretion of the parathyroid hormone, a regulator of calcium and phosphorus metabolism.

2. Progesterone promotes bone formation.

B. At the spine and hips, a 1 SD decrease is associated with a twofold increase in fracture risk.[10]

IV. **Diagnosis**

A. Dual-energy x-ray absorptiometry (DEXA) should be considered.

1. Provides a low-radiation exposure

2. Uses multiple skeletal sites

3. Is unreliable in the presence of vertebral compression

B. A single-dose x-ray absorptiometry measures the bones of the wrist and heel.

C. An absorptiometry, CT scan, and bone biopsy are available but costly and may impose medical risk.

V. **Management**

A. Preventive measures: It is difficult, if not impossible, to replenish bone that is lost; this makes prevention crucial.

1. Exercise

a. Weight-bearing exercise is best to prevent reabsorption.

b. Increased muscle strength, tone, and balance decrease falls and fractures.

2. Nutrition

a. Calcium intake is important, either through diet or supplementation.

(1) The recommended perimenopausal dose is 1000 mg; during pregnancy, 1500 mg is recommended.

(2) Calcium citrate is the most easily absorbed form of calcium.

(3) High-calcium foods include cheese, yogurt, ice cream, milk, sardines, almonds, oranges, tofu, corn tortillas, and broccoli.

b. Calcium should be matched 2:1 with magnesium.

c. The trace minerals manganese, zinc, and copper have been found to be essential.

---

[10]Crandall, p. 259

    d. Vitamin D is essential for calcium absorption and deposition into bone tissue.

        (1) Postmenopausal women should take 800 IU.

        (2) It is found in fatty fish, egg yolks, and fortified foods.

        (3) Vitamin D can also be obtained by exposure to sunlight; twenty to thirty minutes of sunshine should do it.

    e. Dietary changes can prevent increased urinary calcium excretion.

        (1) Decrease animal protein consumption.

        (2) Limit carbonated beverages.

        (3) Limit caffeine to two to three brewed cups per day.

        (4) Limit salt intake.

        (5) Drink alcohol in moderation.

3. Teaching

    a. Make literature available to all.

    b. Target high-risk groups and those with osteopenia.

        (1) Teens: Address junk food, dieting, and cola.

        (2) Postmenopausal women: Check for HRT and exercise frequency.

        (3) Smokers: Advise them that smoking decreases estrogen levels and interferes with vitamin absorption.

        (4) Those with amenorrhea and irregular periods: Regulate blood flow.

        (5) Depo-Provera users: Encourage calcium supplements.

        (6) Those on thyroxine or diuretics: Encourage exercise plus calcium supplements

B. Medical treatment

    1. HRT should be considered for those without contraindications.

    2. If the patient is unable or does not wish to take estrogen or an estrogen-progesterone combination, raloxifene (*Evista*) has estrogenlike effects on bone and lipid metabolism without affecting breast and uterine tissue. Take 60 mg orally every day.

    3. Risedronate (Actonel), 5 mg, can be taken orally, once a day, 30 minutes before the first food of the day.

    4. Alendronate can be taken in the following doses:

        a. 5 mg orally every day for prevention

        b. 10 mg orally every day for treatment of osteoporosis

    5. Calcitonin can be taken as a nasal spray, 200 IU per day, alternating nostrils daily.

 PAP SMEAR OR PAP TEST

I.   **Definition.** The Pap smear or test is a cervical cytologic exam, introduced in 1941, which is instrumental in reducing the incidence and mortality rates for cervical cancer from 35,000 to 5,000 annually. The

Bethesda system is used most often for classifying the results of Pap smears (see Table 4-3).[11]

A. Pap smear: The cervix is visualized, and a wooden spatula is used to scrape the ectocervix. These cells are "smeared" on a glass slide. A Cytobrush is then placed into the cervical os and rotated. The endocervical cells obtained are "smeared" thinly onto the slide, and a fixative is applied.

B. Thin Prep which uses a plastic spatula and Cytobrush, and CytoRich which uses one plastic triangle-shaped brush, are newer methods.

1. The specimen(s) taken are rinsed into the preservative.

2. In the lab, the cells are cleansed of blood, mucus, and other materials.

3. Because the cells are not "smeared," they do not clump together when placed on a slide. This allows visualization of a greater number of cells.

II. Etiology of Abnormalities

A. Cervicitis caused by STDs, yeast, and bacteria

B. Reparative changes from trauma to the cervix from childbirth, therapeutic abortion, or elective abortion

C. Vaginal atrophy seen in menopause and Depo-Provera patients

D. Human papilloma virus (HPV)

1. The virus is found in 98% to 99% of cervical cancers

2. The following contributing factors increase the chance of exposure to HPV:

   a. Unprotected sex

   b. Early age at first intercourse

   c. Multiple sex partners

   d. High-risk male partner

   e. Exposure to other STDs

E. The following contributing factors lower the immune system's protection:

1. Pregnancy

2. Immunosuppression, HIV, or AIDS

3. Cigarette smoking

4. Malnutrition

5. Chronic illnesses

III. Management

A. Prior to making an appointment for a Pap smear, counsel the patient.

1. Midcycle is the best time for a Pap smear.

2. The patient should not have intercourse for 24 hours prior to the test.

3. She should refrain from the use of vaginal creams, suppositories, and douching for 1 to 2 days.

---

[11]For more information on the ThinPrep Pap test, access www.thinprep.com on the Internet.

Table 4-3. Management of Pap Smear by Results

Result	Explanation	Treatment Options
NORMAL RESULTS: May Need Further Follow-up		
No endocervical cells	• Normal Pap smear specimen but an absence of endocervical cells	• If prior Pap smears were within normal limits, perform Pap smear again in 1 year. • Repeat a Pap smear again in 3 to 6 months, if history of prior abnormal Pap smears.
Infection	• Specification of type possibly in results	• Offer an infection check or treatment. Give a Pap smear again in 1 year.
Bethesda System		
ASC (formerly ASCUS)	• Inflammation • Atrophy associated with Depo-Provera use and menopause	• Check for infection. If found, treat only specific infection; give another Pap smear in 3–6 months. • Use vaginal estrogen cream per protocol. Stop cream 1 week before follow-up Pap smear, in 2 to 3 months. If results are normal, place on a maintenance dose of vaginal estrogen cream.
Reactive and reparative changes (optional report in Bethesda System)	• Cell changes associated with inflammation, radiation, and IUD use—*not* an urgent medical problem	• Check for infection and give a Pap smear again in 1 year.
ABNORMAL RESULTS: Recommended Follow-up		
ASC-NOS	• Mildly abnormal cell changes of the cervix (about 50%–60% reverse spontaneously, without treatment)	• Give a Pap smear every 6 months for 2 years; perform a colposcopy, if another Pap smear is abnormal. • Refer patient directly for colposcopy.

Bethesda System

ASC-LSIL/CIN 1	• Negative report for malignant cells	• Give a Pap smear every 6 months for 2 years; perform a colposcopy if the Pap smear is abnormal.
	• Possible evidence of HPV, mild dysplasia	• Triage by HPV testing. Refer patient with positive HPV test for colposcopy. If negative for HPV, schedule Pap smear every 6 months for 2 years.
		• Refer patient directly for a colposcopy.
ASC-HSIL/CIN 2–CIN 3	• Moderate or severe dysplasia (many progress to cancer if left untreated)	• Refer patient for a colposcopy.
AGCs (formerly AGUS)	The following are specified in this category:	• Refer patient for a colposcopy with endocervical curettage as soon as possible.
	• AGCs • Atypical endocervical cells • Atypical endometrial cells	• Request endometrial biopsy if 1) over age 40, or 2) Pap smear shows atypical endocervical cells, or 3) woman has a history of abnormal uterine bleeding.
Adneocarcinoma in situ (AIS)	• Cancerous cells confined to the surface of the cervix	• Refer patient to a specialist for evaluation and treatment.
Adneocarcinoma	Cancer, specified in the report as: • Endocervical • Extrauterine • Endometrial • NOS	• *Urgently* refer patient to a specialist for evaluation and treatment.

ASC = atypical squamous cells; NOS = not otherwise specified; LSIL = low-grade squamous intraepithelial lesion; HSIL = high-grade squamous epithelial lesion.

4. With a vaginal infection or HSV outbreak, it is best to wait until the problem has resolved before getting a Pap smear.

5. The patient should wait at least 4 to 6 weeks after a threatened abortion, elective abortion, or delivery. Sometimes the healing process of the cervix can return a result of abnormal squamous cells (ASC).

B. See Table 4-3, Management of Pap Smear by Results.

C. If patient has a colposcopy, base the therapy on colposcopy and biopsy findings. Therapy may include observation or laser surgery in pregnancy. If the patient is not pregnant, consider these options: observation with Pap smears every 3 to 6 months, LEEP, cone biopsy, cryosurgery, or laser surgery.

 PNEUMONIA

I. **Definition.** Pneumonia is inflammation of the lung parenchyma in which the affected part is consolidated.

II. **Etiology**

A. Pneumonia often follows common viral upper respiratory illness.

B. Two thirds of cases are bacterial.

III. **Clinical Features**

A. Fetal considerations: If any of the following are protracted enough or severe enough, the fetus will be adversely affected; mortality can be up to 30%.

1. Hypoxia secondary to maternal hypoxia: the fetus tolerates it better than the mother because of

a. High glycogen content of fetal tissues.

b. Ability of the fetus to use anaerobic metabolic pathways.

2. Hypoglycemia: there is a decrease in blood glucose in the mother, partly caused by hyperthermia and partly caused by the disease process.

3. Hyperthermia

B. Maternal considerations by type of pneumonia

1. Influenza pneumonia

a. Signs, symptoms, and course of disease

(1) First 6 to 12 hours: prodromal phase

(a) Malaise

(b) Myalgia

(c) Headache

(d) Pain on ocular movement

(e) Chills and fever

(f) Nasal congestion

(g) Mild sore throat

(2) Second or third day: clinical deterioration

   (a) Cough with purulent sputum if bacteria are present

   (b) Diffuse bilateral crepitant basilar inspiratory rales

   (c) Occasional pleuritic chest pain

   (d) Dyspnea

   (e) Hemoptysis .

(3) Fourth day

   (a) Cyanosis secondary to pulmonary decompensation

   (b) Shock secondary to cardiovascular collapse

   (c) Fetal death, then maternal death

b. Diagnosis: Presumptive, based on clinical course and radiograph

2. Varicella-zoster pneumonia

   a. Signs, symptoms, and course of disease

   (1) Respiratory symptoms develop 2 to 5 days after cutaneous lesions appear. The initial and sometimes only manifestation is a dry nonproductive cough.

   (2) In more severe disease, the following symptoms are apparent:

   (a) The cough becomes productive after 36 to 48 hours; mucoid sputum, which may be blood streaked, or frank hemoptysis may occur.

   (b) Bilateral acinar nodular infiltrates appear on the radiograph.

   (c) Dyspnea, tachypnea, cyanosis, and chest pain may occur.

   b. Diagnosis

   (1) Other signs of varicella-zoster virus (chickenpox or shingles) in the woman or family

   (2) Definitive: Serologic confirmation or virus isolation

   (3) Chest radiograph

3. Streptococcus pneumonia

   a. Signs, symptoms, and course of disease

   (1) Dramatically sudden initial onset

   (a) Productive cough: watery sputum at first, which rapidly becomes purulent grayish-green and then a characteristic rust color

   (b) Fever

   (c) Malaise

   (2) Extension of disease

   (a) Pleuritic chest pain

   (b) Chills with tremors

   (c) Shortness of breath, orthopnea, tachypnea, and cyanosis

        (d) Fine crepitant rales

        (e) Tachycardia

   b. Diagnosis

        (1) Presence of encapsulated lancet-shaped diplococci on Gram stain smear of sputum

        (2) Significant expansion of involved pulmonary parenchyma on radiograph

IV. Management

A. See the section on Colds, Flu, and Upper Respiratory Infections in Part IV for management of specific signs and symptoms.

B. If the signs and symptoms listed below are present: Examine the patient in the office or emergency room. Elicit onset, duration, course, and any self-treatment measures.

   1. Fever greater than 101°F

   2. Pain on ocular movement

   3. Severe chest pain

   4. Severe dyspnea, orthopnea, or tachypnea

   5. Purulent or bloody sputum

   6. Severe sore throat that interferes with swallowing or breathing

C. Perform a physical exam.

   1. Inspect the throat for infection, pustules, edema, or abscesses.

   2. Palpate submental, submaxillary, tonsillar, and cervical lymph nodes.

   3. Observe the patient for dyspnea, tachypnea, orthopnea, tachycardia, and cyanosis.

   4. Take the patient's temperature.

   5. Percuss and auscultate the lungs for wheezes, rales, rhonchi, decreased breath sounds, and areas of consolidation.

D. Order the following lab work:

   1. Throat culture, if the throat is infected

   2. Rapid strep test, if strep is suspected

   3. Sputum culture, as necessary

   4. CBC, if there is a fever

E. Initiate penicillin therapy, which is the treatment of choice.

 RUBELLA

I. **Definition and Etiology.** Rubella is an acute exanthematous disease caused by the rubella virus and marked by enlargement of lymph nodes. It is of importance because of the high incidence of fetal abnormalities. It is also called German measles or three-day measles.

II. **Clinical Features**

   A. Course of the disease

1. Rubella is spread by aerosol dissemination from the nasopharynx or oropharynx. The virus is shed for at least 10 to 14 days after a rash appears.
2. The course of infection is as follows:
   a. Incubation period: Presents 11 to 14 days after exposure
   b. Postauricular adenopathy: Presents 7 days before a rash appears and lasts 1 to 2 weeks
   c. Maculopapular rash: Begins on upper thorax of face and spreads downward; presents 11 to 17 days after exposure and lasts 3 days
   d. Virus shedding: Starts 10 to 14 days after a rash appears
   e. Antibody formation: First appears with a rash, peaks 24 to 28 days later, and declines twofold to eightfold after a few weeks
3. Arthralgia and sometimes arthritis are not uncommon complications if the strain is particularly virulent.

B. Characteristics: The rubella virus is well adapted to humans and causes little morbidity or mortality except to the fetus.

III. Management

A. Perform an antibody screen on all prenatal patients at the initial visit, unless there is documentation that one was done during the present pregnancy.

B. If the antibody screen is positive (>1:10), do not treat (not necessary). If the titer is more than 1:1000, repeat the screen as soon as possible to rule out a lab error.
   1. If it is still elevated, repeat the test in 3 weeks to rule out potential convalescent serum.
   2. If the repeat serum is decreased, consult with a physician; a recent rubella infection is indicated.

C. If the antibody screen is negative (<1:10), discuss getting an immunization postpartum.
   1. The patient's informed consent is necessary for immunization.
      a. The woman must not be pregnant at time of vaccination and should not become pregnant for at least 3 months after vaccination.
      b. About 10% of those vaccinated develop a low-grade fever and transient arthritis (aching joints with stiffness). Risks to others in her environment are minimal.
   2. If sterilization is performed immediately postpartum, vaccination is not necessary.

D. If possible exposure or infection occurs during pregnancy, obtain a titer.
   1. If the titer is drawn when or before the rash develops, repeat it 7 to 10 days later. If there is an eightfold increase, infection has occurred.

2. If the titer is drawn within 5 days of the onset of the rash, repeat it 7 to 10 days after the rash onset and compare the two titers. If the second is significantly increased over the first, suspect rubella, even though the increase will not be as much as eightfold.

3. If a titer drawn more than 5 days after the onset of the rash is high in conjunction with postauricular adenopathy, or much higher than the original initial titer, suspect rubella.

4. If uncertain of exposure or physical signs, repeat the titer in 3 weeks. If there is a significant increase, suspect rubella.

E. If there is any suspicion of rubella exposure in a patient who was negative at the initial screening, inform the patient of the potential risks to the fetus. There is an inverse relationship between the age of the fetus at the time of maternal infection and the severity of anomalies.

1. Rubella causes the following effects on the fetus, according to age:

a. If the fetus is 3 to 7 weeks of gestation at the time of exposure, death usually results, caused by serious anomalies.

b. If the fetus is 8 to 13 weeks of gestation at the time of exposure, deafness is the principal defect.

c. Teratogenic manifestations are limited to organ systems with a limited capacity to regenerate in the first trimester.

(1) Cataracts (characteristic)

(2) Congenital heart disease

(3) Hearing problems

(4) Growth retardation

(5) Clotting disorders

(6) Mental retardation

(7) Chromosomal abnormalities

d. Serious manifestations after 13 weeks fetal age at the time of exposure are rare, but growth retardation can occur even though organogenesis is complete. The expanded congenital rubella syndrome includes

(1) Hepatosplenomegaly.

(2) Pneumonitis.

(3) Hepatitis.

(4) Encephalitis.

(5) Lesions of the long bones.

(6) Anemia.

(7) Thrombocytopenic purpura.

2. The fetus does not produce antibodies because the mother's antibody response suppresses that of the fetus. So babies will shed the virus at birth, and 50% will shed the virus until 6 months of age.

SKIN CONDITIONS

I.   Acne

   A. Clinical picture

      1. Skin comedones, papules, and pustules

      2. Severe cases include cysts, abscesses, pits, and scars

   B. Conditions to rule out

      1. Pyoderma

      2. Drug eruptions

   C. Treatment

      1. Wash with medicated soap three times per day.

      2. Apply drying lotions or gels with 5% to 10% benzoyl peroxide, 5% Persa-Gel, or 5% to 10% Desquam-X every day or twice a day.

      3. Use antiseborrheic shampoo, if indicated.

      4. Consider taking certain types of BCPs.

      5. Take 500 mg of tetracycline, orally, four times a day for 7 to 10 days and then take 500 mg every day or twice a day if protected against pregnancy.

      6. Take 50 to 100 mg of doxycycline, orally, twice a day.

      7. Do not use Retin-A while pregnant.

      8. Consult a dermatologist if the acne is severe or not responsive to the previous treatment options.

   D. Patient education

      1. Eat a well-balanced diet.

      2. Do not use oil, grease, or creamy cosmetics on skin.

      3. Avoid hair lotions or creams.

      4. Expect exacerbations during periods of stress and menses.

      5. Keep hands off face.

II. Athlete's Foot (Tinea Pedis)

   A. Clinical picture

      1. Itching, scaling feet

      2. Acute form - vesicles and bullae on soles and sides of feet and between toes

      3. Chronic form - dry and scaly lesions

      4. Thickened toenails with debris under nail

   B. Conditions to rule out

      1. Contact dermatitis

      2. Psoriasis

      3. Bacterial infection

   C. Diagnosis: Use potassium hydroxide on a wet mount to exam skin scrapings for hyphae.

   D. Treatment

1. Snip and drain blisters and trim the edges of blisters to avoid fungi from spreading under the edges.
2. Apply topical antifungal creams once or twice daily.
   a. Oxiconazole (Oxistat) 1% every day for 2 to 3 weeks
   b. Butenafine (Mentax) 1% twice a day for 1 week
   c. Econazole (Spectazole) 1% twice a day for 3 to 4 weeks
3. For severe cases, recommend a 10-day course of a systemic antifungal in addition to antifungal creams.
   a. Itraconazole (Sporanox), 100 mg orally, twice a day
   b. Griseofulvin, 250 to 500 mg orally, twice a day
4. To suppress the acne, treat the patient with the following:
   a. Fluconazole (Diflucan), a 150-mg tablet, taken orally once per month
   b. Itraconazole, 200 mg, taken orally once per month

E. Patient education
1. Air dry the feet for 20 minutes, three times a day.
2. Dry between the toes after bathing.
3. Wear well-ventilated shoes or sandals that expose the feet to the air, when possible.
4. Wear rubber sandals in community showers or bathing places.

III. Contact Dermatitis

A. Clinical picture
1. Contact dermatitis is an allergic reaction, which may be instantaneous or develop over several hours; it may cause pruritus and burning. Poison oak or poison ivy will have the same symptoms and may not erupt for 1 to 2 days after contact.
2. Erythematous papules and vesicles are symptoms of contact dermatitis.
3. Linear streaks of erythema or vesicles are seen where the offending item has been in contact with skin areas.

B. Types
1. Contact dermatitis from an allergic reaction
2. Contact dermatitis from poison oak or poison ivy

C. Treatment
1. Avoid item(s) that caused the problem.
2. Take OTC Benadryl, in 25- to 50-mg oral doses; this works well in most cases. For severe reactions, give 25 to 50 mg of Benadryl IM. Warn the patient that this may drowsiness.
3. As an alternative treatment, try 25 to 100 mg of Atarax, orally, three to four times a day.
4. If there is weeping, soak the area with a cold compress for 20 minutes and apply calamine lotion after each soak.
5. If there is no weeping, apply 1% hydrocortisone cream three times a day until lesions resolve.

D. Patient education

1. Remove the offending item(s).
2. Trim fingernails and keep them clean and short.
3. If the dermatitis is from poison oak or poison ivy, wash all clothing, shoes, and other items that have come in contact with the plant.
4. Wear loose-fitting clothing.
5. Consult with or refer the patient to a physician if there is involvement of the eyes.

IV. Eczema

  A. Patient condition and history

    1. Pruritus

    2. Family history of allergic diseases or atopic dermatitis

    3. History of asthma and allergic rhinitis

  B. Clinical picture

    1. Infancy

      a. Lesions are erythematous and papular to scaly or vesicular, which may progress to oozing and crusting.

      b. Lesions are usually located on the cheeks, scalp, postauricular area, neck, and extensor surface of forearms and legs.

    2. Childhood

      a. Lesions are drier, papular, scaling eruptions with hypopigmentation.

      b. Lesions are located on the flexor surfaces of wrists and on antecubital and popliteal areas.

    3. Adolescence and adulthood

      a. Lesions are dry, thickened skin, with an accentuation of normal lines and folds; they often have hyperpigmentation.

      b. Lesions are usually located on the flexor areas of extremities, eyelids, back of neck, and dorsum of the hands and feet.

  C. Conditions to rule out

    1. Seborrheic dermatitis

    2. Fungal infections of the skin

    3. Contact dermatitis

    4. Irritant contact dermatitis

  D. Treatment

    1. Use an antihistamine for pruritus.

      a. Take 25 to 50 mg of Benadryl, orally, every 6 hours or apply Benadryl lotion or ointment.

      b. Take 25 to 100 mg of Atarax three to four times a day.

    2. After the acute exudative phase has been controlled, apply hydrocortisone cream (0.5% or 1%) four times a day.

    3. Apply Eucerin cream, aqua-aquaphor, or Lubriderm lotion after a bath or shower to seal in moisture.

    4. Take antibiotics (topical or systemic) for a secondary bacterial infection.

   5. If severe, weeping lesions are not improving with treatment, refer the patient to a dermatologist.
E. Patient education
   1. Avoid hot water.
   2. Take short showers and limit baths to one to two per week for no longer than 5 minutes.
   3. Avoid soaps and bubble baths. Use a mild soap like Dove or Neutrogena for cleaning dirty areas.
   4. Avoid wool and starched or rough clothing.
   5. Keep fingernails short.
   6. Pat skin dry and avoid rubbing skin with a washcloth.

V. Folliculitis
A. Clinical picture
   1. Patient complains of mild to severe pain at the site.
   2. Lesions are pinhead sized or slightly larger pustules surrounded by a narrow area of erythema. Many pustules are located in same area.
   3. Lesions are usually seen on the scalp, axilla, extremities, or areas that have been shaved.
   4. *S. aureus* is most often the causative organism.
B. Conditions to rule out
   1. Tinea of the scalp
   2. Contact dermatitis
C. Treatment
   1. Apply warm compresses of tap water four times a day.
   2. Apply topical antibiotics to the site.
      a. Use 2% Mupirocin (Bactroban) twice a day for 7 to 10 days.
      b. Apply Neosporin twice a day for 10 to 14 days.
   3. For severe infections, take systemic antibiotics in addition to using topical cream.
      a. Take 500 mg of amoxicillin/clavulanate potassium (Augmentin) orally twice a day.
      b. Take 600 to 1200 mg of clindamycin phosphate (Cleocin) in two to four equal doses each day.
   4. For folliculitis of the scalp, use Selsun suspension twice per week.
   5. Consult a doctor for cases involving fever and cellulitis.
D. Patient education
   1. Wash the affected area with soap and water. Apply hot compresses for 20 minutes four times a day.
   2. Avoid the use of hair oils, bath oils, or suntan oils.
   3. Return in 1 week if lesions do not clear or return sooner if a fever is present.

VI. Furuncles and Carbuncles
A. Clinical picture

1. The patient complains of mild to severe pain at the site.
2. There is an inflammatory reaction, with pain and tenderness.
3. Lesions may be 2 cm or larger.
4. They may be single or multiple, chronic, and recurrent.
5. They often resolve by necrosis and spontaneous drainage.

B. Conditions to rule out
1. Impetigo
2. Foreign objects with associated infections
3. Insect bites
4. Diabetes
5. Immune deficiency, if there is a recurrence of furuncles or carbuncles

C. Treatment
1. Apply hot moist compresses for 20 minutes, four times a day.
2. Use topical antibiotics.
   a. Apply 2% Mupirocin (Bactroban) twice a day for 7 to 10 days.
   b. Apply Neosporin twice a day for 10 to 14 days.
3. For severe infections, take systemic antibiotics in addition to using topical cream.
   a. Take 500 mg of amoxicillin/clavulanate potassium (Augmentin) orally twice a day.
   b. Take 600 to 1200 mg of clindamycin phosphate (Cleocin) in two to four equal doses each day.
4. Make an incision and drain the nodule when the necrotic white area appears at the top of the nodule. If the lesion is extensive, it may need an incision and drainage plus packing with iodoform or sterile gauze.

D. Patient education
1. Explain general hygiene.
2. If other family members are affected, evaluate them or refer them for evaluation.

VII. Hives (Urticaria)

A. Patient history
1. New foods
2. Medications
3. Family history of allergies
4. Recent illness
5. Previous occurrence

B. Clinical picture
1. The patient complains of itching.
2. Red or raised plaques of welts with sharp borders, which may vary in size and number, are usually located on the trunk and extremities.
3. The lungs are clear, and the patient is not wheezing.

  C. Conditions to rule out
   1. Erythema multiforme
   2. Multiple insect bites (e.g., fleas or mosquitoes)
   3. Contact dermatitis
  D. Treatment
   1. If hives are immediate and severe, check the patient's heart rate and BP, and give 0.3 to 0.5 mL of epinephrine 1:1000, subcutaneously (SQ), for adults. *Consult a physician immediately.* Consider following this treatment with 25 to 50 mg of Benadryl, orally, every 4 to 6 hours.
   2. If hives are mild or moderate, take 25 to 50 mg of Benadryl, orally, every 4 to 6 hours or 10 mg of Zyrtec, orally, every day. A divided oral dose of 5 mg of Zyrtec taken twice a day may provide better 24-hour coverage.
   3. Soaks in a tub of cool water or oatmeal baths will provide an additional antipruritic effect.
  E. Patient education
   1. Instruct the patient on danger signs. Ask her to call if she has difficulty breathing.
   2. Inform the patient of allergic reactions to medication; the rash may worsen over the next 1 to 2 days and take several weeks to resolve.
   3. Observe the patient for recurrence and note commonalities so the source can be identified.

VIII. Impetigo
  A. Clinical picture
   1. Impetigo can occur on any area of the skin. It is often found around the nose and mouth.
   2. Vesicular eruptions contain serous fluid that becomes purulent and surrounded by areas of erythema.
   3. Pustules rupture, dry centrally, and form honey-colored crusted patches of reddened skin.
   4. Lesions vary in size from a few millimeters to several centimeters.
   5. The patient may have anything from asymptomatic skin erosions to itching, stinging, and extremely painful blisters.
  B. Conditions to rule out
   1. Noninfected insect bites
   2. Herpes simplex
   3. Chickenpox
   4. Other vesicular or ulcerating skin lesions
  C. Treatment
   1. Culture a lesion, if necessary, for diagnosis.
   2. Soak crusts with warm water compresses 5 to 10 minutes before removing them at least two to three times a day.

      a. Soak the affected areas with warm water and Betadine or Dial soap.

      b. Apply Neosporin or mupirocin (Bactroban) 2% ointment to lesions after removing crusts.

   3. Give the patient a systemic antibiotic if she has more than a couple of lesions.

      a. Penicillin is often given for 10 days. Staphylococci may be resistant to this medication. Augmentin, in a 500-mg oral dose, taken twice a day for 10 days, is a better choice.[12]

      b. Tetracycline or doxycycline for 10 days is beneficial if the patient is allergic to penicillin.

  D. Patient education

   1. The patient is contagious until 4 days after the initiation of treatment.

   2. No one else should use the patient's washcloth, towel, or bed linen. It should be washed with hot water.

   3. Athletic equipment should be sterilized, whenever possible.

   4. The patient should shower with antibacterial soap.

   5. She should be advised not to scratch and trim her fingernails.

   6. Other family members having skin lesions need evaluation and treatment, if infected.

IX. Molluscum Contagiosum

  A. Clinical picture

   1. Characterized by skin-colored, smooth, waxy, umbilicated papules, 2 to 10 mm in diameter

   2. Transmitted by direct contact

   3. Resolves on its own in 6 to 12 months

   4. Sometimes forms skin-tag-like lesions

  B. Conditions to rule out

   1. Acne

   2. Infected hair follicles and sebaceous glands

  C. Treatment

   1. Remove the core of the papule with a needle.

   2. Wash the area with a medicated drying soap.

   3. Use Neosporin or other antibiotic ointment twice a day and as necessary.

   4. Consider using trichloroacetic acid or cryosurgery to remove large papules and skin tags.

X. Moniliasis

  A. Patient condition and history

   1. Pruritus at site

   2. Monilia vaginitis

---

[12]Basler & Seraly, 2001, p. 55

      3. History of diabetes

      4. History of BCP use

      5. Breast-feeding infant with thrush

  B. Clinical picture

      1. Well-defined, red, eroded patches with scaly, pustular, or pustulovesicular diffuse borders, commonly occurring in the intertriginous areas, such as the axillae, on or around the breasts, and between fingers and toes

      2. White patches on oral mucosa, which usually bleed when removed

  C. Conditions to rule out

      1. Seborrheic dermatitis

      2. Other fungal skin infections

  D. Treatment

      1. Apply antifungal cream such as Monistat or Lotrimin twice a day for 2 weeks.

      2. Use 2 mL of nystatin oral suspension, 100,000 units/mL, four times a day for 1 to 2 weeks. Place 1 mL on each side of the mouth, so the medication is in contact with the lesion for as long as possible. If preferred, take 100 mg of Nizoral orally every day. Continue treatment for 2 weeks after the lesions are gone.

  E. Patient education

      1. Instruct the patient on proper cleaning and drying of affected areas.

      2. Instruct patient on the method of transmission.

XI. Ringworm (Tinea Corporis)

  A. Definition: Ringworm is a superficial fungal infection of the nonhairy skin, excluding the groin, palms of the hands, and soles of the feet.

  B. Clinical Picture

      1. Pruritus

      2. Lesions that are annular scaly plaques with papular borders and some degree of central clearing. They often look like red rings, hence the name.

      3. Lesion size variations, from a few millimeters to several centimeters

      4. Singular or multiple lesions

  C. Diagnosis: Microscopic examination of a potassium hydroxide wet mount of skin scrapings shows yeast hyphae.

  D. Conditions to rule out

      1. Contact dermatitis

      2. Nummular eczema

      3. Scabies

  E. Treatment

      1. Oral or topical fungal agents

    2. OTC white iodine (deodorized iodine) applied to lesions three times per day for 4 to 5 days

  F. Patient education: Teach the patient that ringworm is passed by direct contact or autoinoculation.

XII. Scabies

  A. Definition and etiology: Scabies is a skin eruption caused by the mite *Sarcoptes scabiei*. It is contracted by contact with an infested person or object, such as clothing, bed linen, or upholstered furniture.

  B. Clinical features: The patient presents with an intensely pruritic papular or excoriated erythematous skin rash involving the webs of the fingers and toes, anterior wrist surface, and the backs of the knees, axillae, trunk (especially at the waistline), genitalia, and buttocks (especially gluteal and inguinal folds).

  C. Conditions to rule out

    1. The absence of scaling rules out candidiasis.

    2. The lack of pain and pustules rules out a staphylococcal infection.

  D. Management

    1. Diagnosis

      a. A diagnosis of scabies is confirmed by microscopic findings.

        (1) Scrape the lesions.

        (2) Transfer the scraping to a slide.

        (3) Apply a drop of oil and a coverslip.

        (4) Look for the mite or its eggs or fecal pellets.

      b. Microscopic evidence is frequently difficult to find. Therefore, diagnosis is often made on the basis of the following:

        (1) History, especially of other family members with similar signs and symptoms

        (2) Characteristic appearance and distribution of skin lesions

        (3) Elimination of other dermatologic conditions

    2. Treatment

      a. Pregnant: Use 5% permethrin (Elimite) cream (30 g for an adult).

        (1) Massage it into the skin from the head to the soles of the feet.

        (2) Wash it off after 8 to 14 hours.

        (3) Shampoo it into freshly washed, rinsed, and towel-dried hair. Leave it in for 10 minutes and rinse the hair.

        (4) One treatment is usually sufficient.

      b. Not pregnant

        (1) Permethrin and Kwell creams act at all stages of the parasite's life cycle and, therefore, are the treatments of choice.

      (2) Oral ivermectin has been used successfully, however, it does not eliminate early stages of the parasite. Therefore, it is recommended that it be given in two doses, 8 days apart.[13]

  c. Treatment considerations

      (1) During treatment, all clothing and bed linen should be thoroughly laundered with detergent and hot water and dried in an electric dryer. Clothes that cannot be washed should be dry-cleaned. Also all upholstered furniture should be cleaned.

      (2) Other family members should be treated, especially if they are symptomatic.

      (3) The sexual partner(s) should be evaluated and treated.

      (4) The patient should be advised that itching might continue for several weeks after adequate treatment.

        (a) Apply antipruritic lotion, such as Caladryl.

        (b) Use anesthetic ointment or spray, such as Americaine.

        (c) Apply ice packs to the affected area.

        (d) In severe cases, take 25 to 50 mg of Benadryl orally, as necessary; use this medicine sparingly.

XIII. Seborrheic Dermatitis

  A. Clinical picture

    1. Pruritus

    2. Flaking skin

    3. Redness and scaly skin eruptions, which may be dry or greasy

    4. Location of lesions: often start at the scalp (cradle cap in infants) and progress to eyebrows, eyelids, nasolabial folds, postauricular folds and external auditory canal, presternal area, and diaper area

    5. Association with acne

  B. Conditions to rule out

    1. Tinea capitis or corporis

    2. Psoriasis

    3. Contact dermatitis

    4. Candidiasis

  C. Treatment

    1. Mild cases: Use a nonprescription dandruff shampoo.

      a. Head & Shoulders shampoo

      b. Selsun Blue shampoo

    2. Moderate cases: Apply a selsun suspension twice a week for 2 weeks and then once a week. Leave it on the scalp 15 to 30 minutes before washing it off.

    3. Refer the patient to a dermatologist.

---

[13]Usha & Gopalakrishnan, 2000, p. 236

D. Patient education

1. Instructions should be provided for brushing hair and removing crusts.
2. Vaseline, grease, or oil should not be used on the scalp.
3. Seborrheic dermatitis is not contagious and will not cause baldness; there are seasonal variations.
4. It is a chronic condition; it will get better and worse.
5. It is familial.

XIV. Topical Agents. See Part VIII, Topical Agents.

 SORE THROAT

I. Clinical features

A. History

1. Onset, duration, course, and self-treatment measures
2. Previous history of frequent sore throat or strep throat
3. Associated symptoms
   a. Cough
   b. Nasal congestion
   c. Fever and myalgia
   d. Nausea, vomiting, and diarrhea
   e. Headache
   f. Lung involvement
4. Severity: Interference with eating or drinking

B. Physical exam

1. Inspect throat for infection, swelling, and abscesses.
2. Palpate the submental, submaxillary, tonsillar, and cervical lymph nodes. If they are swollen and tender, suspect infection.
3. Percuss and auscultate the lungs for decreased breath sounds, wheezes, rales, rhonchi, and areas of consolidation. If any of these are present, suspect lung involvement.
4. If the patient's temperature is elevated, suspect an infection.

C. Lab work

1. If the throat is infected, obtain a throat culture.
2. If the patient is febrile, consider a CBC.

II. Management

A. Soothe the throat.

1. Saline or mouthwash gargles
2. Chloraseptic spray
3. Cough lozenges, especially those with a local anesthetic

B. If the throat culture indicates a bacterial infection, treat it with an appropriate antibiotic. Do not prescribe an antibiotic without obtaining the results of a throat culture.

C. If a sore throat is interfering with adequate nutrition, hydration, or both, perform the following activities:

1. Counsel the patient regarding the need for at least eight cups of liquid per day.

2. Advise soft, cool, easily swallowed foods that supply nutritional needs, such as gelatin, custard, or ice cream. Take a nutritional supplement such as Ensure.

 SYPHILIS

I. Definition. Syphilis is an acute and chronic infectious venereal disease.

II. Etiology

A. Syphilis is caused by *Treponema pallidum*, a spirochete that infects the mucous membrane.

B. The length of the incubation period, from the time of exposure to the appearance of the primary chancre, depends on the number of organisms established at the time of infection and how long it takes them to replicate. Spirochetes take 33 hours to replicate, as compared with minutes for bacteria.

1. Incubation for the primary stage is 10 to 90 days after contact, averaging 21 days. Signs and symptoms resolve spontaneously in 3 weeks without treatment.

2. Incubation for the secondary stage is 17 days to 6 months after contact, averaging 2.5 months. If the syphilis is not treated, the signs and symptoms resolve spontaneously in 2 to 8 weeks, with an average of 4 weeks.

3. The latent stage begins after the secondary lesions are gone.

C. A person is contagious when lesions, either primary or secondary, are present.

D. Early antibody response is by IgMs. Within 2 weeks it changes to IgGs.

III. Clinical Features

A. Acquired syphilis

1. The primary stage exhibits the following characteristics:

a. The primary lesion is a chancre: a small papule that forms at the portal of entry and breaks down to form a superficial painless ulcer that lasts about 5 weeks and heals spontaneously. Lesions can be so mild as to escape detection. They may be single or multiple.

b. Dissemination from the portal of infection to the lymph nodes occurs in about 70% of cases, causing satellite buboes, enlarged, tender, firm lymph nodes.

2. The secondary stage results from hematogenous dissemination from drainage of regional lymph nodes. It is characterized by the following:

a. A generalized, bilateral, nonpruritic, painless skin rash appears anywhere on the body, but especially on the mucous membranes, palms of the hands, and soles of the feet. The rash may consist of either or all of the following:

        (1) Flat, coppery-colored maculae

        (2) Erythematous, scaly papules

        (3) Pustules

    b. Involvement in the mouth appears as white erosions called "mucous patches."

    c. Intertriginous confluent condyloma latum forms in moist areas of the body, such as the vulva and perianal region. It looks like a group of small, flat warts covered with a grayish exudate; these are highly infectious. These should not be confused with condylomata acuminata, the external warts caused by HPV.

    d. Systemic symptoms are common.

        (1) Generalized adenopathy

        (2) Fever, malaise, lethargy, and headache

        (3) Anorexia and weight loss

        (4) Alopecia anywhere on the body

  3. The latent stage takes place after the manifestations of secondary syphilis disappear without treatment. The spirochete lies dormant in the body and manifests itself several years later as multiorgan degeneration. It can be diagnosed by lab tests in the absence of clinical manifestations, especially with a history of known exposure or history of primary or secondary lesions.

B. Congenital syphilis

  1. It is primarily a reflection of inadequate prenatal care.

  2. The placenta appears pale gray, large in relation to the baby's weight, and often fibrotic.

  3. Congenital syphilis causes the following fetal and neonatal effects:

    a. An increase in spontaneous abortion, stillbirth, and neonatal death

    b. Effects in relation to treatment

        (1) If not treated, heart defects and "snuffles" are the main defects.

        (2) If the is mother treated before 16 weeks, infection of baby is probably preventable because the spirochete does not usually cross the placental barrier before that time.

        (3) If the mother is treated after 16 weeks, the course of syphilis is arrested in the baby, but defects that already exist will remain.

        (4) If mother has latent syphilis, the baby can be infected, but infectivity decreases with the duration of the mother's infection. If the mother has had latent syphilis more than 4 years, the baby will probably not be affected.

IV. Lab Tests

  A. Rapid plasma reagin (RPR)

    1. The RPR test is not a titer; it does not give an antibody level.

    2. Once positive, it remains positive for life.

3. It is more sensitive than VDRL in picking up active infection during the early stages.

4. A false positive may occur because of viruses, vaccinations, immunizations, and some diseases, such as malaria and yaws.

5. A positive test should be considered presumptive for syphilis, until a second, different test is performed.

B. VDRL

1. Once positive, it remains positive for life.

2. A false positive may occur because of viruses, vaccinations, immunizations, and some diseases, such as malaria and yaws.

3. A positive test should be considered presumptive for syphilis, until a second, different test is performed.

4. False-positive results are usually less than one in eight.

5. A VDRL test is reported as a titer, unlike the RPR test.

6. A low level indicates effective treatment; a high level indicates active infection.

7. Once a patient has had syphilis, all the blood tests will be positive. The VDRL is most useful for follow-up or rediagnosis.

C. Fluorescent treponema antibody (FTA)

1. Direct FTA tests of lesion exudate or tissue provide specific evidence to diagnose syphilis, because they identify the *Treponema* organism.

2. Once positive, the test remains positive for a long time, possibly for life.

D. Dark-field microscopic exam: Examining serum from a lesion with a dark-field microscope is a definitive method for diagnosing early-stage syphilis, as it also identifies the *Treponema* organism.

V. **Management**

A. Order an RPR or VDRL for all patients at the initial prenatal visit.

1. If the RPR test is positive, the patient may or may not have syphilis.

a. Order an FTA test, if there is no previous history of syphilis.

(1) If the FTA test is negative and no clinical signs or symptoms are present, assume the patient does not have syphilis.

(2) If the FTA is positive, obtain a VDRL test. The patient may need a series of VDRLs to follow the titers. Also obtain specific cultures for gonorrhea and chlamydia.

b. Question the patient regarding possible exposure, history, or presence of signs and symptoms.

(1) Assure the patient that a positive RPR does not necessarily indicate syphilis. In order to rule out a false-positive RPR result, await FTA or VDRL results.

(2) If any of these factors apply, ask patient to come in for a physical exam for signs of primary or secondary lesions.

B. Make an accurate diagnosis of syphilis at other times.

1. Indicators that a patient may have syphilis

    a. Signs and symptoms of syphilis

    b. Diagnosis of gonorrhea, chlamydia, or both

    c. A patient-expressed concern that she may have an STD

C. Treat the patient as follows:

    1. Prescribe penicillin, which is the only treatment for syphilis during pregnancy, because it crosses the placenta.

       a. For a patient with early syphilis—primary, secondary, or latent—of less than 1 year's duration, treat the patient as follows:

          (1) Ensure the patient has had a documented nonreactive RPR or VDRL within the last year. Otherwise, treat it as syphilis of more than 1 year's duration.

          (2) Give 2.4 MU of penicillin G benzathine IM in a single dose as a standard treatment.

       b. For syphilis of more than 1 year's duration give 2.4 MU of penicillin G benzathine, IM, in three doses, given at 1-week intervals.

    2. Treat patients who have a history of allergy to penicillin as follows:

       a. Pregnant—Send the patient for a penicillin allergy skin test and consult a specialist on hospitalization, desensitization, and treatment with the appropriate penicillin regimen for her stage of syphilis.

       b. Not pregnant

          (1) In early syphilis, give either doxycycline 100mg orally twice a day for two weeks or tetracycline 500mg orally four times per day for 2 weeks.

          (2) In late syphilis or syphilis of unknown duration, give either 100 mg of doxycycline, orally, twice a day for 4 weeks or 500 mg of tetracycline, orally, four times a day for 4 weeks.

    3. Repeat a follow-up VDRL monthly while pregnant and at least 3 to 12 months after treatment. Patients with syphilis of more than 1 year's duration should have a repeat VDRL done 24 months after treatment.

    4. Do not retreat patients with documentation of adequate treatment who have a positive VDRL, unless there is a fourfold rise in titer from 1:4 to 1:16 or from 1:8 to 1:32.

    5. Tell the patient her diagnosis, how the disease is acquired, and the necessity of completion of treatment and follow-up.

    6. Inform the health department for epidemiologic follow-up; the department will make every effort to contact the patient's sexual partner(s) and confirm his treatment.

D. Consider the CDC recommendations for management of sex partners.[14]

    1. Persons exposed sexually to a patient who has syphilis in any stage should be evaluated clinically and serologically.

---

[14]CDC, 1998, p. 30

2. If exposed within the past 90 days, the partner may be infected even if he or she is seronegative; treat the partner presumptively.

3. Notify the pediatrician or neonatal nurse practitioner, as well as the nursery, of the problem at the time of delivery.

 THROMBOPHLEBITIS

I. **Definition.** Thrombophlebitis is venous inflammation with thrombus formation.

II. **Etiology**

A. The condition of thrombophlebitis in pregnancy may reflect an extension of infection through the veins originating from infected thrombosed veins at the placental site. This extension is either into the pelvic veins (e.g., ovarian or renal inferior vena cava) or into the femoral vein from the uterine veins through the iliac veins.

B. Thrombophlebitis has an unknown etiology but is associated with the following:

1. Preexisting varicosities

2. Pregnancy

3. Trauma

III. **Clinical Features**

A. General signs and symptoms

1. An unexplained elevation of pulse often occurs as a first sign.

2. Repeated severe chills are characteristic.

3. Extreme swings in temperature occur, climbing from subnormal to 105°F and then falling precipitously within an hour's time.

4. Hypotension results from bacterial shock.

5. Small pulmonary emboli cause pleurisy and pneumonia.

B. Venous thrombosis

1. Superficial

   a. Slight temperature

   b. Slight pulse elevation

   c. Leg pain

   d. Local heat, extreme tenderness, and redness at site of vein inflammation

2. Deep

   a. High fever with tachycardia and chills that may be severe

   b. Presence of Homans' sign—pain at the site of the thrombosis when the foot of the affected leg is dorsiflexed

   c. Abrupt onset with severe leg pain

   d. Discolored, pale, or cool extremity, with a decrease in pulse pressure below the affected area

C. Pulmonary embolism

1. Most likely with deep venous thrombophlebitis

2. Unlikely with superficial thrombophlebitis

IV. Management

   A. Manage the patient in collaboration with a physician.

   B. Advise bed rest.

   C. Elevate the affected extremity.

   D. Apply hot packs to the affected extremity.

   E. Initiate analgesia, as needed.

   F. Make a cradle for bedclothes if the leg is tender to the touch.

   G. Consider anticoagulant or antibiotic therapy.

   H. Suggest taking a low-dose aspirin daily.

   I. *Never massage the leg*; massage may release a thrombus into the circulation, which can cause a pulmonary embolism.

 THYROID DISEASE

I. **Definition.** Thyroid disease is an abnormality of the thyroid gland, which is the largest endocrine gland. It produces hormones that are vital in maintaining normal growth and metabolism.

II. **Etiology**

   A. The thyroid gland becomes more vascular and enlarges slightly during pregnancy.

   B. The iodine uptake by the thyroid is increased. This change is caused by a large increase in serum proteins, to which thyroid hormones are bound. The blood level of free, active thyroxine is actually slightly reduced during pregnancy.

   C. The basal metabolic rate increases steadily during pregnancy, but most of the increase is due to the metabolism of the fetus and placenta.

III. **Clinical Features**

   A. Hyperthyroidism

     1. Prominent eyes

     2. Increased appetite and weight loss

     3. Tachycardia

     4. Increased bowel movements and diarrhea

     5. Heat intolerance

     6. Amenorrhea or oligomenorrhea

   B. Hypothyroidism

     1. Fatigue

     2. Constipation

     3. Weight gain not accounted for by excessive food intake

     4. Edema

     5. Hoarse voice

     6. Dry and thin hair

     7. History of abnormal uterine bleeding

     8. History of infertility or amenorrhea

IV. **Differential Diagnosis**

    A. Palpable nodules indicate a focal enlargement; cancer of the thyroid must be ruled out.

    B. A diffuse enlargement or goiter is usually benign but may become obstructive.

    C. Inflammation of the thyroid indicates the following:

        1. A pain in the neck that worsens upon swallowing

        2. Possible transient hyperthyroidism or permanent hypothyroidism

V. **Management**

    A. Obtain a patient history.

        1. When was the last thorough medical evaluation for patient's thyroid condition?

        2. Is the patient currently on thyroid medication? If so, what type and how much?

        3. When did the person who prescribed the medication last examine the patient?

    B. If the patient is pregnant and an endocrinologist or physician of long standing is managing her thyroid condition, instruct the patient to inform this physician of her current pregnancy and seek a projected plan of thyroid management throughout the pregnancy. Send a letter to the managing physician.

    C. Routinely palpate the thyroid at the initial physical exam, 6-week postpartum exam, and other times, as indicated.

    D. Obtain T3, T4, and TSH levels if any of the following situations exist:

        1. The patient has been on chronic thyroid medication since before pregnancy and is not currently being managed by a physician for her thyroid condition.

        2. The patient gives a history of being on thyroid medication in the past.

        3. Any abnormality of the thyroid is discovered on exam.

        4. There are any signs or symptoms of the disease.

 TRICHOMONAS VAGINITIS

I.   **Definition.** Trichomonas vaginitis is an STI caused by *Trichomonas vaginalis*, pear-shaped one-celled protozoa, which are slightly larger than WBCs, with several flagella that make them extremely motile.

II. **Etiology**

    A. Although it is usually sexually transmitted, trichomonas vaginitis has been shown to survive for 90 minutes on a wet sponge, suggesting that transmission could occur from a bath, toilet seat, washcloth, or douche equipment.

    B. Although trichomonas vaginitis is not usually symptomatic in men, they harbor it in their urethra and can transmit it to women.

C. The disease may involve the paraurethral Skene's glands and occasionally the lower urinary tract.

D. Trichomonas prefers a pH higher than that of the normal vagina, and therefore, may multiply more rapidly during or immediately following menstruation or during pregnancy.

E. Trichomonads can carry bacteria to the fallopian tubes and cause PID.

III. Clinical Features

A. Signs and symptoms

1. Fifty percent of affected women may be asymptomatic.

2. Severe vulvar and vaginal edema, excoriation, itching, and burning may be present.

3. Frothy thin greenish-yellow discharge is characteristic, although discharge may be thin, white, relatively scanty, and nonfrothy.

4. Red patches on the cervix and vaginal mucosa (the characteristic "strawberry patches") occur in 10% of women.

5. Malodorous discharge occurs.

6. Dyspareunia and dysuria are common.

B. Microscopic examination of a wet mount

1. Motile, colorless, pyriform, flagellated trichomonads, which are readily seen in most cases. The specimen must be kept warm to preserve the organisms' motility; nonmotile trichomonads are indistinguishable from WBCs.

2. Numerous WBCs

3. Absence of lactobacilli

C. Nitrazene paper applied to discharge: The pH may be 5.5 or more with trichomonas vaginitis. A normal pH of 4 to 4.5 virtually rules out trichomonas vaginitis.

D. Pap smears or urinalysis: Trichomonads can occasionally be observed in these tests.

IV. Management

A. See Vaginal Discharge guidelines later in Part IV for extensive differential diagnoses and management.

B. In the first trimester of pregnancy, perform the following actions:

1. Avoid treatment in the first trimester whenever possible.

2. If the patient is symptomatic and needs to be treated, give the following:

   a. MetroGel vaginal cream should be taken at bedtime for 7 days.

   b. Cleocin 2% vaginal cream should be taken at bedtime for 7 days.

   c. Flagyl (metronidazole) is not recommended during the first trimester, but it has been used without any known adverse effects. Dosing should be 500 mg, orally, twice a day for 5 days.[15]

C. Treat pregnancies over 12 weeks' gestation with 500 mg of Flagyl, taken orally, twice a day for 5 to 7 days or 2 g of Flagyl, taken orally,

---

[15]Caro-Paton et al., 1997

one time. One dose of Flagyl, while convenient, is less effective than a smaller dose over a longer period of time.

D. If the patient is not pregnant, treat her with 2 g of Flagyl one time, unless the infection is severe. Then treat her with 500 mg of Flagyl, taken orally, twice a day for 5 to 7 days.

E. Also treat the partner(s). Urge abstinence during the course of treatment to avoid reinfection. Use condoms if abstinence is not carried out.

F. Warn the patient of the following:

1. The patient and her partner should be advised to avoid alcohol during the course of the treatment to avoid nausea and vomiting from the Flagyl.

2. The patient should be warned that monilia vaginitis might develop secondary to Flagyl therapy.

3. If the patient is allergic to Flagyl, she can be treated with 2% Cleocin vaginal cream; she should take one vaginally every night for 7 nights.

 TUBERCULOSIS

I. Definition. Tuberculosis (TB) is an acute or chronic infection caused by the bacterium *Mycobacterium tuberculosis*. It is acquired from a person with active TB through airborne transmission.

II. Incidence

A. The incidence of TB in the United States had been declining since the 1900s, but in 1985, the trend reversed. At present, 10 million new cases occur annually, resulting in 3 million deaths.

B. Recent appearances of strains resistant to multiple anti-TB drugs are cause for concern.

III. Clinical Features

A. TB is usually asymptomatic at first until the lesions are large enough to be visible on a radiograph.

B. The first signs are fever, general malaise, and weight loss.

C. A chronic cough will be more frequent in the morning.

D. Sputum will increase in amount and may be blood tinged.

E. TB can become systemic; signs and symptoms will depend on the location.

IV. Management

A. Diagnosis

1. Skin tests are effective 10 weeks after exposure.

a. Mantoux test: A purified protein derivative (PPD) is injected intradermally in the forearm and read 48 to 72 hours later.

(1) A test is positive with a 15-mm or larger induration.

(2) It is safe to use in pregnancy.

b. Tine Test

(1) Prongs are coated with the PPD.

(2) A 2-mm area of induration is considered a positive result.

c. False-negative PPDs can occur in the following cases:

(1) The test is given incorrectly.

(2) The person's immune system is compromised (e.g., HIV, malnutrition, corticosteroid use).

(3) Less than 10 weeks have passed since exposure.

d. False positives often occur with allergies or if the person has been given bacillus Calmette-Guérin (BCG), a live bacterial vaccine often used in third-world countries to protect against TB.

2. Chest radiographs should be done on all patients with positive PPDs and on any patients with negative PPD tests who have symptoms of the disease or have been exposed to TB.

a. Use an abdominal shield in pregnancy and wait, if possible, until the second trimester.

b. A radiograph will help distinguish between latent and active TB.

c. Sputum cultures can be used to confirm active TB.

B. Treatment

1. There is a 10% chance that latent TB will become active.

a. Taking 300 mg of isoniazid hydrochloride (INH) orally every day for 6 months reduces the incidence of latent disease becoming active.

b. HIV patients should complete a 12-month course of INH.

c. Pregnant women need 25 to 50 mg of vitamin B6, taken orally every day, to prevent the development of peripheral neuropathy associated with INH.

2. A patient with active TB should be referred for treatment.

a. Medications are usually ordered for 6 to 12 months. These may include INH, rifampin, ethambutol, and pyrazinamide.

b. Sputum should return to negative in 3 to 4 weeks.

3. The patient's family and contacts need to be tested.

C. Teaching

1. The patient needs to wear a mask when active TB is present or cover her mouth when coughing. Good hygiene is mandatory because TB is airborne.

2. The patient needs to comply with all medical treatment for as long as necessary.

3. Latent TB is not contagious. To prevent it from becoming active, it is important to take daily medication, according to recommendations, for 6 to 12 months.

URINARY INCONTINENCE

I. **Definition.** Urinary incontinence is involuntary loss of urine that is objectively demonstrable and that is severe enough to constitute a social or hygienic problem, as defined by the International Incontinence Society.

II. **Etiology**
    A. Pelvic floor relaxation (dysfunction)
    B. Infection
    C. Atrophy
    D. Drugs
    E. Excess urine
    F. Immobility
    G. Bowel dysfunction

III. **Clinical Features**
    A. Urge incontinence: Uncontrolled detrusor muscle contraction, causing urinary leakage, overactive bladder, or detrusor instability
        1. Neurologic dysfunction
        2. Cystitis
        3. Bladder outlet obstruction
    B. Stress urinary incontinence: Urine loss without a detrusor contraction
        1. Poor pelvic muscle tone
        2. Urethral sphincter deficiency, congenital or acquired
        3. Overweight
    C. Mixed incontinence: A combination of symptoms from A and B above
    D. Overflow Incontinence
        1. Neurologic dysfunction
        2. Endocrine diseases
        3. Decreased bladder wall compliance
        4. Bladder outlet obstruction

IV. **Management**
    A. Obtain a complete history.
        1. Assess the patient's symptoms.
            a. Urge incontinence
                (1) Urgency
                (2) Frequency more than 7 times a day
                (3) Large amount of urine loss
                (4) Waking at night to urinate
            b. Stress incontinence
                (1) Urine leakage during physical activity
                (2) Small amount of urine loss with incontinence
                (3) Difficulty reaching the toilet in time, following the urge to void

    c. Mixed incontinence—Some symptoms of both urge and stress incontinence mentioned previously

  2. Obtain a complete list of medications that the patient is taking, looking for those that might affect incontinence.

    a. Urgency—Diuretics and caffeine

    b. Frequency—Diuretics

    c. Urinary retention—Anticholinergics, narcotics, alpha- and beta-adrenergic antagonists, and calcium channel blockers

    d. Overflow incontinence—Anticholinergics and calcium channel blockers

    e. Stress incontinence—Alpha-adrenergic antagonists

B. Perform a complete physical exam.

  1. Observe the patient's gait, affect, and mental status.

  2. Perform a complete gynecologic exam.

    a. Check for lesions, masses, cervical and uterine position and size, pelvic floor tone, fecal impaction, and condition of vaginal tissue.

    b. Observe the urethral tone.

    c. Check the intactness of the pudendal nerve.

  3. Laboratory tests

    a. Routine urine test and C&S

    b. Diabetes screen

    c. Urine volume

C. Treat the patient as follows:

  1. Behavioral therapy

    a. Pelvic floor exercises: See the section on Kegel Exercises in Part I.

    b. Fluid management: Avoid fluids 4 hours prior to bedtime.

    c. Irritants: Avoid bladder irritants such as soda, caffeine, and alcohol.

    d. Bladder training: Increase bladder capacity through training, which has been shown to be 67% effective in curing overactive bladder syndrome.[16]

    e. Biofeedback: Use this for stress incontinence, urge incontinence or mixed incontinence. Improvement has been reported in 85% of patients.

  2. Functional electrical stimulation (FES): Patients start by performing voluntary contractions with stimulated contractions and then progress to voluntary contractions with the device. FES has been used with mixed results.

  3. Vaginal cones: Weighted cones are used to improve the tone of the vagina.

  4. Pessaries: Used to control stress incontinence, these incontinence rings or Introl prostheses must be individually fitted. The patient must be able to insert and remove them.

---

[16]Winkler & Sand, 1998, p. 286

5. Occlusive devices: These devices are used to occlude the urethra in women with stress incontinence.

   a. Impress: A soft, one-time-use patch with adhesive, which is applied after each voiding

   b. FemAssist: A reusable cap that fits over the urethra and should be changed on a weekly basis

   c. Reliance catheter: An intraurethral catheter with a small balloon and a blind end. It must be removed and discarded prior to voiding.

6. Medications

   a. Estrogen: Either a 0.3- to 1.25-mg oral dose, taken on a daily basis, or vaginal cream improves the estrogen status of the urethra. Its efficiency is unclear for urge incontinence.

   b. Alpha-adrenergic agonists such as pseudoephedrine—A 15- to 30-mg oral dose, taken twice a day, produces smooth muscle contractions, improving maximal urethral closure pressure. It works best with stress incontinence.

   c. Anticholinergic drugs

      (1) Ditropan or Ditropan XL (oxybutynin) prevents spontaneous detrusor contraction. Side effects include dry mouth, irritability, anxiety, and urinary retention.

      (2) Detrol or Detrol LA (tolterodine) has fewer side effects because it has a higher selective affinity for muscarinic receptors in the bladder. However, it is contraindicated in patients with glaucoma, urinary or gastric retention.[17]

   d. Tricyclic antidepressants such as imipramine - These have been used to successfully treat both stress and urge incontinence. They have both anticholinergic and alpha-adrenergic properties.[18]

   e. Antimuscarinic agents: Because they indirectly reverse sympathetically mediated smooth muscle relaxation, these are used for an overactive bladder. See the previous information on Anticholinergic Drugs.

URINARY TRACT INFECTIONS (UTI)

I. **Definition**

   A. An asymptomatic bacteriuria colony count of more than 100,000 bacteria per mL of urine

   B. Urethritis: Inflammation of the urethra

   C. Cystitis: Inflammation of the bladder

   D. Pyelonephritis: Inflammation of the kidney

II. **Etiology**

   A. Antepartum: Urinary stasis caused by the effects of progesterone

---

[17]Roberts, 2001, p. 28
[18]Krissovich, 1998

      1. Ureteral dilation

      2. Slowed ureteral peristalsis

      3. Increased pressure from an enlarging uterus

  B. Intrapartum

      1. Catheterization secondary to regional anesthesia - While catheterization does not otherwise significantly lead to UTI, the incidence of UTI secondary to catheterization at delivery is 20%.

      2. Trauma and swelling of the urethra secondary to the use of forceps or other traumatic delivery

  C. Postpartum

      1. Diuresis after delivery, which can lead to overdistention and stasis

      2. Use of oxytocin, which causes antidiuresis until it is metabolized; then there is a surge of diuresis, which rapidly distends the bladder.

  D. Interconceptional

      1. Sexual activity: Introduction of bacteria to the urethra caused by intercourse

      2. Physiologic: Congenital causes, prolapsed bladder, relaxation of the pelvic floor muscles, and diabetes

      3. Poor hygiene habits

        a. Not washing enough or changing underwear or peri pads often enough, thus allowing bacteria near the urethra to multiply

        b. Wiping from back to front, thus introducing bacteria from the rectum into the urethra.

      4. Health habits

        a. Not emptying the bladder often enough, which results in stasis of urine

        b. Excessive use of caffeine, which causes urinary irritation and diuresis

III. Clinical Features

  A. Asymptomatic bacteriuria: No symptoms

  B. Cystitis

      1. Symptoms

        a. Urinary frequency

        b. Urinary urgency

        c. Dysuria

        d. Suprapubic pain

        e. Hematuria

      2. Signs

        a. A bacteriuria colony count greater than 100,000

        b. Nitrates, by-products of bacteria in the urine

        c. WBCs greater than 50 per mL or 25 per HPF spun urine

        d. RBCs in urine

    C. Pyelonephritis

        1. Fever over 100°F or more with shaking chills

        2. Low back pain

        3. Anorexia, nausea, and vomiting

        4. Urinary urgency, frequency, and dysuria

        5. Costovertebral angle (CVA) tenderness

        6. Suprapubic pain

        7. Bacteria, nitrates, WBCs, RBCs, and protein in the urine

IV. Differential Diagnosis

    A. Urethritis, especially that caused by chlamydia

    B. Vaginitis, vulvitis, or trauma, which may mimic dysuria

    C. Urinary frequency, which may be normal for pregnancy

V. Management

    A. At the initial OB visit, obtain a history of UTIs and a clean-catch urinalysis and urine C&S to check for an asymptomatic UTI.

        1. If the history for UTIs is negative, proceed as follows:

            a. If the initial culture is also negative, no further testing is needed unless symptoms develop.

            b. If the initial culture is positive, treat the patient and repeat the urine culture 1 week after treatment and at 28 weeks' gestation.

    B. Do a urine test at each prenatal visit.

        1. If it is positive for bacteria, nitrates, or blood, perform a clean-catch urinalysis.

        2. If there is more than a trace of proteinuria, follow these steps:

            a. Obtain another clean-catch urine sample and recheck it.

            b. If protein is still present, rule out preeclampsia and pregnancy-induced hypertension (PIH).

            c. If there is no hypertension, obtain a urine C&S to rule out an asymptomatic UTI.

            d. If proteinuria is 1+ or higher at two office visits, consider doing a 24-hour urine test to evaluate the total protein. Consult a specialist, as necessary.

    C. Any time a patient presents with signs and symptoms of cystitis, follow these steps:

        1. Perform a clean-catch urinalysis and urine C&S.

            a. If the tests are negative in the presence of symptoms, consider doing a GC culture and a chlamydia culture.

            b. If the urinalysis is positive and classic symptoms are present, consider initiating treatment before the results of the culture are obtained.

        2. Check the patient for CVA tenderness.

        3. Consider prescribing 200 mg of Pyridium, to be taken orally, three times a day for 3 days to relieve dysuria.

    D. Treat the patient according to these steps:

1. Treat the patient with antibiotics, if that is indicated by the results of the urinalysis or urine C&S. If the patient has two or fewer UTIs in 1 year, consider prescribing a 3-day regimen. If she has three or more in a year, a longer regimen is indicated.

   a. Sulfa drugs, which are the most effective for treating UTIs

      (1) Sulfa drugs are contraindicated in the following situations:

         (a) Allergy to sulfa

         (b) After 36 weeks' gestation, because sulfa can lead to kernicterus of the newborn

         (c) G6PD anemia, because sulfa can lead to hemolytic anemia

      (2) If sulfa drugs are used, one choice is Bactrim DS (trimethoprim and sulfamethoxazole) orally twice a day for 3 to 10 days.

   b. Nitrofurantoin (Furadantin, Macrodantin), 100 mg orally, twice a day for 3 to 10 days

   c. Amoxicillin (Amoxil), 500 mg orally, three times a day for 7 to 10 days

   d. Norfloxacin (Noroxin), 400 mg orally, twice a day for 3 to 10 days

   e. Fosfomycin tromethamine (Monural), 3 g orally; mix one packet with water and give it in a single dose.

2. Inform the patient that response to antibiotics is usually rapid. Symptoms disappear 1 to 2 days after starting treatment. The patient may feel the infection is gone and discontinue treatment. Instruct the patient to take the antibiotic for the full 3 to 10 days to prevent relapse.

3. Warn the patient that monilia vaginitis may develop secondary to antibiotic therapy. She should be alert for signs and symptoms.

   a. Consider acidophilus tablets to prevent against infection.

   b. Consider 150 mg of Diflucan to be taken orally at the completion of the antibiotic - except during pregnancy.

4. If the patient is pregnant, repeat the urine culture 1 week after treatment. Cultures should be negative within 24 hours of starting antibiotic therapy.

5. Teach self-help and self-prevention measures.

E. Any time the patient presents with signs and symptoms of pyelonephritis, follow these steps:

   1. Obtain a clean-catch urinalysis, urine culture, and CBC.

   2. Perform a physical exam for CVA tenderness and discomfort over the symphysis.

F. If the patient is pregnant and has a UTI twice or more,

   1. Consider screening for

      a. Sickle-cell anemia if the patient is African American (should have been done routinely at the initial OB visit).

  b. G6PD anemia if the patient is African American, Asian, or of Mediterranean descent.

  c. Diabetes.

  2. Initiate prophylactic prevention with 50 to 100 mg of Macrodantin, orally, every day.

  3. Consider a urology consultation.

G. Suggest these self-help measures:

  1. Drink at least 6 to 8 glasses of liquid daily to encourage adequate kidney function and prevent urinary stasis.

  2. Avoid caffeine, which is irritating to the urinary system and acts as a diuretic. Excess vitamin C is also an irritant.

  3. Use proper perineal hygiene to prevent urethral contamination from rectal bacteria.

  4. Urinate frequently throughout the day to prevent urinary stasis.

  5. Urinate immediately after intercourse to wash away bacteria that may have been moved to the urethra.

  6. Take cranberry juice or tablets at the first indication of an infection.

 ## VACCINATIONS

I. **Live Virus.** *Vaccination with live virus is never recommended in pregnancy.* Killed virus may be considered if the risk of disease outweighs the risk of exposure to a vaccination during pregnancy.

II. **Specific Types of Vaccination**

A. Influenza vaccine

  1. The CDC recommends flu vaccinations for women who have an underlying high-risk condition.

  2. Vaccines should be avoided until the second or third trimester, if at all possible.

B. Rubella vaccine—See the Rubella guidelines previously included in this chapter.

  1. This vaccine is not recommended during pregnancy or sooner than 3 months before conception because of possible teratogenic effects.

  2. If the patient is rubella negative, she should be vaccinated in the immediate postpartum period to prevent possible exposure and resultant teratogenic effects in subsequent pregnancies.

  3. Informed consent should be obtained before vaccination. About 10% to 12% develop transient arthritis. Risks to others in her environment are minimal.

C. Hepatitis vaccines (Heptovax and Havrix)—See the Hepatitis guidelines previously included in this chapter. These vaccines consist of killed virus, so logically, they should be safe in pregnancy. However, they have not been widely used. Weigh the potential risk of contracting hepatitis against the potential risk of the vaccine.

VAGINAL DISCHARGE

I. **Incidence.** Vaginal discharge is the most frequent complaint of women seeking gynecologic care.

II. **Etiology and Management**

   A. Extravaginal disease simulating vaginal discharge

      1. Vulvar or perineal lesions

         a. Syphilis chancre

         b. Chancroid

         c. Herpes

         d. Condylomata

         e. Cancer

         f. Miscellaneous (e.g., psoriasis, dermatitis, and parasitic infestations)

      2. Bartholinitis or Bartholin's cyst

      3. Vaginal fistulae

   B. Physiologic discharge—A normal discharge that is cervical in origin

      1. Most apparent in high estrogen states

         a. At the time of ovulation

         b. During pregnancy

         c. During oral contraceptive use

      2. Changes in cervical mucus during the menstrual cycle

         a. Just after menses, hormone levels are low, causing mucus to be scant.

         b. As estrogen increases, mucus increases in amount and becomes thinner.

         c. At midcycle, the mucus is clear, slippery, and stretchy, like raw egg white. This mucus heralds ovulation and the fertile period.

         d. After ovulation, progesterone dominates, making the mucus cloudy. The discharge slowly decreases in amount, becoming white to white-yellow until menses begins.

   C. Noninfectious vaginal discharge

      1. Local irritation or allergic response

         a. Usual causative agents

            (1) Douche chemical

            (2) Feminine hygiene products

            (3) Sexual aid products

            (4) Contraceptive creams, foams, and jellies (nonoxynol 9)

         b. Diagnosis

            (1) This diagnosis is confirmed by finding large numbers of eosinophils in the discharge via a wet prep.

      (2) The discharge, under this diagnosis, will clear up when use of the offending agent is stopped.

2. Foreign object in the vagina
   a. Usual causative agents: A forgotten tampon or diaphragm
   b. Pathology
      (1) Discharge
         (a) Often scanty but may be purulent, brown tinged, or frankly bloody
         (b) Possible offensive odor
      (2) Possible signs of infection
   c. Management
      (1) Place double gloves on the examining hand, remove the foreign object, fold the top of glove of the examining hand over the object, tie a knot in the end, and discard it.
      (2) If there are signs of significant irritation or infection, order a vaginal cream or an oral antibiotic.

3. Atrophic vaginitis
   a. It is caused by a low estrogen state.
      (1) Prepuberty
      (2) Lactation
      (3) Postmenopause
   b. The high pH of the vagina changes the normal flora.
   c. The vaginal mucosa is thin and, therefore, susceptible to infection and trauma.
   d. The following symptoms may occur:
      (1) Dyspareunia
      (2) Postcoital spotting
      (3) Vulvar irritation
   e. A wet prep will reveal the following:
      (1) Immature epithelial cells
      (2) Large numbers of WBCs
   f. The patient should be treated following this procedure:
      (1) Rule out a secondary infection.
      (2) Consider using topical estrogen cream, which works well. Use Estrace 0.1% or 0.625 mg of Premarin at bedtime for 1 week, four times a day for 1 week, twice a week for 2 weeks, and then a maintenance dose of 1 to 2 days per week.
      (3) Insert one Vagifem tablet vaginally every night for 2 weeks and then use them one or two times per week for maintenance.
      (4) Place the Estring vaginal ring (2 mg of estradiol) in the vagina. Wear it continuously for 90 days before replacing it.

4. Cervicitis: An infection of the endocervix
   a. Cause of 30% of all vaginal discharge

      b. Clinical picture

        (1) Mucopurulent discharge from os

        (2) Inflamed, friable, bleeding, or edematous cervix.

      c. Symptoms

        (1) Mucopurulent discharge

        (2) Intermenstrual or postcoital spotting

      d. Causes

        (1) STDs

        (2) Cervical cap

        (3) Cancer (cause or secondary effect)

    5. Neoplasia: Gradual onsets of discharge, similar to the pattern seen in foreign body irritation. Consult a specialist.

  D. Infectious vaginal discharge

    1. *Trichomonas vaginalis*—See the Trichomonas Vaginitis guidelines in this chapter. The discharge is frothy, thin, yellow-green or gray, irritating, and malodorous.

    2. *Candida albicans*—See the Monilia Vaginitis guidelines in this chapter. The discharge is cheesy, curdy, yellow-white, irritating, yeasty smelling.

    3. *Gardnerella*—See the Bacterial Vaginitis guidelines in this chapter. The discharge is minimal, creamy, yellow or gray, and malodorous.

    4. *Neisseria gonorrhoeae*—See the Gonorrhea guidelines in this chapter. There may be no discharge, or it may be green or yellow-green and irritating.

    5. *Treponema pallidum*—See the Syphilis guidelines in this chapter. This does not usually cause discharge, although chancres or condylomata may be weepy or infected.

    6. *Herpes virus*—See the Herpes Simplex guidelines in this chapter. There may be a grayish exudate or thin discharge from weepy lesions or superinfection.

    7. *Chlamydia trachomatis*—See the Chlamydia guidelines in this chapter. There may be no discharge, or there may be mucopurulent, foul-smelling discharge.

III. Clinical Features

  A. History

    1. Age

      a. Women in their sexually active years are most likely to present with STDs.

      b. Older women are most likely to have neoplasms, although young women get them too.

      c. Any vaginal discharge is unlikely in a prepubescent girl and warrants a vigorous workup.

    2. Mode and time of onset

      a. Mode: A woman who can say exactly which day her discharge began is likely to have an infection.

        b. Relationship to menstrual cycle

          (1) An onset of discharge in the premenstrual period may indicate monilia vaginitis.

          (2) Discharge beginning at the time of the menses is likely to be trichomonas vaginitis or gonorrhea.

          (3) Discharge at midcycle and up to a week after may be physiologic.

  3. Presence of other diseases

        a. Diabetes and hypoparathyroidism are associated with an increased frequency of monilia vaginitis.

        b. Impaired resistance to infection, such as leukemia, chronic renal or hepatic disease, or collagen-vascular disease, can predispose the patient to vaginitis.

        c. HIV not only predisposes the patient to *Candida* infection, but treatment is difficult.

  4. Contraceptive history

        a. Oral contraceptives may predispose the patient to *Monilia* infection.

        b. An IUD may predispose the patient to PID.

        c. The cervical cap may cause a cervical ulcer or local cervicitis.

        d. Spermicides may cause a chemical irritation or allergy.

  5. History of current and prior medications

        a. Locally applied chemicals can cause vaginitis.

        b. Antibiotics, including Flagyl, steroids, and oral contraceptives can lead to a *Candida* infection.

        c. Low-dose or broad-spectrum antibiotics can mask tests for gonorrhea and syphilis and result in an antibiotic-resistant strain.

  6. Sexual history

        a. Ask the question, "Do you have a reason to suspect that you may have a sexually transmitted disease?"

        b. Discover dates and treatment of previous conditions.

        c. Determine if previous condition is not resolved or is recurring.

        d. Ask about new sexual partners, number of partners, and whether they are steady or casual.

  7. Hygiene habits that may be causing local irritation

        a. Poor hygiene

        b. Frequent use of douches, chemicals, sprays, and other hygiene products

        c. Use of perfume, powders, and scented toiletries

B. Physical exam

  1. Inspect the external genitalia for the following:

        a. Erythema, edema, or excoriation

        b. Lesions—Note whether they are draining.

        c. Presence of discharge at the introitus

d. Discharge from Bartholin's or paraurethral Skene's glands; purulent discharge is indicative of gonorrhea.

2. Palpate for an inguinal lymphadenopathy, which would indicate an infectious process, such as syphilis or herpes.

3. Perform a speculum exam.

   a. Inspect the vaginal walls and cervix for irritation, lesions, and discharge.

   (1) Monilia: White patches on vaginal or cervical mucosa

   (2) Trichomonas: Red, inflamed, "strawberry patch" appearance of vaginal or cervical mucosa

   (3) Herpes: Cervicitis usually only in primary episodes and ulcers usually only on the endocervix

   b. If indicated, gather specimens.

   (1) Swab for a wet prep.

   (2) Take culture samples.

   (a) Do a GC or chlamydia culture of the cervix and lesions.

   (b) Do a herpes culture of the cervix and lesions.

4. Perform a bimanual exam.

   a. Palpate the cervix for cervical motion tenderness, which is indicative of PID and gonorrhea.

   b. Palpate the uterus and adnexa for

   (1) Masses.

   (2) Enlargements.

   (3) Abnormal shape, consistency, or position.

   (4) Tenderness.

IV. Management

A. Lab work

1. Evaluate a wet prep.

   a. A positive whiff test is indicative of bacterial vaginosis (*Gardnerella*).

   b. Clue cells are indicative of bacterial vaginosis.

   c. Trichomonads are diagnostic of trichomonas vaginitis.

   d. Filaments with budding spores or pseudohyphae are diagnostic of monilia vaginitis.

   e. Immature cells and numerous WBCs are indicative of infection and possible atrophic vaginitis.

   f. Numerous eosinophils are indicative of an allergic response.

   g. Numerous Döderlein's bacilli (lactobacilli) are indicative of physiologic discharge.

2. Evaluate the vaginal pH.

   a. The normal pH of vaginal discharge is 4.5, plus or minus 0.5.

   b. A pH under 4.5 indicates a high estrogen state, such as pregnancy.

    c. A pH over 5 indicates the following:

        (1) A low estrogen state, as in atrophic vaginitis

        (2) Monilia, trichomonas, or gardnerella vaginitis

3. Order blood work: Request a CBC with differential if there are signs of a systemic infection or PID.

4. Perform a Pap smear to diagnose any of the following:

    a. Dysplasia or carcinoma

    b. Monilia vaginitis

    c. Bacterial vaginitis

    d. Herpes simplex

    e. HPV

    f. Low-estrogen states (atrophic vaginitis)

    g. Possible trichomonas vaginitis or chlamydia (but do not treat the patient until specific tests are done to confirm or rule out the diagnosis)

B. Treatment

1. Diagnose the disease according to the patient's history, physical exam, and lab work.

2. Manage and treat the patient according to specific guidelines.

3. Educate the patient on the following general points:

    a. Discuss characteristics of normal vaginal discharge.

    b. Avoid the use of irritating products.

    c. Practice good hygiene.

    d. Avoid douching.

    e. Use treatment measures to prevent monilia vaginitis from occurring or becoming a superinfection (common) when broad-spectrum antibiotics are taken.

    f. Inform the patient that with each new partner or multiple partners, the risk of vaginal infection increases.

    g. Avoid intercourse with active symptoms of infection, until the infection is treated.

    h. If the infection is sexually transmitted, inform the partner(s), who may need to be treated.

    i. While undergoing treatment, avoid intercourse or use condoms if the infection could be sexually transmitted.

    j. Explain examination and laboratory tests, which are necessary for diagnosis.

    k. Urge the patient to use all the medication prescribed, not just until the symptoms are gone.

    l. Inform the patient that a vaginal infection may cause an abnormal Pap smear.

    m. Inform the patient that menopausal women with vaginal atrophy have a higher rate of atypical squamous cells on a Pap smear. Treat them with local or systemic hormones and repeat the Pap smear in 6 months.

    n. Expect a follow-up examination to test for cure.

PART 5

Management of Common Problems and Procedures Specific to Pregnancy

Geri Morgan, CNM, ND

Carol Hamilton, BSN, MA, CNM

ABORTION

I. Definition. Abortion is the termination of an unwanted pregnancy by medical or surgical methods.

II. Safety. Legally induced abortion is safer than continuing a pregnancy to term. "The risk of death from abortion in the first twelve weeks of pregnancy is approximately 1 in 100,000 to 1 in 400,000. From this perspective, abortion is 10–40 times safer than having a baby."[1]

III. History. In 1970, several states, including New York and California, passed laws legalizing abortion. In 1973, the U.S. Supreme Court in the landmark ruling of *Roe v. Wade* effectively legalized abortion nationwide. It was setup by trimesters. In the first trimester, the ruling allowed the decision to be made between the woman and her physician. In the second trimester, each state was allowed to regulate abortion procedures. In the third trimester, the viability of the fetus had to be considered. States could prohibit, or severely limit, access to abortion.

IV. Counseling

    A. Counseling should begin at first contact, whether the woman comes to the office for a pregnancy test or initial exam. It is unfortunate, but regardless of her decision to terminate the pregnancy or continue it, time becomes an important factor. If termination is desired, the options for terminating a pregnancy decrease as the days of pregnancy increase.

    B. Give information and make referrals as necessary to counselors, clinics or physicians for prenatal care, adoption, abortion clinics and agencies providing financial assistance.

    C. Care must be exercised to insure that the decision the woman makes is not subject to duress or to coercion, expressed or implied, and that all decisions are reached on the basis of full information and free discussion.

    D. If abortion is selected, every effort should be made by history and exam to determine the length of the pregnancy. The length of the pregnancy will determine the termination options available. Give oral and written information on the available options. Allow for free discussion and questions. Be sure to use language and terminology best understood by the patient.

V. Pre-Abortion Physical

    A. History: In addition to a routine history, the following information is needed:

        1. Menstrual history, including the date of the last menstrual period (LMP), normal number of days between periods, amount, length and spotting that occurred after menses, if any.

        2. Past Contraceptive methods.

        3. Method in use at the time of conception.

        4. Future contraceptive method desired.

        5. Any abdominal or pelvic problems, including surgery.

[1]Benson, Michael. Gynecological Pearls. 2000. p 64

6. Drugs currently being used. Include over the counter and recreational drugs, as well as prescribed.

7. Any allergies or intolerances to drugs. Include a list of anesthetics, analgesics and other medications that may be used.

B. Clinical exam: Perform a thorough physical exam with particular attention to

1. Blood pressure and pulse

2. Pelvic speculum exam to check for any abnormalities or infections

3. Bimanual exam, including size of the uterus, position of the uterus and cervix, any adnexal masses or other problems.

C. Laboratory tests

1. Hemoglobin or hematocrit

2. An Rho(D) determination

3. Other tests as indicated (e.g. pap smear, chlamydia, gonorrhea, urine or serum pregnancy test)

D. Ultrasound (U/S) evaluation

1. Should be performed as close to the procedure date as possible.

2. An intrauterine sac should be seen after 35 days from LMP. If there is no clearly visible gestational sac on U/S, a pregnancy test or a beta hCG must be done and the patient evaluated for possible ectopic pregnancy.

VI. Medical Abortion

A. Definition. Termination of a pregnancy by medical means

B. Effectiveness: A termination rate of 95% for early pregnancies has been reported.[2] The success rate declines rapidly after 49 days and is contraindicated after that date.[3]

C. Advantage

1. May be emotionally easier

2. Avoids surgery

3. May be less painful

4. Seen as more natural

5. Often can be completed at home with support of family and significant other

6. Methotrexate, if used, is an effective treatment for ectopic pregnancies.

D. Disadvantages

1. There have been reports of fetal malformations after administration of the medicines currently in use. *Once the medicine is given, the abortion must be completed, either medically or surgically.*

2. May have nausea, vomiting, diarrhea, headache, fever, chills, back pain, bleeding and cramping. Most of these side effects will be of a short duration.

---

[2]Spitz, I.M., et al. New England Journal of Medicine. 1998. p. 338, 1241

[3]Mifeprex Medication Guide, Danco Laboratories, p 2

3. Must wait for the medications to work
   a. Mifepristone day one/Misoprostol day three—90% will abort within 24 hours of taking misoprostol
   b. Methotrexate may take longer and be less effective.
4. Extra office visits are required.

E. Patient Selection
   1. The patient must have freely chosen to terminate her pregnancy and be capable of giving voluntary informed consent.
   2. Appear psychologically prepared.
   3. Be willing to have a surgical abortion, if indicated.
   4. Have a confirmed intrauterine pregnancy of no more than 49 days gestation.
   5. Have no physical contraindications to the procedure.
   6. Be without logistical problems (e.g. has access to transportation, a telephone, and is able to return to the affiliate for follow up or if medically indicated.
   7. Contraindications:
      a. Over 49 days gestation by LMP and U/S
      b. Allergic to any medications
      c. Taking anticoagulants
      d. Long term corticosteroid use
      e. Chronic adrenal failure
      f. Poorly controlled inflammatory bowel disease
      g. Severe anemia
      h. IUD in place
   8. If patient is breast-feeding, she must stop for 72 hours as medications may cause diarrhea in her infant.

F. Medications
   1. Mifepristone is supplied as Mifeprex 200 mg tablets. Mifepristone blocks progesterone binding sites in the uterus and elsewhere. Uterine activity results in bleeding and cramping.
   2. Methotrexate is a folic acid antagonist that affects trophoblastic cells so they are unable to divide and multiply. The development of the placenta is halted and is, therefore, unable to support the embryo.
   3. Misoprostol (Cytotec) is a prostaglandin that acts on the uterus increasing activity and causing it to cramp and bleed. Note: Misoprostol is widely used as an abortive and for labor induction. It only has FDA approval for prevention of NSAID induced gastric ulcers.
   4. Mifepristone/Misoprostol
      a. Danco Laboratories recommends the following:[4]
         (1) Day 1—Mifepristone 600 mg (three 200 mg tablets) orally

---

[4]www.earlypill.com

        (2) Day 3—If abortion is suspected, it must be confirmed. If still pregnant, give misoprostol 400 mcg (two tablets) orally.

        (3) Day 14—If the patient has not returned prior, the patient must return to the office for confirmation. If the patient is still pregnant, a surgical abortion is recommended.

    b. Planned Parenthood asks patients to return to clinic if no bleeding has occurred after the first dose of misoprostol; by 48 hours, one additional does of misoprostol may be given.[5]

    c. Rh negative women should be given Rh immune globulin on Day 1.

    d. Studies are finding that mifepristone given as a 200 mg oral dose may be as effective as a 600 mg dose.[6]

  5. Methotrexate/misoprostol: The schedule for the administration of methotrexate/misoprostol is similar to mifepristone/misoprostol. The dosage of methotrexate is calculated based on body surface area and is given on Day 1. If abortion has not occurred by Day 5 to Day 7, misoprostol is given. The patient needs to be seen on Day 14, if not seen prior, to confirm a complete abortion.

  6. Medications during/after abortion

    a. Cramping: NSAID such as IBP 600 mg orally every six hours may be backed or alternated with Tylenol #3.

    b. Excessive bleeding after expulsion of products of conception —Methergine (Ergotrate) 0.2 mg, one orally every six hours

G. After the abortion is complete, contraception should be started as soon as allowed by the method chosen.

H. See VIII, Postabortion Complications.

VII. Surgical Abortion

A. Definition. Termination of an intrauterine pregnancy by surgical means.

B. Effectiveness: 99%–99.5%

C. Advantages

  1. Quicker

  2. Can be asleep or medicated for the procedure

  3. Does not require active participation

D. Disadvantages

  1. Invasive surgical procedure with a chance of reaction to the medications, anesthetics and procedure itself

  2. Cervix may be damaged

  3. Uterus may be punctured

  4. The procedure may lead to an incomplete abortion and a second vacuum aspiration or a D&C may need to be done.

---

[5]Planned Parenthood of Central and Northern Arizona Manual of Medical Standards Guidelines, p 10

[6]Hatcher, R et al, Contraceptive Technology, 1998, p 610

E. Patient Selection—With the exception that surgical abortions may be done during the first and second trimester and are not limited to 49 days or less of pregnancy, the counseling, education, physical exam, ultrasound and medical screening are the same as for those undergoing a medical abortion.

F. Vacuum aspiration (suction curettage): Almost all first trimester abortions are performed using this procedure.

1. A bimanual is performed noting uterine size and cervical placement.

2. A paracervical block may be used after cleansing the cervix.

3. A tenaculum is placed on the cervix and it is pulled to straighten the cervix.

4. The suction curettage is introduced into the uterus and the contents are aspirated by an electrical vacuum pump or manually.

5. The contents in the suction jar should be checked to be sure that it contains the products of conception (POC).

G. Dilation and evacuation (D&E): This method is preferred between 13 and 16 weeks, but may be done up to 20 weeks.

1. Synthetic osmotic dilators (Lamicel, Dilapan) or Laminaria (dried seaweed) are placed in the endocervical canal to dilate both the internal and external os.

2. After dilation, the dilators are removed and the procedure is the same as with vacuum extraction except that larger POC may require forceps.

H. Medications

1. Infection: A prophylactic antibiotic such as doxycycline 100 mg orally twice a day for seven days may be used to prevent infection.

2. Bleeding: After 13 to 14 weeks gestation the uterus is larger and there may be more uterine atony and bleeding. Methergine (Ergotrate) IM or 0.2 mg orally every four hours times six will facilitate contractions and decrease bleeding.

3. Pain/cramping

   a. Motrin or another IBP product is recommended. It may be taken 400 to 600 mg orally every four to six hours to decrease the discomfort from the Methergine.

   b. Tylenol #3 works well especially if alternated every two to four hours with IBP.

VIII. Postabortion Complications

A. Infection

1. Counsel patient to call if she has a temperature over 100°, chills, uterine tenderness to pressure or foul smelling discharge.

2. Rule out retained POC.

3. A prophylactic antibiotic is often given postabortion. May need to treat or retreat as necessary.

B. Retained Products of Conception: Incomplete Abortion

1. Suspect if history of continuous bleeding

    2. The uterus will be subinvoluted and the cervix not fully closed.

    3. Confirm by U/S

    4. Consult for a vacuum aspiration or D&C

  C. Bleeding

    1. Second trimester abortions often receive oxytocin IV or Ergotrate IM or orally to encourage contractions and minimize bleeding.

    2. Bleeding longer and heavier than a typical menstrual period may be excessive.

      a. Less than 1% have heavy bleeding and less than 1 in 500 to 1000 require a D&C or blood transfusion.

      b. Has she soaked through four maxi pads in two hours?

      c. Is she passing numerous large size clots?

      d. Does she feel faint, dizzy, excessively tired (this may result from pain medication or stress)?

      e. Bring in for exam—Do Hgb/Hct

  D. Undiagnosed ectopic pregnancy

    1. Suspect by history, serum hCG levels, exam and ultrasound

    2. Methotrexate is 90% effective

  E. Continuing pregnancy

IX. **Contraception.** Fertility can return in as little as ten days postabortion. For this reason, it is important to start contraception as soon as possible after her abortion.

  A. Consider past methods used, those liked and those rejected

  B. What method was being used when pregnancy occurred? Why did that method fail?

  C. See methods of contraception for counseling and information on individual methods.

 ABRUPTIO PLACENTAE

I. **Definition.** Abruptio placenta is the premature separation of the normally implanted placenta at any time before delivery of the baby. It varies from a small area to complete separation. Types are:

  A. Marginal sinus: A small margin of the placenta separates.

  B. Mild: Includes marginal, very small area separated.

  C. Moderate: At least one fourth but less than two thirds separated.

  D. Severe: More than two thirds of the placenta is separated.

II. **Incidence.** About one in 150 births

III. **Etiology**

  A. More frequent in multiparas

  B. More frequent in women over age 35

  C. More frequent if hypertension is present

  D. Trauma to the abdomen may contribute

        1. Direct blow to the uterus

        2. Forceful external version

        3. Needle puncture at amniocentesis

    E. Rapid reduction of uterine size and pressure after rupture of membranes in polyhydramnios

    F. Malnutrition

    G. Short umbilical cord

    H. Smoking

IV. Clinical Features: See Table 5-1.

V. Complications

    A. Hemorrhage and resulting shock

    B. Hemorrhage may shear off remaining attached placenta.

    C. Force of collecting blood in uterus may cause:

        1. Rupture into amniotic sac

        2. Extravasation between muscle fibers of the myometrium (Couvelaire uterus) causes irritable uterus and inability to relax its tone.

    D. Disseminated intravascular coagulation due to myometrial damage and large amount of blood clotting

    E. Renal disturbances secondary to shock and/or clotting disturbances

    F. Fetal distress due to hemorrhaging

    G. Renal failure secondary to ischemia

    H. Pituitary necrosis (Sheehan's syndrome) secondary to ischemia

    I. Hepatitis secondary to massive blood transfusions

VI. Management

    A. Consult with physician immediately for *all* cases.

    B. Rh(D) negative patients: All unsensitized Rh(D) negative patients should receive a RhoGAM injection after each uterine bleeding episode to prevent sensitization from possible mixing of Rh(D) positive fetal blood with maternal blood. The usual dose is one vial, which is adequate for a transfusion of up to 15ml of fetal blood into the maternal circulation. The dosage should be larger if it is possible that more than 15ml was transfused. A Betke-Kleihauer test can be ordered to determine the amount of fetal blood in the maternal circulation.

 ANTIPHOSPHOLIPID ANTIBODY SYNDROME

I.   **Definition.** Antiphospholipid Antibody Syndrome (APS) is a recognized cause of thromboembolitic events, thrombocytopenia, and adverse pregnancy outcomes. Antiphospholipid antibodies are immunoglobulins that act against phospholipids on plasma membranes and plasma proteins, and bind to circulating phospholipids involved in coagulation causing APS, a serious hypercoagulability condition. There are two types.

    A. Primary: Diagnosed in the absence of associated systemic disease and comprises 50% of cases. In pregnancy there may be no symp-

Table 5-1. Clinical Features of Abruptio Placentae

Symptoms	Mild	Moderate	Severe
Bleeding	Dark, none to moderate	Scant to moderate; may be up to 1000 mL behind placenta	Moderate to profuse
Fetus	No distress	Distress	Severe distress, dead
Uterine tone	Poor uterine relaxation between contractions	Little relaxation between contractions	Extreme rigidity
Pain	None or vague lower abdomen discomfort	Tender	Agonizing, tearing, knifelike, unremitting
Shock	None	Varies	Severe
Psychologic	No change	Vague to moderate anxiety	Extremely anxious
Other	Uterine irritability	Fetal heart tones hard to hear with external monitor	Fetal heart tones may be absent; uterine size increases as it fills with blood

toms until complications arise. Testing is positive for antiphospholipid antibodies such anticardiolipin antibodies and lupus anticoagulant.

- **B.** Secondary: The above antibodies associated with positive criteria of systemic lupus erythematosus (SLE), other autoimmune diseases or certain infections or drugs such as procainamide (Procanbid), Fansidar, phenothiazines, and chlorpromazine (Thorazine).

II. Etiology

- **A.** This is an acquired rather than a genetic disease; how the disease develops is as yet unclear.
- **B.** Ten percent of woman with unexplained recurrent pregnancy loss test positive for APS. This percentage increases to 41% after three spontaneous abortions.[7]

III. Clinical Features

- **A.** Thrombocytopenia
- **B.** Recurrent pregnancy loss; recurrent spontaneous miscarriage or second/third trimester fetal loss.
- **C.** Positive anticardiolipin antibodies and/or lupus anticoagulant antibodies with medium or high titers.
- **D.** Lupus anticoagulant antibodies may occur with 10% of SLE.

E. May be associated with other autoimmune diseases such as scleroderma.

F. Antiphospholipid antibodies cause narrowing and thrombi of blood vessels, 50% of which occur during pregnancy.

G. Severe preeclampsia is associated with APS in 48% of women.[s]

H. Fetal growth restriction occurs in up to 30% of APS women.

I. Some women have a postpartum event at about two to ten weeks postpartum consisting of chest pain, fever, dyspnea or cardiomyopathy.

IV. Management

A. Preconceptual counseling if prior history of a problem

B. ANA, ACA, Anti-ssa and Anti-ssb laboratory tests are used for screening for APS on patients who have a history of SLE, repeated fetal loss, thromboembolic events, thrombocytopenia, or severe or early onset of preeclampsia.

C. Women who are pregnant and are positive for APS are high risk and should be evaluated by a perinatologist.

D. Expected management will be as follows:

1. Heparin throughout pregnancy and for six weeks postpartum.

2. Warfarin may be substituted for heparin postpartum.

3. Monitor carefully for preeclampsia and preterm labor.

4. Monitor fetal well being with serial ultrasounds and biophysical profiles beginning at 20 weeks EGA.

5. Doppler flow studies to identify abnormal uteroplacental flow.

E. Consider early delivery.

F. Treatment of these pregnancies present a dilemma as some women do well with treatment using heparin, prednisone or low dose aspirin while others continue to have pregnancy losses.

 BACKACHE

I. Etiology

A. Softening of the pelvic ligaments during pregnancy

B. Increasing weight of the uterus changes the woman's center of gravity, causing postural changes, which result in increased lumbar lordosis.

C. Back strain due to

1. Excessive bending

2. Excessive walking

3. Improper lifting

D. Lax abdominal muscle tone, especially in multiparas.

II. Management

[7]Lash, Ayhan, Mertens, Diana and Okumus, Hulya. Advance for Nurse Practitioners. June 2001. p 55

[8]Chang, Elizabeth and Ramsey-Goldman, Rosiland. Women's Health Gynecology Edition. Vol 1-2. April 2001

A. Use good body mechanics when reaching for something on the floor or lifting: bend the knees, keep the back straight rather than bending from the waist.

B. Good posture when sitting or standing; avoid exaggerated lordosis. OTC inserts or Rx orthotics may help posture.

C. Avoid excessive bending, lifting, or walking without rest periods.

D. Pelvic rock exercises to strengthen the lower back and relieve tension.

E. Use flexion and stretch exercises to strengthen muscles.

F. Wear supportive low-heeled shoes; avoid high-heeled shoes, which further exaggerate the lordosis.

G. For sleeping,
   1. Use a firm mattress.
   2. Use pillows for support, to straighten out the back, and alleviate pulling and strain on the back.

H. If the problem is due to lax abdominal muscles, a maternity girdle may help.

I. Heat to the area.

J. Massage may be of help.

K. Offer referral to chiropractor

L. Offer referral to physician if:
   1. The problem persists despite above measures
   2. Persistent muscle spasm
   3. Severe or significant hindrance to activities of daily living

III. **Differential Diagnosis**

A. Rule out UTI (see Guidelines). If any question, get urine C&S.

B. Rule out labor. Question regarding timing of backache (e.g., rhythmicity, associated with uterine hardening). If any question, assess with external fetal monitor, ascertain if cervical changes occur over time.

BLEEDING IN PREGNANCY UNDER 20 WEEKS' GESTATION

I. **Definition and Etiology.** Approximately 20% of pregnant women experience vaginal bleeding during the first trimester. Less than half of these women will have a spontaneous abortion (SAB). Causes of bleeding under 20 weeks' gestation include:

A. Implantation bleeding

B. Threatened spontaneous abortion

C. Inevitable spontaneous abortion

D. Incomplete spontaneous abortion

E. Complete spontaneous abortion

F. Missed spontaneous abortion

G. Ectopic pregnancy

    H. Molar pregnancy

    I. Cervicitis—See Chlamydia and Gonorrhea Guidelines

    J. Cervical polyps

    K. Cervical carcinoma

    L. Normal hyperemia of the cervix

    M. Unknown etiology

II. Clinical Features

    A. Implantation bleeding

        1. Occurs one to two weeks after conception.

        2. It is caused by blood escaping from blood vessels in the uterine epithelium that have been eroded by the implanting fertilized ovum.

        3. Bleeding is usually scant, light pink, unaccompanied by pain, and lasts only one to two days.

    B. Threatened abortion

        1. Vaginal bleeding with or without pelvic cramping and backache during the first trimester

        2. No cervical changes observed.

        3. Approximately 50% of threatened SABs do progress to complete SABs.

    C. Inevitable spontaneous abortion

        1. Increase in vaginal bleeding, accompanied by increasingly severe pelvic cramping

        2. Evidence of cervical dilatation, and/or effacement with or without the presence of fetal membranes or placenta at the cervical os

        3. It is impossible to halt the progress of the SAB at this point.

    D. Incomplete spontaneous abortion

        1. Part of the products of conception remain within the uterine cavity, causing persistent, sometimes profuse, vaginal bleeding.

        2. Passage of tissue and clots, with a history of vaginal bleeding and cramping will persist until all the products of conception have been evacuated from the uterus.

    E. Complete spontaneous abortion

        1. The uterus spontaneously evacuates itself of all the products of conception.

        2. Usually occurs before the 6th week or after the 14th week of pregnancy

    F. Spontaneous missed abortion

        1. Products of conception are retained in the uterus after the embryo or fetus has died.

        2. May have previously had signs and symptoms of a threatened SAB, which appear to resolve except for occasional brown spotting.

        3. Eventually the symptoms of pregnancy disappear and the uterine size becomes smaller.

    4. The term "missed AB" is usually applied to retention of a dead embryo or fetus for at least four to eight weeks.

  G. Ectopic pregnancy: See Ectopic Pregnancy guidelines.

  H. GTN or molar pregnancy

    1. Rapid enlargement of uterus during the first and early second trimester.

    2. Passage of grape-like clusters

    3. No FHTs heard by 12 weeks' of pregnancy

  I. Cervicitis (See Chlamydia and Gonorrhea Guidelines)

  J. Cervical polyps

    1. Painless bleeding, especially after coitus

    2. Bleeding appears early in gestation

    3. Appear as bright red pedunculated growths protruding from the cervical os

  K. Cervical carcinoma

    1. Painless vaginal bleeding, often after coitus

    2. Cervical erosion often is seen on routine speculum exam

    3. Abnormal Pap smear results

  L. Normal hyperemia of the cervix

    1. Spontaneous light vaginal spotting or bleeding, which may or may not be related to coitus

    2. Caused by the increased vascularization of the cervix that normally occurs during pregnancy

III. Clinical Features

  A. History

    1. Reports having, or having had, the symptoms of pregnancy

    2. Vaginal bleeding that can be scant, profuse; brown, pink, or bright red in color

    3. Abdominal pain, ranging from mild cramping to severe, sharp, unilateral pain

    4. Passage of tissue, blood clots, or grape-like vesicles (GTN)

    5. Bleeding that occurs at specific times (e.g., postcoitally) or is unrelated to activity

    6. Exposure to and symptoms of STD

    7. History of pelvic inflammatory disease (PID), previous ectopic pregnancy, intrauterine device (IUD) use, infertility, or adnexal surgery

    8. Disappearance of subjective signs and symptoms of pregnancy (missed SAB)

  B. Signs and symptoms

    1. Uterine size

      a. Normal for dates in threatened SABs

      b. Size less than dates in incomplete and missed SABs and ectopic pregnancies

    c. Size will decrease in complete SABs.

    d. Size greater than dates in 50% of GTN cases

  2. Cervical dilatation and effacement in inevitable SABs

  3. Presence of products of conception at cervical os or in the vaginal vault in incomplete SABs

  4. Nitrozine-positive fluid in vaginal vault in some cases of inevitable and incomplete SABs

  5. Unilateral sausage-like enlargement of adnexa, usually accompanied by tenderness, is sometimes palpable in ectopic pregnancies.

  6. Bright red, pedunculated growth, protruding from the cervical os, may be observed if cervical polyp is causing the bleeding.

  7. Cervical inflammation, erythema, friability, and leukorrhea may be seen in cervicitis.

  8. Suspect SAB if absence of fetal heart tones (FHTs) with Doppler in a pregnancy over 12 weeks by size and dates; 14 weeks in obese patients

C. Diagnostic tests

  1. Sonogram may indicate the presence or absence of a fetal sac, fetal heart pulsations, or "snowstorm" pattern (GTN). Fetal heart activity should be seen on a sonogram by four to six weeks of pregnancy.

  2. CBC or hemoglobin and hematocrit (H&H), serial quantitative hCG type and Rh(D) if unknown

  3. Cervical cultures for gonorrhea, chlamydia, and beta strep as necessary

  4. Coagulation studies in patients with missed SABs due to the potential of disseminated intravascular coagulation developing. This is especially important if it has been five or more weeks since the death of the fetus, or five months after last menstrual period.

IV. Management

A. Threatened SAB

  1. Bedrest until bleeding subsides

  2. Pelvic rest for at least two weeks after the bleeding has stopped

  3. Refrain from sexual intercourse.

  4. If bleeding continues or is accompanied by the passage of clots or tissues, do an ultrasound and refer to a physician.

B. Inevitable, incomplete, complete, or missed abortion

  1. Ultrasound

  2. Quantitative beta human chorionic gonadotropin (QBHCG) (PRN)

  3. Refer to physician's care as indicated.

C. Ectopic pregnancy

  1. Ultrasound

  2. Consult with or refer to physician as soon as suspected.

    D. If a patient with threatened SAB has resolution of her symptoms, continue routine prenatal care at 2-week intervals until normal uterine growth and FHTs are confirmed.

    E. If patient is Rh(D) negative and she has a threatened SAB, incomplete or complete SAB, or ectopic pregnancy, she should have an injection of Rh(D) immune globulin (RhoGAM) within 72 hours after the completion of the SAB or termination of ectopic pregnancy.

    F. If cervical polyps are present, consultation/referral to physician for treatment is indicated. Or a trained practitioner if comfortable and the stock is visible, may remove the polyp and send to pathology.

    G. Transfer to physician care all patients with vaginal bleeding during the first trimester when GTN is suspected or diagnosed.

    H. Follow-up includes:

        1. If threatened SAB resolves, then patient is seen routinely.

        2. Appropriate documentation on problem list and progress notes.

        3. For patients who have aborted, contraception needs to be discussed. It is best to wait for two to three menstrual cycles before becoming pregnant again.

V. Education

    A. Discuss the diagnostic tests that will be ordered and interpretation of results.

    B. If a threatened SAB, inform the patient that she has a 50% chance of maintaining the pregnancy.

    C. Inform the patient that she should call if she develops a fever, has foul-smelling discharge, has profuse or prolonged bleeding, has passage of tissue or clots, or develops abdominal or low back pain. She should save any tissue passed.

    D. If an SAB has occurred, educate the patient regarding the normal course of recovery from a SAB, and the need to have follow-up evaluation of her physical and psychological status.

    E. If an SAB has occurred, help the patient and her partner to work through any guilt or grief regarding their loss. Refer as necessary.

    F. Give information on the administration of RhoGAM if patient is Rh(D) negative.

BLEEDING IN PREGNANCY OVER 20 WEEKS' GESTATION

I. **Etiology.** Vaginal bleeding in a pregnancy that is over 20 weeks' gestation can be due to:

    A. Abruptio placenta (see guidelines)

        1. If bleeding is present, blood is usually dark, moderate in amount.

        2. Pain may range from vague to intense discomfort.

        3. Uterus increases in size as bleeding continues, ranges from mild irritability to extreme rigidity.

        4. Uterine tenderness may be absent, mild and localized, or marked and diffuse.

      5. FHT may be absent or difficult to auscultate.

  B. Placenta previa

      1. Painless hemorrhage

      2. Does not usually appear until near the end of the second trimester

      3. Blood usually bright red, may be slight to copious

      4. There is no uterine irritability, rigidity, or tenderness

  C. Cervical lesions

      1. Bleeding usually light

      2. History of vaginitis, cervicitis, polyps, condylomata, and so on

      3. Recent intercourse, which may cause spotting

  D. Bloody show

      1. Always a possibility at term

      2. Usually scant in amount, pinkish rather than bright red, and accompanied by mucous

  E. Uterine rupture

      1. Those at risk include:

         a. Women with a history of previous cesarean section or other uterine surgery

         b. Women with cephalopelvic disproportion (CPD) allowed to labor too long—the lower uterine segment continues to thin out as long as contractions continue and may rupture

         c. Improper use of oxytocin for induction or augmentation of labor—tetanic contractions may result in rupture

         d. Attempt at external or internal version

      2. The classic symptom is severe pain at time of a contraction, followed by sudden absence of pain and contractions.

II. **Management**

  A. History

      1. Type of bleeding

         a. Bright red—most likely with previa

         b. Dark brown—old blood, may be from earlier abruption or bloody show

         c. Serous—may indicate rupture of membranes

      2. Amount: If soaking more than two pads in an hour, needs immediate attention. Watch for shock.

      3. Weeks gestation

      4. Any pain? Most likely with abruption. Previa is characteristically painless.

  B. Physical exam

      1. Assess color and amount of bleeding.

      2. Do not do manual vaginal exams until the cause of the bleeding is determined. An exam may rupture a placental vessel if there is a placenta previa, and cause instant severe hemorrhage. Use ultrasound.

3. Assess vital signs, FHT, and signs of shock. Use external fetal monitor if bleeding significant.

4. Order CBC, clot tube to hold, pro time, platelets, and fibrinogen if bleeding is excessive.

5. Placenta previa and abruptio placenta can be diagnosed by ultrasound.

6. If the patient is not in labor and placenta previa has been ruled out, a careful speculum exam may be done to assess the condition of the cervix. If cervical infection/lesions are present, treat according to guidelines.

C. Consult with physician if:

1. There is any frank bleeding.

2. There are signs of fetal compromise or maternal shock.

3. The cause of the bleeding cannot be determined and/or treated by the nurse-midwife or practitioner.

D. If the situation is urgent:

1. Summon physician immediately.

2. Prepare for immediate cesarean section.

3. Start IV of lactated Ringer's solution with large-bore Intracath.

4. Treat signs of shock (See Postpartum Hemorrhage guidelines).

5. Keep flow sheet of vital signs, events, actions taken. Maintain continuous recording of FHT per monitor.

E. Treatment of the unsensitized Rh(D) negative patient

1. Give RhoGAM injection after each uterine bleeding episode.

2. Usual dose is one vial Rh(D) immune globulin, which is adequate for a transfusion of up to 15ml of fetal blood into the maternal circulation.

3. Dosage should be larger if it is possible that more than 15ml was transfused.

5. A Betke-Kleihauer test can be ordered to determine the amount of fetal blood in the maternal circulation.

 BREECH PRESENTATION

I. **Definition.** The presentation of the fetus in the uterus in which it is breech. The types are frank breech, complete breech, or footling breech.

II. **Etiology.** A breech presentation may be caused by some circumstance that prevents the normal version from taking place.

III. **Management**

A. Before 30 to 32 weeks: Insignificant

B. At 30 to 32 weeks: Incidence—14% of fetuses present breech

1. Discuss with the patient the implication of breech presentation now and at term.

    2. Discuss danger signs.

    3. Be sure patient knows that she should inform care providers that the baby is breech.

    4. Instruct patient in doing breech turning exercises.

C. At 36 weeks

    1. In most pregnancies, the fetus has assumed its final position by the 34th week.

    2. At term, only 3% to 4% of fetuses present in any position other than cephalic.

    3. Discuss pros and cons of vaginal breech delivery versus cesarean section.

    4. Refer to a physician to discuss options and make plans. An external version may be attempted at 37 weeks if primipara, and from 38 weeks to term in the multiparous patient. This needs to be done in the hospital, under ultrasound, with proper monitoring of patient and fetus.

 DIABETES MELLITUS IN PREGNANCY

I. **Definition.** A chronic disorder that is characterized by hyperglycemia, associated with major abnormalities in carbohydrate, fat, and protein metabolism. Patients with diabetes have a tendency to develop renal, ocular, neurologic, and premature cardiovascular diseases.

II. **Incidence.** Approximately 3 in 100 pregnancies

III. **Etiology**

A. Glucose metabolism in pregnancy

    1. The baby uses glucose from the mother's bloodstream at a constant rate. The pregnant woman may have hypoglycemia symptoms.

    2. The normal fasting blood sugar (FBS) in pregnancy is 65.

    3. One hour postprandial blood sugar (PP BS) is elevated after 20 weeks' because of the elevation of certain hormones that antagonize insulin and make it less effective.

    a. Human placental lactogen

    b. Cortisol

    c. Estrogen

    d. Progesterone

B. Insulin requirements change throughout pregnancy.

    1. In the first 20 weeks, insulin requirements drop because:

    a. The baby is using glucose from the mother's bloodstream at a constant rate, yet the hormones that antagonize insulin are not yet being produced in significant amounts.

    b. Nausea and vomiting are common, so the woman's food intake may be less than normal.

2. There is an ever-increasing need for insulin in the last 20 weeks. If the woman's pancreas cannot produce this extra insulin, the glucose from the food she eats cannot be used by her cells, resulting in hyperglycemia and ketosis.

C. Effect on the fetus

1. Because of hyperglycemia in the diabetic mother, the baby's pancreas is stimulated to hyperinsulinism, which enhances glycogen synthesis, lipogenesis, and protein synthesis, leading to macrosomia.

2. The woman may be relatively asymptomatic because it is common for pregnant women to complain of hunger, thirst, and polyuria. Yet without treatment, the baby is in jeopardy. Besides macrosomia, there is an increased incidence of perinatal complications, such as:

a. Stillbirths

b. Birth trauma

c. Neonatal hypoglycemia

IV. Clinical Features

A. Classification

1. Class A: Gestational

a. Diabetes mellitus induced by pregnancy, diagnosed on the basis of an abnormal glucose tolerance test (GTT)

b. Blood sugar returns to normal after the pregnancy ends.

c. 20% of average weight and 60% of overweight patients with gestational diabetes will develop diabetes mellitus later in life.

2. Class B: Overt, adult onset

a. Onset after age 20

b. Duration less than ten years

c. No evidence of vascular disease

3. Class C: Overt, teen onset

a. Duration 10 to 19 years

b. No evidence of vascular disease

4. Class D: Overt, childhood onset

a. Onset under age 10

b. Duration more than 20 years

c. Calcification of the vessels of the leg

d. Benign retinopathy

e. Hypertension

B. History

1. Family history of diabetes

2. Two or more spontaneous abortions

3. Stillbirth or unexplained neonatal death

4. Giving birth to a baby with macrosomia (>9.6 lb, 4500 g)
5. Giving birth to a baby with congenital anomalies
6. Polyhydramnios in a previous pregnancy
7. Hypertensive disorders in a previous pregnancy
8. Predisposition to infections, especially UTIs and monilia vaginitis

C. Contributing factors in present pregnancy:
   1. Obesity—any of the following:
      a. Being more than 30% overweight at the beginning of the pregnancy
      b. Reaching 200 lb at any time in the pregnancy
      c. A weight gain > 50 lb
   2. Glycosuria
   3. Polyhydramnios
   4. Hypertension
   5. Multiple gestation
   6. Frequent infections, especially UTIs and monilia vaginitis

V. **Diagnosis**

A. Fifty percent of class A diabetics can be diagnosed by history.
   1. Presence of one or more predisposing factors
   2. Signs and symptoms of diabetes
      a. Polyuria (excessive urinary output)
      b. Polydipsia (excessive thirst)
      c. Polyphagia (excessive hunger)
      d. Unexplained weight loss, especially in the presence of a large food intake. Or may see unexplained weight gain in the presence of a normal food intake.
      e. Weakness

B. The other 50% can be picked up by lab tests.
   1. Glycosuria on two consecutive occasions not related to carbohydrate intake warrants further investigation.
      a. One in ten such women have class A diabetes.
      b. The other nine in ten have glycosuria of pregnancy due to decreased kidney threshold for glucose.
   2. FBS and 2-hour PP BS, one-hour post 50 g Glucola load BS, and 3-hour GTT are other lab tests to assess carbohydrate metabolism. Abnormal levels are diagnostic of diabetes.
      a. When done at 20 weeks, 60% to 80% of women with class A diabetes will be detected.
      b. When done at 26 weeks, an even greater percentage will be detected.
      c. If only one test can be done, 24 to 26 weeks' gestation is the optimum compromise time.

    C. Overt diabetes is diagnosed on the basis of two or more FBSs of 105 or greater, two or more elevated values on a GTT, or 1-hour Glucola above 200.

VI. Management

  A. Lab tests

    1. Test the urine at each routine prenatal visit.

      a. If there is glycosuria, question the patient about her recent intake of refined carbohydrates.

      b. If only a trace of glycosuria and positive diet history:

        (1) Counsel regarding avoidance of refined carbohydrates.

        (2) Recheck at next visit.

      c. If more than trace of glycosuria times two, not diet-related, schedule for either a FBS and 2-hour PP BS or a 1-hour post 50 g Glucola load BS (see section A-3 below).

    2. On all pregnant patients, order a Glucola load BS or a 2-hour PP BS after a 50- or 100 g high carbohydrate diet for patients unable to do 50 g loading dose.

      a. Preferably between 24 and 28 weeks

      b. Immediately in the following situations:

        (1) History of stillborn or unexplained neonatal death

        (2) History of gestational diabetes

        (3) Sibling or parent with insulin-dependent diabetes

        (4) Two consecutive episodes of glycosuria unrelated to carbohydrate intake

        (5) Strong suspicion of diabetes, based on two or more predisposing factors, presence of symptoms, or both

    3. Order a 3-hour GTT and a hemoglobin A_1C if abnormal results are obtained from either a FBS, 2-hour PP BS or a 1-hour post 50 g Glucola load BS as ordered in #2 above. Results are considered abnormal if the following values are met or exceeded.

      a. FBS: 105 mg glucose/100 ml plasma

      b. 2-hour PP: 120

      c. 1-hour post 50 g Glucola: 140

      d. GTT

        (1) FBS: 105

        (2) 1-hour: 190

        (3) 2-hour: 165

        (4) 3-hour: 145

  B. Diagnosis is made on the basis of an abnormal GTT.

    1. If the GTT is grossly abnormal, the patient should be referred for physician management.

    2. If the GTT is mildly abnormal (two abnormal values, none above 200) consult with physician. Collaborative management is possible. Usual course:

    a. Put the patient on a 2200 to 2400 caloric diabetic diet. Offer referral to a dietitian. Tips for diet:

        (1) Eat 150 to 200 g carbohydrates (CHO) per day.

            (a) Eat only complex CHO: starches, bread, pasta, beans, potatoes.

            (b) Avoid all refined CHO: eat very little fruit.

            (c) Divide food evenly throughout the day; eat regular meals and snacks. Eat two sevenths of CHO in morning, two sevenths at lunch, two sevenths at dinner, and one seventh at bedtime.

        (2) Eat 100 to 150 g protein per day.

        (3) Eat 45 to 90g fat per day or about 35% of total calories.

C. Continuing management

    1. When possible, refer for home glucose/urine monitoring.

    2. Schedule the patient for a FBS and 2-hour PP BS after two weeks of being on the diet. The meal for the 2-hour PP BS should be the usual diabetic meal, not a high carbohydrate meal.

        a. If the blood sugars are normal, the patient can continue to be co-managed. About two thirds of women will be in this category.

        b. If the blood sugars are abnormal, consult. Physician referral is probably indicated.

        c. Start strict fetal activity count at 30 weeks.

        d. Nonstress test (NST) weekly after 32 to 34 weeks, biweekly after 36 weeks

        e. Plan to deliver baby at 37 to 39 weeks, before it is too large.

VII. Complications (seldom seen in class A diabetes)

  A. Maternal

    1. Polyhydramnios is common for unknown reasons; it can lead to premature rupture of membranes, respiratory distress.

    2. The likelihood of pre-eclampsia is increased times four.

    3. Infection occurs more often and is likely to be more severe.

    4. Cesarean section is much more common due to fetal macrosomia, fetal distress, and worsening of condition in the last weeks of pregnancy.

    5. Postpartum hemorrhage is more common.

    6. Vascular complications (e.g., proliferating retinopathy and nephropathy), especially in diabetics of long duration

  B. Fetal

    1. Intrauterine fetal death: Incidence is 3% to 12%.

    2. Neonatal morbidity

        a. Incidence is 4% to 7%.

        b. Causes

            (1) Hyperbilirubinemia: possibly due to prematurity

            (2) Macrosomia: may cause birth injury if delivery is vaginal.

(3) Hypoglycemia: due to sudden withdrawal of maternal hyperglycemia

(4) Hypocalcemia: due to asphyxia, prematurity, or a variety of other possibilities

(5) Idiopathic respiratory distress: Contributing factors are

   (a) High incidence of cesareans

   (b) Desirability of delivery before term to lessen mortality

   (c) Babies of diabetic mothers make a different, less efficient type of surfactant. The lecithin/sphingomyelin (L/S) ratio, which normally indicates lung maturity at 2:1, may be unreliable.

3. Fetal morbidity: 5% to 10% of those above class A have congenital malformations versus 3% normally; most common are ventral septal defects and neural disorders.

ECTOPIC PREGNANCY

I. **Definition.** Implantation of the blastocyst anywhere besides the endometrium. The site is usually in the most distal part of the fallopian tube.

II. **Incidence.** Occurs in one in 200 pregnancies in white women, one in 120 pregnancies in nonwhite women. Recurs in 7% to 20% of cases.

III. **Etiology**

A. Conditions that prevent or retard passage of the fertilized ovum to the uterus:

   1. Endosalpingitis (PID)
   2. Developmental anomalies
   3. Adhesions in the tube from previous surgeries, infections, IUD
   4. Tumors that distort the shape of the tube.
   5. Menstrual reflux
   6. Hormonal factors that slow peristalsis of the tube.

B. Increase in receptivity of the tubal mucosa of the fertilized ovum (e.g., endometriosis)

IV. **Clinical Course.** If not diagnosed and removed, will eventually rupture. Signs and symptoms are as follows:

A. Before rupture

   1. Amenorrhea, then continuous intermittent spotting. May be subtle, so that the spotting appears to be a normal menstrual period.
   2. Pelvic, abdominal pain, sometimes neck/shoulder pain
   3. Soft pliable mass palpated in adnexa. Mass may be firm if distended with blood.
   4. Uterus does enlarge due to the placental hormones, may be normal size for gestation. May be displaced to one side.
   5. Nausea, vomiting less common than usual. Diarrhea more common than usual.

6. Positive pregnancy test but may be negative up to 50% of the time due to suboptimal placental function.

7. Acute abdominal pain—may be anywhere in the abdomen.

B. After rupture

1. Sudden, severe, sharp, lower abdominal pain

2. Hypotension and signs of shock depending on amount of internal bleeding; can lose large amounts quickly.

3. Abdominal pain and cervical motion tenderness

4. Blood in the cul-de-sac

5. Pain in the neck and shoulder, especially on inspiration, due to irritation of diaphragm from blood in the peritoneal cavity

V. Differential Diagnosis

A. Spontaneous abortion

1. More bleeding

2. Less pain

3. No adnexal mass palpated

4. Lower incidence of shock

5. Products of conception may be expelled and found on speculum exam or in the toilet.

B. PID

1. History of previous infection

2. Amenorrhea rare

3. Pain is bilateral, not unilateral

4. Fever usually greater than 101°F

C. Ovarian cyst

1. Normal menses

2. Pain uncommon

3. Mass smooth and mobile

4. Uterus feels nonpregnant.

D. Appendicitis

1. Nausea, vomiting, fever almost always present

2. No signs and symptoms of pregnancy

3. Pelvic exam normal

4. Pain in epigastrium, not neck and shoulder

5. Presence of McBurney's sign

VI. Management

A. See guidelines for Bleeding Under 20 Weeks' Gestation.

B. Ultrasound

C. See that all unsensitized Rh(D)-negative patients receive Rh(D) immune globulin, one vial, IM within 72 hours of rupture or removal to prevent possible sensitization from an Rh(D) positive fetus.

D. Refer to physician. Treatment is usually surgical. Methotrexate may be tried in early pregnancies.

    E. Inform patient that there is a 7% to 20% risk for repeat ectopic pregnancy.

 EDEMA IN PREGNANCY

I. Etiology

    A. High estrogen levels make the blood vessels more fragile and "leaky."

    B. Impaired venous circulation and increased venous pressure in the lower extremities due to:

        1. Pressure of the enlarging uterus on the pelvic veins when sitting or standing.

        2. Pressure of the enlarging uterus on the vena cava when supine.

    C. Increased venous pressure may also be due to the expanding blood volume of pregnancy.

II. Clinical Features

    A. Physiologic edema is dependent.

        1. Usually seen in the feet and ankles after being upright, and decreases with leg elevation or bedrest.

        2. May be seen in the sacrum if on bedrest

        3. Not usually seen in the face or hands

    B. Very common in pregnancy and may be a sign of well-being because it indicates an expanding blood volume

III. Differential Diagnosis

    A. Pre-eclampsia

        1. Usually more severe than physiologic edema

        2. Sudden onset

        3. Generalized body edema, particularly in face and hands

        4. Present even after bedrest, limb elevation, or both

        5. Look for other signs and symptoms:

            a. High blood pressure

            b. Proteinuria

            c. Brisk deep tendon reflexes (DTRs)

            d. Elevated hematocrit, decreased platelets

    B. High sodium intake: Salt should not be restricted during pregnancy, but consuming an excessive amount may result in edema.

        1. May see generalized, nondependent edema

        2. History of high sodium intake from foods such as ham, potato chips, pretzels; habit of oversalting food

IV. Management

    A. When a patient presents with edema, make a differential diagnosis.

        1. Assess characteristics of edema.

            a. Onset

            b. Severity

    c. Relieved by bedrest, limb elevation, or both

  2. Diet history: recent high sodium intake

  3. History of prolonged standing or sitting

  4. Habit of wearing tight waistbands or stockings, which further constrict the circulation

  5. Look for signs and symptoms of pre-eclampsia.

B. If diagnosis is physiologic edema:

  1. Avoid constrictive clothing.

  2. Lie down and elevate legs periodically throughout the day to aid venous return.

  3. Elastic stockings may aid venous return. Put them on before arising in the morning.

  4. Take rest periods lying on the left side to keep the uterus off the vena cava and aid venous return.

  5. Avoid excessive sodium in the diet.

  6. Call office if edema suddenly becomes more severe or generalized, in spite of the above measures.

ENDOMETRITIS

I. **Definition.** Endometritis is the infection of the endometrium, decidua, and myometrium of the uterus after delivery.

II. **Etiology**

A. Bacteria invade the area after delivery and spread rapidly.

B. Sources of bacteria may be any one or a combination of:

  1. Endogenous vaginal bacteria, usually pathogenic only when tissue is damaged or devitalized

    a. Beta hemolytic streptococcus

    b. *Streptococcus viridans*

    c. *Neisseria gonococcus*

    d. *Gardnerella*

  2. Contamination by normal bowel bacteria

    a. *Clostridium welchii*

    b. *Escherichia coli*

    c. *Proteus mirabilis*

    d. *Aerobacter aerogenes*

    e. *Enterococcus*

    f. *Pseudomonas aeruginosa*

    g. *Klebsiella pneumonia*

  3. Contamination from environment. Staphylococcus is a common organism.

III. **Clinical Features**

A. Predisposing causes

  1. Extensive tissue edema

2. Prolonged labor
3. Prolonged rupture of membranes
4. Numerous vaginal exams in labor
5. Breaks in aseptic technique
6. Careless hand washing
7. Any intrauterine manipulation: placement of intrauterine catheter, internal rotation, or manual removal of the placenta.
8. Retained placental fragments or membranes
9. Operative delivery
10. Improper perineal care, leading to contamination by gastrointestinal bacteria
11. Malnutrition, debilitation, anemia, excessive blood loss
12. Pre-existing infection

B. Signs and symptoms
1. Fever and chills
   a. Fever between 100.4°F and 104°F, depending on severity of infection
   b. Temperature is often low grade for several days then spikes.
   c. Chills indicate severe infection.
2. Tachycardia between 100 and 140, depending on severity of infection
3. Uterine signs and symptoms
   a. Tenderness extending laterally
   b. Prolonged or recurrent afterbirth pains
   c. Subinvolution
   d. Slight abdominal distention
   e. Abnormalities of lochia
      (1) May be scant and odorless if anaerobic infection
      (2) May be moderately heavy, foul, bloody, seropurulent if aerobic infection
4. Onset usually three to five days after delivery unless caused by beta hemolytic streptococcus. Then onset is earlier and more precipitous.
5. Elevated WBC more than usual for postpartum; greater than 25,000

IV. **Differential Diagnosis** (See Puerperal Infection guidelines)

V. **Management**
A. If history/signs/symptoms consistent with endometritis:
1. Perform sterile speculum exam.
   a. Observe character and odor of lochia.
   b. Obtain cultures as necessary of cervix and to rule out STDs.
2. Perform sterile bimanual exam.
   a. Assess uterus for unusual tenderness

        b. Assess uterus for bogginess.

   3. Obtain CBC if febrile.

   4. Antibiotic treatment pending culture results:

        a. Ampicillin 500mg orally four times a day for ten days if not allergic

        b. If allergic to penicillin and not breast-feeding, doxycycline 100mg orally every 12 hours for seven days

        c. If allergic to penicillin and breast-feeding, Keflex 500mg orally four times a day for seven days.

   5. If uterus boggy and/or bleeding excessive, prescribe Methergine 0.2mg orally every four hours for six doses. *Do not* give Methergine if patient is hypertensive.

   6. Instruct patient to take temperature four times a day for the next week. It should be below 100°F within 48 hours of starting antibiotics.

   7. Instruct patient to drink three liters of fluid daily and increase rest.

   8. Obtain results of cultures, both preliminary and final. Patient needs to be on antibiotic to which organism is sensitive. Check safety of antibiotic during breast-feeding.

   9. Patient should be instructed to call if symptoms do not resolve within 24 hours, or if they worsen. If no significant improvement within two to three days, patient may need to be admitted to hospital for treatment. Otherwise, follow up by telephone or office visit within three days.

B. Consult with physician in the following situations:

   1. Symptoms do not resolve or worsen within 24 hours.

   2. Temperature does not go below 100°F after 48 hours on antibiotics.

C. Prevention and early detection of endometritis

   1. Encourage good nutrition during pregnancy.

   2. Prevent or treat anemia.

   3. Try to avoid overexhaustion in labor.

   4. If membranes have ruptured:

        a. Confirm with a sterile speculum exam unless in active labor.

        b. Do not perform vaginal exams if there is no labor.

        c. Minimize vaginal exams as much as possible if the patient is in active labor.

   5. Avoid unnecessary vaginal exams whether membranes are ruptured or not.

   6. Take patient's temperature at least every four hours in active labor, every two hours if membranes are ruptured.

   7. Observe careful aseptic technique.

        a. Keep field as sterile as possible.

        b. Place a sterile drape under patient's hips before delivery.

        c. Avoid rectal contamination of the vaginal area.

    d. Change gloves between delivery of the baby and internal inspection and suturing.

8. Assess placenta for intactness.

    a. Watch for signs of infection if possible retained fragments or membranes.

    b. Do uterine exploration if probable retained fragments or membranes.

9. Avoid extensive manipulation of tissue while suturing.

10. Instruct patient in good perineal care.

    a. Wipe from front to back.

    b. Remove peri pad from front to back.

    c. Change peri pad at least every four hours.

    d. Wash vulva daily and as necessary.

11. Instruct patient in postpartum care.

    a. If patient feels she has a temperature, have her take temperature. Call if temperature reaches 101°F or exceeds 100.4°F twice four hours apart.

    b. Instruct patient to call if lochia begins to smell foul, uterine tenderness develops, or cramping increases.

ESTABLISHING THE ESTIMATED DATE OF CONFINEMENT (EDC)

I. **Definition.** The estimated date of confinement (EDC) is usually 280 days, or 40 weeks after the last normal menstrual period (LNMP). It also may be calculated as 266 days, or 38 weeks from the last ovulation in a normal 28-day cycle. The EDC can be determined mathematically by using Nägele's rule: subtract three from the month of the LNMP and add seven days.

II. **Clinical Features**

    A. History

        1. Menstrual history

            a. Length of cycles

            b. Regularity of cycles

            c. Recent menstrual history affected by:

                (1) Recent previous pregnancy, cycles not yet re-established

                (2) Breast-feeding

                (3) BCPs, DMPA

                (4) Disease, trauma

                (5) Malnutrition, eating disorders

        2. First day of last menstrual period

            a. Was it a normal period? If not, was the previous period normal?

            b. Is the exact date known, or is only a general time frame known?

        3. Contraceptive history

       a. Contraceptive method patient was using

       b. Was this method being used correctly and consistently?

   4. Sexual history

       a. Has there been regular sexual intercourse in the recent past?

       b. Have there only been isolated incidences of intercourse that could pinpoint a possible conception date?

       c. Does the patient have any idea when conception might have occurred?

   5. Fertility history

       a. Was this pregnancy planned?

       b. If so, how long did she try to conceive?

       c. What is her past pregnancy history?

   6. Symptoms of pregnancy

       a. Nausea/vomiting

       b. Breast changes, tenderness

       c. Urinary frequency

       d. Fatigue

       e. Unexplained weight gain

       f. Fetal movement

B. Physical signs

   1. Bimanual palpation of uterine size, shape, consistency in first trimester

   2. First documented FHTs expected at ten to 12 weeks with fetal Doptone and 18 to 20 weeks with fetoscope

   3. Uterine measurements and growth trend

III. Lab and Adjunctive Studies

A. Was a pregnancy test done? If so:

   1. When was it first positive?

   2. If ever negative, when was it last negative?

   3. Was it a urine test or a blood test?

B. Order a sonogram if dates are unclear by the above evaluation.

C. Indications for change of menstrual EDC to ultrasound EDC:

   1. Unsure of LNMP, or had abnormal LMP

   2. Size agrees with ultrasound

   3. Ultrasound EDC is different from EDC indicated by LNMP by seven days first trimester and ten days until 28 weeks.

 FETAL HEART TONES

I. **Definition.** Heart tones of the fetus normally heard through the mother's abdomen. The normal rate is between 120 and 160 beats per minute.

II. **Clinical Features**

   A. FHTs can first be heard via Doptone at 10 to 12 weeks.

1. If the FHT cannot be heard with the Doptone at 12 weeks by size and dates, the patient should return at 14 weeks. If at that time the FHTs are not heard, an ultrasound scan should be done to confirm fetal viability. If any abnormal results are obtained, consult with physician.

2. FHT should be taken and recorded at every prenatal visit.

B. FHT can first be heard via fetoscope at about 18 to 20 weeks, verifying the EDC.

III. Management: Monitoring FHT in Labor

A. All patients should have a 10- to 15-minute fetal monitor strip on admission.

B. Fetal monitoring should be used in the following situations:

1. Patient request
2. Postdates
3. Polyhydramnios
4. Intrauterine fetal growth retardation
5. Hypertension
6. Significant anemia (Hct <27%, HBG <9.0)
7. Unusual vaginal bleeding
8. Abnormal fetal-placental tests (e.g., low estriols, positive OCT, etc.)
9. Premature labor
10. Twins
11. Abnormal FHT per auscultation or Doptone
12. Prostaglandins, misoprostol or Prepidil for cervical ripening
13. Pitocin induction or augmentation of labor
14. Vaginal birth after cesarean (VBAC)

C. The internal scalp electrode (ISE) monitor is more accurate than the external monitor.

1. Situations in which the external monitor is adequate include:

   a. When the FHT reading via the external monitor is adequate and within normal limits

   b. Until the membranes have ruptured or until it is reasonable to rupture them to apply the internal monitor

2. Situations in which the ISE is recommended:

   a. Non-reassuring fetal heart patterns

   b. After membranes are ruptured in all situations in section III B

3. Situations in which the ISE is *not* recommended, unless benefits outweigh risks:

   a. Bleeding disorders, for example, potential for hemophilia in the fetus, factor IX deficiency in the mother, etc.

   b. History of group B streptococcus, genital herpes, untreated vaginitis

   c. Individuals with HIV/AIDS

D. A Doptone may be used to listen to FHT in all laboring women.

    1. According to the guidelines of the American College of Obstetricians and Gynecologists, FHT should be assessed in labor according to the following schedule:

        a. Every 15 minutes in first stage of active labor

        b. Every five minutes in second stage of active labor

        c. More often if abnormalities are heard

    2. Listen to FHTs for at least one minute just before and just after a contraction.

 FETAL MOVEMENT

I. **Definition.** The movement of the fetus starting as early as six weeks. Most women do not detect it until 16 to 20 weeks gestation. Another name for the first perception of fetal movement is quickening.

II. **Clinical Features**

    A. Fetal movement should be detected by the 18th week of gestation by a multipara and by the 22nd week gestation by a primigravida.

    B. Fetal movement is highly idiosyncratic; some babies are more active than others.

    C. Babies normally have activity cycles in utero, which may correspond to sleep–awake cycles. By paying attention to the time and number of movements, the mother may become aware of a pattern of alternating stillness and activity.

    D. Smoking decreases baby's movements.

    E. Fetal movement may slow normally in amount and/or strength in the last month of pregnancy due to decreased room in the uterus, but should still occur in regular patterns and at more than ten movements per day.

III. **Management**

    A. Near the beginning of the second trimester, ask patients if they have perceived fetal movement.

        1. If so, attempt to determine the date of quickening.

        2. If not, instruct the patient to note the date movement is first felt.

    B. The date of the first perceived fetal movement can be used to help assess the EDC.

    C. If the patient is over 24 weeks and expresses concern that the baby is not moving enough:

        1. Educate her regarding the physiologic principles of fetal activity.

        2. Have the patient count movements for one hour or until ten movements have been reached.

        3. If the patient is a smoker, she needs to refrain for one hour.

        4. The best time to count is from seven to ten o'clock PM when baby is usually the most active.

        5. If the baby moves four times or more in 60 minutes, well-being is assured.

6. If the baby moves less than four times in 60 minutes, the patient should have something to eat, drink two to three glasses of cold water, and recount for another hour. If the baby still does not move four times in 60 minutes, the patient should call.

7. The patient should have an NST. If reactive, well-being is assured. If nonreactive, consult with physician.

D. High-risk patients should be advised to keep a fetal movement log in the following situations:

1. Postdates

2. Hypertension

3. History of stillbirth or intrauterine fetal growth retardation

4. Gestational diabetes

5. FHTs heard below 120 in the office

6. At any time the patient expresses concern about fetal movement

 GRAND MULTIPARITY

I. **Definition.** A grand multipara is a woman who has given birth to five or more children.

II. **Clinical Features**

A. Potential antepartum complication

1. Anemia, especially if pregnancies spaced less than a year apart

2. Obesity

3. Hypertension

4. Placenta previa

B. Intrapartum and postpartum

1. Abnormal presentation

2. Precipitous labor, delivery, or both

3. Dystocias of labor due to poor muscle tone

4. Large-for-gestation-age infant with attendant problems at delivery (e.g., shoulder dystocia)

5. Postpartum hemorrhage

III. **Management**

A. At the initial visit, ascertain gravidity and parity. Ask specifically whether any of the complications in section II above were present with previous pregnancies.

B. Usual management plan

1. Antepartum

a. Be alert for potential problems.

b. Plan for birth in hospital, not birth center.

c. If previous history of large babies, plan delivery at term to avoid macrosomia.

d. If previous history of precipitous labor and/or delivery:

      (1) Instruct patient/couple to go to the hospital at the first sign of labor.

      (2) Instruct patient/couple in emergency childbirth management.

    e. Discuss family planning with patient/couple.

2. Intrapartum

    a. Be sure on-call physician is notified of patient's admission to the hospital.

    b. Prophylactic IV or heparin lock recommended

3. Postpartum

    a. Be alert for potential postpartum hemorrhage in first 24 hours.

    b. Consider prophylactic oxytocin IV immediately after delivery of the placenta.

 HELLP SYNDROME

I. **Definition.** A syndrome in pregnancy that includes hypertension with hemolysis, elevated liver enzymes and low platelets.

II. **Etiology.** Arteriolar vasospasm is considered the underlying factor. Lesions develop in the endothelial layer of the small blood vessels as a result of vasospasm. Platelets aggregate at the site of the lesion. Red blood cells are forced through the sieve-like structure due to increased pressure, resulting in red blood cell fragments and hyperbilirubinemia. Thrombocytopenia is seen as platelets are consumed in the microcirculation.

III. **Clinical Features**

  A. Arteriolar vasospasm

    1. Decreased cerebral blood flow

      a. Headaches

      b. Scotoma

    2. Hypertension

    3. Decreased uterine blood flow

      a. Intrauterine fetal growth retardation (IUFGR)

      b. Intrapartum fetal hypoxia

      c. Fetal demise

  B. Endothelial damage

    1. Microangiopathic hemolytic anemia

      a. Platelet consumption

      b. Thrombocytopenia

    2. Red cell destruction

      a. Decreased Hct

      b. Hyperbilirubinemia

    3. Glomerular damage

       a. Proteinuria

       b. Oliguria: increased blood urea nitrogen and creatinine

    4. Hepatic congestion

       a. Right upper quadrant pain

       b. Increased serum glutamic-oxaloacetic transaminase (SGOT), decreased serum glutamic-pyruvic transaminase (SGPT)

       c. Decreased blood glucose

C. Incidence: Occurs in 4% to 12% of severe pre-eclamptic and/or eclamptic patients and is associated with poor maternal and fetal outcome

D. Occurrence: Often rapid onset after 28 weeks' of pregnancy

E. Signs and symptoms

    1. Hypertension

    2. Edema

    3. Proteinuria

    4. Fatigue

    5. Nausea, vomiting. or both

    6. Epigastric or right upper quadrant pain

F. Lab work

    1. CBC with platelet count. Decreased hematocrit and thrombocytopenia are diagnostic.

    2. SMAC-20, lab values will show hyperbilirubinemia, increased SGOT, increased blood urea nitrogen and creatinine and a decreased blood glucose.

    3. Urine dip and catheterized specimen will reveal proteinuria, 24-hour urine will have excessive protein.

G. Management

    1. Refer to physician.

    2. Conservative approach is contraindicated in a patient with HELLP; she must be delivered expeditiously to prevent potentially irreversible complications for the mother or fetal demise.

 ## HYDATIDIFORM MOLE

I. **Definition.** A developmental tumor of the placenta, originating in the trophoblastic cells that develop into the placenta. The trophoblastic cells are fast growing and invasive, like cancer. It is believed that most spontaneously abort in the first trimester.

II. **Incidence**

    A. Occurs in 1 in 200 pregnancies in the United States

    B. Recurs in 2% of women who have had them

    C. Women over 45 have a ten times greater incidence.

    D. Two to eight percent of molar pregnancies are malignant.

III. **Clinical Features**

A. Signs and symptoms

1. Can appear to be a normal pregnancy

2. Great increase in human chorionic gonadotropin (hCG) levels due to rapid proliferation of placental cells, which excrete hCG

3. Hyperemesis gravidarum in 30% of these patients because the increased placental tissue overstimulates the corpus luteum and there is increased hormone production.

4. Uterus often large for dates because mole grows fast

5. Often enlarged, tender ovaries

6. No FHT

7. Irregular painless bleeding in most by 12th week. May be continuous or intermittent, usually brownish, not heavy.

8. Pre-eclampsia before 24 weeks

9. May be anemic secondary to blood loss and/or poor nutrition due to hyperemesis

B. Diagnosis

1. Can be diagnosed by ultrasound

2. Passage of pieces of mole-the chorionic villi, which have developed into grape-like vesicles and can break off and be expelled vaginally

IV. **Management**

A. See section on first-trimester bleeding.

B. Refer to physician. Mole needs to be removed.

C. Hydatidiform mole is usually benign but can become malignant trophoblastic disease.

1. Types of malignant trophoblastic disease

a. Choriocarcinoma: Metastasizes quickly early in pregnancy. Fastest growing cancer known; therefore, highly responsive to chemotherapy.

b. Chorioadenoma: Does not metastasize fast. Curable with hysterectomy if still confined to uterus.

2. Follow-up treatment of hydatidiform moles after removal:

a. Monitor serum hCG levels biweekly till negative, then monthly for one year. The woman should be encouraged not to become pregnant again until after a year of negative levels.

b. If patient is Rh(D) negative, she needs RhoGAM.

c. If malignant, refer for chemotherapy.

 HYPEREMESIS GRAVIDARUM

I. **Definition.** Persistent nausea and vomiting during pregnancy that interferes with fluid intake and nutrition; onset usually before the 20th week of gestation; is severe enough to produce weight loss, fluid and electrolyte imbalance.

II. **Etiology.** Occurrence in 1.3% of pregnant women. Unknown etiology despite numerous studies.

III. **Clinical Features**

   A. History: Usually occurs in first trimester; may continue throughout the entire pregnancy

   B. Sign and Symptoms
   1. Dysgeusia (bad taste in mouth)
   2. Ptyalism (Excess saliva)
   3. Nausea
   4. Emesis
   5. Weight loss greater than 5%

   C. Lab tests
   1. Ketonuria
   2. Elevated hematocrit
   3. Metabolic Alkalosis
   4. Hyponatremia, hypokalemia, hypochloremia
   5. Mild to moderate hepatic and renal abnormalities

IV. **Management**

   A. IV Fluids D5 1/2NS with 10 mEq KCL and 100 mg Pyridoxine (B_6) —first liter to run rapidly then run at 250 cc per hour. Reassess in 24 hours.

   B. NPO for 24 to 48 hours

   C. Diet after 24 to 48 hours
   1. Clear fluids: start with 1/4 cup every 15 minutes and increase as tolerated
   2. Bratt/bland diet: Start with dry toast, crackers, rice or dry potato and increase as tolerated

   D. Laboratory tests
   1. Complete blood count
   2. BUN, creatinine, electrolytes and thyroid panel, hectobacteria, pylori screen, liver panel
   3. Other tests as needed
      a. Amylase, lipase to rule out pancreatitis
      b. Hepatitis panel to rule out hepatitis
      c. Toxicology screen to rule out substance abuse

   E. Ultrasound to rule out molar pregnancy

   F. Antiemetics
   1. Phenergan, 25 mg IM IV or orally
   2. Zofran 4 to 8mg IV orally or titrated subcutaneously
   3. Reglan 10mg IV, orally or titrated subcutaneously

   G. Hyperalimentation: May be used as needed for severe cases.

HYPERTENSION DURING PREGNANCY

I. **Definition**

   A. An increase of 30 mmHg systolic or 15 mmHg diastolic over base-line BP readings

   B. A BP reading of greater than 140/90

   C. The elevated readings occur on two occasions at least six hours apart.

II. **Clinical Features**

   A. Classification

   1. Chronic hypertensive disease: The presence of persistent hypertension, BP greater than 140/90 before pregnancy or before the 20th week of gestation

   2. Pregnancy-induced hypertension (PIH): The development of hypertension during pregnancy or within the first 24 hours after delivery in a previously normotensive woman. No other evidence of pre-eclampsia or hypertensive vascular disease is seen. The BP goes no higher than 150/100 with activity, rapidly returns to normal with rest, and returns to normotensive levels within ten days postpartum.

   3. Pre-eclampsia: The development of hypertension with proteinuria, excessive edema, or both. It occurs after 20 weeks' gestation. More common with:

      a. Primigravidas, especially if under 17 or over 35

      b. Family history of pre-eclampsia

      c. Multiple gestation

      d. Hydatidiform mole

   4. Eclampsia: The occurrence of convulsions in a patient with pre-eclampsia

   5. Superimposed pre-eclampsia or eclampsia: The development of pre-eclampsia or eclampsia in a woman with chronic hypertensive vascular disease or renal disease.

   6. HELLP syndrome (See HELLP Syndrome)

   B. Signs and symptoms of pre-eclampsia

   1. Hypertension: Increase of 30 mmHg systolic or 15 mmHg diastolic

   2. Marked hyperreflexia, especially with transient or sustained ankle clonus

   3. Edema of the face

   4. Visual disturbances

   5. Drowsiness or severe headaches (forerunner of convulsion)

   6. A sharp increase in the amount of proteinuria (5 g or more in a 24-hour specimen or 3 to 4+ dipstix)

   7. Oliguria: Urine output less than 30 mL/hr or less than 500 ml/24 hours

   8. Epigastric pain due to liver distention

III. Management

A. Initial history

    1. Be alert to any history of:

        a. Previous abruption

        b. Premature labor

        c. IUFGR

        d. Stillbirth

        e. Hypertension when on BCPs

        f. Family history of hypertension

        g. Pre-eclampsia in a previous pregnancy

        h. Previous hypertension, now resolved

    2. Consult with physician if history reveals any of the following:

        a. Two or more consecutive episodes of premature labor, IUFGR, or stillbirth

        b. Chronic hypertension

        a. Severe pre-eclampsia or eclampsia

B. Any patient with a questionably elevated BP at the prenatal visit

    1. Position the patient on her left side for 5 minutes.

    2. Retake the BP before a diagnosis is assumed.

C. If a patient's BP starts rising, institute the following:

    1. Advise rest on the left side four to six hours a day in addition to her regular night's sleep.

    2. Stop work if still working.

    3. Recommend daily BP checks. If patient, her family, or a friend cannot do, refer for home BP monitoring.

    4. Give fetal movement log and instruct in use.

    5. Schedule for biweekly NST.

    6. Inform of danger signs with instructions to call if any appear:

        a. Headache unrelieved by Tylenol and rest in a dark room

        b. Visual changes

        c. Sudden severe increase in weight and/or edema

        d. Drastic decrease in urine output despite usual intake.

        e. Epigastric pain

    7. Diet counseling

    8. Increase frequency of office visits; see weekly or biweekly.

D. If hypertension (by definition) develops:

    1. Review history, question regarding presence of any abnormal symptoms.

    2. Conduct physical exam.

        a. Check DTRs for clonus.

        b. Check retinal fundi.

        c. Observe for excessive edema, especially of the hands and face.

3. Obtain blood workup.
   a. SMAC
      (1) Uric acid: elevated in pre-eclampsia but not in chronic hypertension. Significant if greater than 6.
      (2) Elevated SGOT
   b. CBC
      (1) An elevated Hct may be caused by hemoconcentration
      (2) Platelet count, if low, may indicate vascular damage.
4. Urine workup
   a. Dipstix of 3+ to 4+ protein is significant and needs further study.
   b. If catheterized specimen has any protein, further study is required.
   c. Twenty-four-hour urine will test kidney function.
      (1) Total volume should never be less than 500 ml if collected correctly.
      (2) Total protein should not be over 5 g.
      (3) Creatinine, creatinine clearance
5. Consult with physician to develop a plan of management. Treatment of choice is delivery if near term.
6. If patient has seizure:
   a. Have someone summon physician immediately.
   b. Protect woman from harming herself.
   c. Give Valium 10 mg IV slowly (over one to two minutes).
   d. Give $MgSO_4$ 2 g IV push, slowly over two to three minutes.
   e. Monitor vital signs immediately after.

E. Prevention
   1. Good prenatal care
      a. Encourage regular visits.
      b. Check weight, BP and urine at each prenatal visit.
   2. Encourage a good diet including:
      a. Adequate weight gain: 20 to 40 lb
      b. Well-balanced, high-protein diet

 INTRAUTERINE FETAL GROWTH RETARDATION (IUFGR)

I. **Definition.** A condition in which a fetus shows clinical evidence of abnormal or dysfunctional growth

II. **Etiology**
   A. Maternal: Alcoholism or drug abuse
   B. Heavy smoking greater than one pack per day
   C. Hypertension or renal disease

    D. Systemic disease, such as cardiac disease

    E. Rubella or other viral infection

    F. History of previous small-for-gestational-age baby

    G. Severe malnutrition

    H. Poor weight gain pattern

III. Clinical Features

    A. Types

        1. Symmetric growth retardation: growth is proportional but slow.

        2. Asymmetric: To protect itself, the fetus shunts more food to the brain and other vital organs. The biparietal diameter is at least 2 cm larger than the chest.

    B. Inadequate maternal weight gain: less than ten lb in the first half of pregnancy and less than two lb per month in the second half

    C. Size/date discrepancy of concern

        1. If size seemed consistent with dates earlier in the pregnancy and dates are thought to be reliable

        2. If fundal height is 2 cm below the estimated gestational age in weeks

    D. Suspect trisomy 18 if IUFGR is found in first half of pregnancy.

IV. Differential Diagnosis

    A. Inaccurate fundal measurement

    B. Inaccurate dates

    C. Oligohydramnios (can be diagnosed by ultrasound)

    D. Transverse lie

    E. Small but normal fetus. Suspect this if patient is small-boned, five foot tall, with a prepregnant weight of less than 100 lb.

V. Management

    A. If suspect

        1. Will need serial ultrasounds to confirm

        2. If initial ultrasound shows size appropriate for dates and no body-head discrepancy, reassure family that all is within normal limits and no further action is needed.

        3. If initial ultrasound shows size small for dates or other discrepancy, such as mild oligohydramnios or low total intrauterine volume, repeat ultrasound in one to two weeks.

        4. Doppler flow studies can be used to check maternal–fetal–placental unit.

    B. If IUFGR is suspected or confirmed by ultrasound, consult with physician. Collaborative management is possible.

    C. Management after diagnosis of IUFGR

        1. Treat underlying cause if known.

        2. If patient is a smoker, urge her to quit.

        3. Evaluate diet for adequate protein, calories.

        4. Increase rest, fluids.

5. Instruct patient to keep daily fetal movement log and call if movements not adequate.

6. Biweekly nonstress tests with office visits

7. Obtain fasting blood sugar and 2-hour PP blood sugar to assess carbohydrate metabolism.

8. May need serial ultrasounds to monitor fetal growth.

9. Consult with physician regarding the best time to induce this patient. Early delivery is preferred.

10. Fetal monitor is mandatory in labor.

11. Notify pediatrician or neonatal nurse practitioner of admission to labor and delivery.

 ISOIMMUNIZATION

I. **Definition**

A. Rh isoimmunization is caused by maternal antibody production in response to exposure to fetal RBC antigens of the Rh group, including C, D, and E. The maternal antibody response may cross the placenta, potentially destroying fetal RBCs, causing anemia, and may result in erythroblastosis fetalis.

B. ABO group O–positive women have anti-A and anti-B isoagglutination, which may cause hemolytic disease in the newborn. Group O–negative women have neither A nor B and their newborns are born without problems.

C. Over 400 other red cell antigens have been identified. While most have little clinical importance, some are significant and in pregnancy may affect the developing fetus. Some are:

1. Moderate to severe disease

   a. Kell system: K,k antigens

   b. Duffy system: FY2 (Fyb does not cause problems)

   c. Kidd system: Jka, Jkb antigens

2. Mild hemolytic disease

   a. Kell system: K, Ko, Kpb antigens

   b. Diego system: Dia, Dib antigens

   c. MNSs system: M, N antigens

3. Without problems: Lewis system—All antigens

II. **Incidence**

A. Rh or D isoimmunization has been reported in 2% of primiparous patients at the time of delivery. Seven percent more will have anti-D six months postpartum, and 7% more will go on to develop sensitization in subsequent pregnancies. RhoGAM has reduced these figures when given at the recommended times.

B. The CDE antigen groupings have racial differences.

1. Thirteen percent of white Americans are negative.

2. Seven percent of African Americans are negative.

      3. One percent of Native Americans, those of Chinese descent, and other Asians are negative.

  C. ABO: The mother is O positive, the fetus is A, B, or AB.

      1. Twenty percent of all infants have an ABO incompatibility.

      2. Five percent of newborns will show signs of hemolytic disease.

      3. The later the onset of signs and symptoms, the less severe the problem for the newborn

III. Clinical Features

  A. Maternal and fetal blood rarely mix, however, mixing can occur during the following incidents, which can result in sensitization:

      1. At time of delivery, especially if accompanied by manual removal of the placenta or other manipulative procedures that result in increased mixing of maternal and fetal blood

      2. During pregnancy, probably due to breaks in the fetal and/or maternal circulation, which result in transfusion of fetal blood to the maternal circulation. It should be suspected if an amniocentesis is performed and in any case of uterine bleeding in pregnancy, such as placenta previa or abruptio placenta.

      3. Induced and spontaneous abortions

      4. Ectopic pregnancy

      5. Trauma

  B. If natural antibodies gain access to the fetal circulation, they act as hemolysins to the fetal erythrocytes. Danger to the fetus varies with degree of severity.

      1. In less severe cases, the fetus has jaundice either at birth or soon after due to erythroblastosis with possible resulting kernicterus and/or anemia.

      2. In severe cases, the fetus develops hydrops fetalis, a condition of severe anemia and edema and may die in utero or soon after birth from circulatory collapse and/or anemia and dyspnea.

      3. ABO incompatibility seldom causes hydrops fetalis, but does sometimes cause jaundice.

IV. Management

  A. Initial obstetrics (OB) visit

      1. Ask about a history of blood transfusions, blood disorders, or problems with previous pregnancies or deliveries, and determine if the patient is known to be Rh(D) negative.

      2. If sensitization is confirmed by an antibody titer, refer the patient to a perinatologist.

  B. Routine lab work

      1. At the initial visit, all pregnant patients need to have blood drawn for lab work to determine the D factor and antibody titer.

        a. If the antibody titer is positive, order a repeat titer and an antibody identification. Ask if the patient has recently received a RhoGAM injection, because this may cause the titer to be positive. If the problem continues, refer the patient to a specialist.

    b. If the patient is Rh(D) negative, be sure to counsel her and chart her status in a prominent place.

  2. A repeat antibody titer should be performed on all Rh(D)-negative patients between 24 and 28 weeks' gestation. Note if the patient has received RhoGAM because of a bleed, amniocentesis, or other reason. This will cause the titer to convert to a positive status.

C. RhoGAM administration

  1. RhoGAM is a passive immunoglobulin that prevents the Rh(D)-negative person from producing antibodies against the D antigen, thus preventing sensitization.

  2. RhoGAM should be administered to all unsensitized Rh(D)-negative patients.

    a. RhoGAM should be given prophylactically at 28 to 30 weeks' gestation.

    b. It should be administered within 72 hours of the following:

      (1) Removal of an ectopic pregnancy

      (2) Amniocentesis

      (3) Removal of hydatidiform mole

      (4) An episode of uterine bleeding in pregnancy

      (5) Delivery of an Rh(D)-positive baby, whether or not RhoGAM had been given prophylactically at 28 to 30 weeks' gestation

    c. RhoGAM should be given in the following doses and routes.

      (1) It is always given intramuscularly.

      (2) The standard dose is one vial, although micro or macro doses may be given, depending on the amount of mixing of maternal and fetal blood that potentially occurred.

      (3) One MICRhoGAM dose appears adequate for abortions up to 12 weeks' gestation.

      (4) One vial of Rh(D) immune globulin is adequate to cover up to 15 mL of fetal blood in the maternal circulation.

      (5) A Betke-Kleihauer test may be ordered to determine the amount of fetal blood in the maternal circulation, and thus the dose of RhoGAM needed.

  3. RhoGAM *should not* be administered in the following situations:

    a. Rh(D)-positive woman

    b. Sensitized Rh(D)-negative woman

    c. Rh(D)-negative woman who has given birth to a Rh(D)-negative baby

    d. *Never* give RhoGAM to a baby.

V. **Teaching**

A. All Rh(D)-negative patients should be counseled regarding the physiology and implications of being Rh(D) negative, and the importance of receiving RhoGAM in situations when sensitization may occur.

B. After the patient has been given a dose of RhoGAM, be sure the patient is given the lab slip that indicates she has had RhoGAM with the date and dose given.

C. Patients with other blood group incompatibilities should be counseled/referred as appropriate for that particular antigen.

 MULTIPLE PREGNANCY

I.   Definition. A multiple pregnancy is one involving two or more fetuses.

II.   Incidence

    A. Approximately 2% of births in the United States are multiple.

    B. Most involve twins; triplets occur naturally in 1 of 7,600 pregnancies.

    C. Multiple births higher than triplets are rare, but the incidence is rising due to the increasing use of gonadotropins to treat women with ovulatory failure and new methods of returning fertilized eggs (zygotes) to the uterus.

III. Etiology. Racial or family tendency to twinning increases the likelihood of dizygotic pregnancy; this is not true in monozygotic pregnancy.

IV.   Clinical Features

    A. History

        1. History of recent infertility problem treated with fertility drugs

        2. History of introducing several zygotes into the uterus

        3. Familial history of twins

    B. Signs and symptoms

        1. Large-for-dates uterine size, fundal height, and abdominal girth associated with rapid uterine growth during the second trimester. Especially significant if early uterine size was consistent with dates.

        2. Inexplicable excessive weight gain

        3. Abdominal palpation reveals three or more large parts and/or multiple small parts, especially in the third trimester when these are more readily felt.

        4. Auscultation of more than one FHT

    C. Potential complications

        1. Polyhydramnios is more common.

        2. The incidence of pre-eclampsia is increased fivefold.

        3. Anemia is prevalent.

        4. May get twin to twin transfusion, slower growth of one baby over the other.

        5. Congenital malformations are more common.

        6. Prematurity is greatest cause of fetal morbidity and mortality in multiple gestations.

        7. Fetal mortality is quadrupled in twin pregnancy. Risk to the second twin is twice that of the first.

        8. Malpresentation, premature rupture of membranes (PROM), and cord prolapse are more common.

9. Dystocia in labor and cesarean section are more likely.
10. Postpartum hemorrhage (PPH) is more common due to overdistention of the uterus.

D. Discomforts

1. Discomforts associated with large intrauterine volume
   a. Dyspnea
   b. Heartburn
   c. Abdominal pain and/or itching
2. Excessive weight gain due to:
   a. Increased volume of uterine contents
   b. Increased water retention
   c. Polyhydramnios
   d. Overeating
3. Complaints of fetal overactivity are frequent.
4. Increased fatigue and hunger

V. Management

A. At initial visit, ask about personal or family history of twins.

B. If at any time signs and symptoms develop, confirm or rule out with sonogram.

C. If diagnosed, consult; collaborative management is possible for twins.

D. Usual antepartum management

1. Increase oral iron to 120mg elemental iron per day.
2. Increase folic acid to 1mg per day.
3. Offer referral to dietitian. Increase protein intake to 120gm/day and add 500 extra calories to diet.
4. Office visits every two weeks after 24 weeks
5. Weekly NST after 32 weeks
6. Consider vaginal exam at every office visit after 24 weeks to check for cervical changes that would indicate impending premature labor.
7. Advise patient to stop work outside the home by 24 weeks and to restrict travel.
8. Advise frequent rest periods after 30 weeks.
9. Provide support, reassurance, and teaching regarding associated discomforts and potential dangers.
10. Monthly sonogram for growth, positions and to measure the length of the cervix.

E. Management during labor and delivery

1. Collaborative management
   a. Management is the physician's prerogative
   b. Certified nurse-midwife may deliver first baby if vertex.
   c. Certified nurse-midwife may assist with second infant as necessary.
2. Obtain ultrasound on admission to hospital for fetal position.

3. IV or heparin lock is mandatory in labor.
4. Fetal monitoring of both babies is mandatory in labor.

 NON-STRESS TEST

I. **Definition.** A non-stress test is a test of fetal condition in which fetal movements are recorded and concomitant fetal heart rate changes are monitored.

II. **Indications.** All patients at risk for placental insufficiency

   A. Hypertension: At 32 weeks, at least weekly as long as hypertension is a concern, then biweekly at 36 weeks

   B. Gestational diabetes: Weekly after 32 weeks

   C. Possible IUFGR biweekly after diagnosis

   D. Postdates: Biweekly after 40 weeks

   E. Marked decrease in fetal movements: at once, then as indicated depending on results

   F. Previous stillbirth: Weekly after 32 to 34 weeks, if undelivered, biweekly after 40 weeks.

   G. Any other combination of factors suggesting an increased risk of placental insufficiency, such as total weight gain below 15 lb at 36 weeks EGA, heavy smoker, drug abuse, etc.

III. **Management**

   A. Reactive test
      1. Baseline heart rate between 120 and 160 beats per minute
      2. Four or more fetal movements within a 20 minute tracing
      3. Heart rate acceleration of at least 15 beats per minute with a duration of 15 seconds or more above the baseline rate two times in 20 minutes

   B. Nonreactive test
      1. Physician should be consulted for any non-stress test that does not meet the criteria designated above.
      2. Depending on the situation, the patient could be sent out to eat and return later for another test or she may be sent to the hospital to:
         a. Try another NST
         b. Do a nipple stimulation test
         c. Do a contraction stress test (CST)
         d. Induction of labor

 PLACENTA PREVIA

I. **Definition.** Placenta previa is a condition in which the placenta is implanted in the lower pole of the uterus. This implantation can be:

   A. Total or complete: The placenta covers the entire cervical os.

    B. Partial: Only a portion of the os is covered.

    C. Marginal: Edge of placenta is at the edge of os.

    D. Low-lying: Edge of placenta is almost at edge of os.

II. **Incidence.** 1 in 200 births

III. **Etiology**

    A. Factors that affect the localization of implantation:

        1. Early or late fertilization

        2. Variability in the implantation potential of the blastocyst

        3. The receptivity and adequacy of the endometrium

    B. In multiple pregnancies because the placental surface is increased in size

    C. Tendency to avoid implantation on uterine scar, for example, previous cesarean section

    D. Rate increases proportional to increase in parity. The endometrium is changed at previous placental site; the blastocyst tries to attach where no placenta has been before.

    E. Rate increases in older women.

    F. Rate increases in diabetes, possibly because the placenta is larger than usual.

IV. **Clinical Features**

    A. Signs and symptoms

        1. Painless vaginal bleeding

        2. Sudden onset of bleeding without warning

        3. Occurs during third trimester

        4. Malpresentation or malpositions because the fetus must accommodate itself to the presence of the placenta

    B. Complications

        1. Hemorrhage and resulting shock

        2. Prematurity of the fetus

        3. Increased fetal mortality

        4. Postpartum hemorrhage due to bleeding at the site of placental implantation where the uterine muscle fibers contract less effectively.

        5. Sheehan's syndrome and clotting defects may occur but are more common in placental abruption.

V. **Management**

    A. Do not do vaginal exams! A placental vessel may be ruptured and result in massive hemorrhage.

    B. Diagnosis can be made by ultrasound.

    C. If diagnosis is made early in pregnancy, placenta may migrate up in the uterus as the uterus enlarges.

        1. Follow-up with serial ultrasounds until the placenta is well away from the cervical os. If the placenta still encroaches on the os at 32 weeks, refer to a physician.

        2. Instruct the patient to call at the first sign of any vaginal bleeding.

D. Consult with physician immediately upon diagnosis of total, partial, or marginal placenta previa after 20 weeks of pregnancy.

E. See that any unsensitized, Rh(D)-negative patient receives a RhoGAM injection after each bleeding episode to prevent sensitization from possible mixing of D-positive fetal blood with maternal blood.

    1. The usual dose is one vial, which is adequate for a transfusion of up to 15 mL of fetal blood into the maternal circulation.

    2. The dosage should be larger if it is possible that more than 15 mL was transfused.

    3. A Betke-Kleihauer test can be done to determine the amount of fetal blood in the maternal circulation.

F. Order limited activity or bed rest for a woman with diagnosed total or partial placenta previa.

    1. Observe the patient closely until the baby is mature or until a serious bleeding episode occurs that necessitates immediate delivery.

    2. Plan for a delivery by cesarean section, because the placenta is blocking the cervical os and preventing vaginal descent of the fetus.

VI. Patient Education

A. Explain the causes, location of the placenta, and possible problems.

B. The patient is to call at the first sign of bleeding. She should inform the hospital or person she talks to of the previa diagnosis.

C. Patients with a total or partial previa should remain at home on limited activity.

D. No intercourse

E. Information should be given on cesarean section in case this is or becomes necessary.

 POLYHYDRAMNIOS

I. **Definition.** Polyhydramnios is an excessive amount of amniotic fluid.

II. Etiology

A. Multiple gestations, especially with monozygotic twins

B. Diabetes

C. Erythroblastosis

D. Fetal malformations

    1. Gastrointestinal tract, for example, esophageal atresia or some other abnormality that would prohibit fetal swallowing of amniotic fluid

    2. Central nervous system anomalies, for example, anencephaly, meningomyelocele

III. Clinical Features

A. Complications

    1. Fetal malpresentation

2. Placental abruption
3. Problems in labor
   a. Premature labor
   b. Premature rupture during labor
   c. Uterine dysfunction during labor
   d. Cord prolapse
   e. Postpartum hemorrhage secondary to atony from uterine overdistention
4. Baby small for gestational age

B. Signs and symptoms
   1. Uterine enlargement, abdominal girth, and fundal height far beyond that expected for gestational age.
   2. Tenseness of the uterine wall, making it difficult or impossible to:
      a. Auscultate fetal heart tones.
      b. Palpate the fetal outline and parts.
   3. Auscultation of a uterine fluid thrill
   4. If severe, mechanical problems such as:
      a. Severe dyspnea
      b. Lower extremity and vulvar edema
      c. Pressure pain in back, abdomen, and/or thighs
      d. Nausea and vomiting

IV. **Management**
   A. Ultrasound for definitive diagnosis
   B. If diagnosis confirmed by ultrasound, consult with physician. Collaborative management is possible. Usual management:
      1. Advise patient of associated conditions and complications.
      2. Order repeat scan to observe for fetal abnormalities.
      3. Do daily fetal activity counts (FAC) and biweekly non-stress test (NST).
      4. Advise restriction of activities (bedrest if severe).
      5. Plan delivery at hospital with level III nursery if labor starts before 35 weeks.
      6. Instruct patient to call at first sign of labor.
      7. If moderate to severe: Consult, consider induction of labor.
      8. Notify physician if patient is hospitalized for labor.
      9. Avoid artificial rupture of membranes (AROM) in labor unless vertex -1, -2 and well applied to the cervix.
      10. IV or heparin lock is mandatory in labor because of increased likelihood of cord prolapse with ROM or postpartum hemorrhage.
      11. Fetal monitor is mandatory in labor.
      12. Notify pediatrician or neonatal nurse practitioner when delivery is imminent.

POSTMATURITY

I. Definition. Any pregnancy that goes to the end of the 42nd week. Currently many define postmaturity as any pregnancy beginning the 41st week.

II. Incidence
   A. If not induced, 12% of all pregnancies would reach the 43rd week.
   B. If not induced, 4% of all pregnancies would reach the 44th week.

III. Etiology
   A. Malfunction in the labor-starting mechanism
   B. A variation in the time it takes for fetus to mature
   C. More common with anencephaly
   D. Question method(s) of determining EDC.
   E. Unknown

IV. Clinical Features. Problems associated with postmaturity are as follows:
   A. Fetal dysmaturity syndrome
       1. Cause: Placental insufficiency
       2. Signs and symptoms
           a. Low weight in relation to length
           b. Little subcutaneous fat, baggy skin
           c. Vernix scant or absent
           d. Hair and nails long
           e. Skin dry and peeling, especially on hands and feet
           f. Skin, nails, and cord gold- or green-colored from meconium staining
           g. Reduced amount of amniotic fluid, thick with meconium
   B. Dystocia
       1. Risk of shoulder dystocia in labor because of fetal macrosomia
       2. The suture lines of the head are closing and do not give as well, which results in a larger biparietal diameter presenting.
   C. Increased perinatal mortality from:
       1. Anoxia secondary to placental insufficiency
       2. Difficult birth due to dystocia
       3. Higher incidence of meconium aspiration

V. Management
   A. Establish clear EDC as early in pregnancy as possible.
       1. Both the known LMP and length of her cycles need to be considered when determining EDC.
       2. Ultrasound before 12 weeks, especially of the crown-rump length, tends to be more accurate for dating purposes and should be given more weight in decision making.
   B. Discuss labor stimulation and post-dates management at 40 to 41 weeks. Labor stimulation includes:

Table 5-2. Bishop's Score

	0	1	2	3
Dilation (cm)	0	1–2	3–4	5–6
Effacement (%)	0–30	40–50	60–70	80+
Station	−3	−2	−1	+1 or +2
Consistency	Firm	Medium	Soft	
Position	Posterior	Mid	Anterior	

A score of four or greater is considered positive and yields a successful induction rate of 80% to 90%. A score of nine is almost fail proof.

    1. Increase walking and other activity.

    2. Sexual excitement-intercourse/orgasm

  C. Advise patient to keep fetal movement log beginning at 39 weeks.

  D. At 39 to 40 weeks:

    1. Begin biweekly NSTs.

    2. Evaluate cervix for ripeness according to Bishop's score (Table 5-2). If ripe:

      a. Consider stripping the membranes.

      b. If Bishop score greater than 9, consider induction.

      c. Consider prostaglandin gel or misoprostol (although not approved for this use) if cervix is unripe.

    3. If patient desires to go into labor naturally and is greater than 41 weeks EGA, consider biophysical profile.

  E. Consult with physician for any of the following:

    1. Abnormal NST or oxytocin challenge test (OCT)

    2. Ultrasound showing oligohydramnios

    3. Biophysical profile less than 8

    4. Induction

 POSTPARTUM HEMORRHAGE

I. Third Stage Hemorrhage

  A. Definition. Third stage hemorrhage is defined as blood loss of 500 ml or more between the time the baby is delivered and the time the placenta is delivered.

  B. Etiology. Partial separation of the placenta

  C. Management

    1. Prevent by managing third stage properly.

      a. Do not massage the uterus during third stage.

b. Do not pull the placenta. Allow physiologic separation, which may take up to 30 minutes.

2. If third stage hemorrhage occurs:

a. Thoroughly massage the uterus to contract and complete placental separation, while applying mild cord traction to effect delivery (Brandt-Andrews maneuver).

b. Instruct assistant to start IV or insure patency if already in place. (Ringer's lactate is best.)

c. If there is difficulty delivering the placenta and/or hemorrhage continues, have assistant call for physician immediately.

d. If physician has not yet arrived and hemorrhage continues, perform manual removal of the placenta. If time and conditions permit, have epidural re-dosed or give patient 2 mg Stadol or Demerol 50 mg IV before manual removal is attempted.

e. If the placenta is out but bleeding continues, explore the uterus for retained placenta fragments (premedicate if time allows) and perform bimanual compression.

(1) Order 10 to 20 units Pitocin to current IV if not already given.

(2) If not improving, see Fourth Stage Hemorrhage Management guidelines below.

f. If signs and symptoms of shock develop:

(1) Infuse Ringer's lactate solution (RL) rapidly.

(2) Place patient flat with legs slightly elevated.

(3) Give oxygen per mask.

(4) Keep patient warm, cover with warm blankets.

(5) Continue monitoring vital signs.

II. Fourth Stage Hemorrhage

A. Definition. Fourth stage hemorrhage is defined as blood loss of 500 ml (some references use 650 ml) or more between the time the placenta is delivered and 24 hours after.

B. Etiology

1. Uterine atony due to:

a. Primary atony

b. Overdistended uterus

(1) Multiple gestation

(2) Large baby

(3) Polyhydramnios

c. Exhaustion of uterine muscle

(1) Multiparity

(2) Prolonged labor

(3) Use of oxytocin in labor

d. Inability of the uterus to contract properly:

        (1) Precipitous labor, delivery, or both

        (2) Uterine myomas

        (3) Full bladder

  2. Trauma and lacerations

    a. Episiotomy. Blood loss can reach 200 cc normally. When arterioles or large veins are cut or torn, the amount of blood loss can be considerably more.

    b. Lacerations of the vulva, vagina, or cervix

    c. Ruptured uterus, possibly from a previous cesarean scar

    d. Uterine inversion

    e. Puerperal hematomas

  3. Retained placental fragments or clots

C. Management

  1. Preventive techniques

    a. Clamp bleeding vessels immediately to conserve blood.

    b. Avoid an episiotomy if possible. If an episiotomy is necessary, avoid a prolonged interval between performance of episiotomy and delivery of the baby.

    c. Avoid undue delay from birth of the baby to repair of episiotomy or lacerations.

    d. Routinely inspect upper vaginal vault and cervix.

    e. Start repair above apex to avoid failure to secure a bleeding vessel there.

    f. Routinely inspect placenta for missing parts and broken vessels. Be aware of trailing membranes at time of delivery of the placenta. Remove them slowly.

    g. If there is reason to believe placental fragments are retained, medicate as necessary, manually explore uterus, inform physician as necessary.

    h. Give 10 mg of Pitocin in current IV or 200 mg of Cytotec orally to aid with uterine contractions.

  2. Consult with physician if:

    a. Physician was not notified during the emergency

    b. Bleeding persists or returns

    c. Symptoms of hypovolemia, such as dizziness, faintness, tachycardia, are unrelieved with hydration.

    d. There is a significant drop in the hematocrit

  3. If there is a significant drop in hematocrit, start patient on iron supplements and educate regarding dietary sources of iron and folic acid.

  4. Prophylactic antibodies should be given if the uterus was explored.

  5. Be alert for signs of postpartum infection.

  6. Blood or blood products should never be given except as a last resort and after consulting.

III. Late Postpartum Hemorrhage

A. **Definition.** Blood loss of 500 ml or more after the first 24 hours of delivery and within six weeks.

B. **Etiology**

1. Retained fragments of placenta; infection usually follows.
2. Subinvolution of the uterus and placental site
3. Uterine myoma, especially when submucosal
4. Hematoma or reproductive tract laceration
5. Idiopathic, tendency to recurrence
6. Late detachment of thrombi at the placental site with reopening of the vascular sinuses
7. Abnormalities in the separation of the decidua vera
8. Intrauterine infection, leading to dissolution of the thrombosis in the vessels

C. **Clinical Signs**

1. The first clinical sign is a rapid pulse. A blood pressure drop will follow later.
2. She will feel week, cold and may have a headache.
3. Going through four maxi pads in two hours or passing clots that total the size of a lemon every hour times two is considered excessive.
4. Orthostatic hypotension: When placed in a sitting or standing position, patient gets lightheaded, dizzy and my pass out.

D. **Management**

1. Usual treatment
   a. Oxytocics
      (1) Methergine 0.2 mg orally every four hours for six doses. Back with a pain medication for cramping.
      (2) May need to be admitted to hospital for D&C if presently hemorrhaging.
   b. Antibiotics if infection exists
2. Immediate management
   a. Support the lower uterine segment and express clots.
   b. Check the consistency of the uterus.
      (1) If atonic, massage it.
      (2) If no response, do bimanual compression.
      (3) Give oxytocics and/or ergots listed here in order of preference:
         (a) Pitocin 10 to 20 units to 1000 cc IV fluids
         (b) Methergine 0.2 mg intramuscularly if no history of hypertension
         (c) Prostin suppositories per vagina, uterus, or rectum
         (d) If still bleeding administer Hemabate one amp IM every five minutes three times. Give first dose 10 minutes post Prostin.

(4) Send someone to call physician.

(5) Continue bimanual compression.

(6) Have assistant monitor vital signs and watch for signs of shock.

c. If bleeding is not under control, have assistant get type and cross if not already done.

d. If uterus is well-contracted and bleeding continues, look for lacerations.

(1) If first or second degree lacerations of vagina or perineum, repair.

(2) If lacerations of cervix or third or fourth degree lacerations of vagina or perineum:

(a) Clamp any bleeders and wait for physician.

(b) If physician still has not arrived and hemostasis is not attained, repair as necessary to attain hemostasis.

e. If signs of shock develop:

(1) Infuse LR rapidly.

(2) Place patient flat with legs slightly elevated.

(3) Give oxygen per mask.

(4) Keep patient warm, cover with blankets.

(5) Have assistant monitor vital signs.

f. In extreme cases, consider the following:

(1) Injection of oxytocin directly into the uterus with Iowa trumpet

(2) Aortic compression

(3) Alert OR in case a D&C or hysterectomy are necessary

3. Follow-up management

a. Obtain hematocrit:

(1) Twelve hours after delivery

(2) Twenty-four hours after delivery

b. Consider ordering supplemental iron

 ## PREMATURE RUPTURE OF MEMBRANES (PROM)

I. **Definition.** PROM is rupture of the membranes before the onset of labor.

II. **Etiology**

A. Preterm labor

B. Chorioamnionitis twice as frequent in PROM

C. Malposition or malpresentation of fetus

D. Factors due to cervical damage

1. Prior cervical instrumentation (e.g., therapeutic abortion (TAB), LEEP, etc.)

2. Increasing parity with possible damage to the cervix during previous deliveries

        3. Incompetent cervix

  E. Previous history of PROM twice or more

  F. Factors due to maternal weight

        1. Overweight before pregnancy

        2. Low weight gain during pregnancy

  G. Cigarette smoking during pregnancy

  H. Advanced maternal age possibly because the membranes are less strong than in young mothers

  I. Recent coitus

III. Management

  A. Prevention

        1. Treat gonococcus, chlamydia, and bacterial vaginosis.

        2. Discuss smoking in pregnancy and support efforts to cut down or quit.

        3. Encourage adequate weight gain in pregnancy.

        4. May discuss abstaining from coitus in the last trimester if any of the predisposing factors are present.

  B. Anticipatory guidance: Inform the following patients prenatally that they should call immediately if membranes rupture.

        1. Conditions in which ruptured membranes could result in cord prolapse

            a. Presenting part other than vertex

            b. Polyhydramnios

        2. Active herpes

        3. Previous history of beta hemolytic streptococcus

  C. If membranes have ruptured:

        1. Instruct patient to go to hospital or office.

        2. Document rupture.

            a. Obtain careful history. Attempt to establish a time of rupture

            b. If gross rupture:

                (1) While patient is lying supine, apply fundal pressure to see if it elicits a gush of fluid from the vagina.

                (2) Wet a cotton swab with fluid and smear on a slide to assess ferning under a microscope.

                (3) Apply some fluid to Nitrazene paper. If positive, consider diagnostic if patient has not had recent sex, is not bleeding, and has not been examined vaginally using K-Y Jelly.

            c. If uncertain of rupture and/or signs of possible infection, perform sterile speculum exam.

                (1) Assess Bishop score of cervix (see Bishop Score, Table 5-2).

                (2) Do culture of cervix only if signs of infection.

                (3) Obtain another specimen of fluid with a sterile swab to smear on slide to assess ferning under microscope.

            d. If gestation is less than 37 weeks or patient has a herpes II outbreak, refer to physician.

D. Conservative management

    1. Most labor starts within 24 to 72 hours of rupture.

    2. Possibility of infection is less if nothing is put into the vagina but sterile speculum; *no vaginal exams.*

    3. Waiting involves close monitoring of patient.

        a. Take temperature four times a day; if it rises significantly and/or reaches 100.4°F, two antibiotics are necessary and delivery needs to be accomplished.

        b. Observe vaginal discharge: foul odor, purulent or yellowish appearance indicates infection.

        c. Note uterine tenderness and irritability and report any changes.

E. Aggressive management

    1. Prostaglandin gel or Misoprostol (although, not approved for this use) may be used after consulting with physician

    2. May require serial Pitocin induction if cervix is unfavorable

    3. Some wait 12 hours for labor. If none, Pitocin is started.

    4. Involves need for IV, fetal monitor

    5. Increased risk of cesarean if induction ineffective

    6. If decision depends on inducibility of cervix, assess Bishop score (see Table 5-2) after speculum exam. If decision is then made to wait for labor, *no more exams* are to be done, either digital or speculum, until labor starts or an induction is started.

    7. Obtain CBC if rupture documented. Repeat every other day until delivery or more often if signs of infection.

    8. Obtain NST following rupture; be alert for fetal tachycardia, which is one of the first signs of infection.

    9. Begin induction after consult with physician if:

        a. Significant rise in maternal temperature

        b. Fetal tachycardia develops

        c. Foul lochia

        d. Significant uterine irritability or tenderness

        e. Vaginal culture shows beta hemolytic streptococcus

        f. CBC indicates elevated white count (shift to left).

F. Management of labor more than 24 hours after rupture

    1. Spontaneous labor

        a. Obtain patient's temperature every two hours, initiate antibiotics if fever develops.

        b. Internal monitoring suggested

        c. Notify obstetrician and pediatrician or neonatal nurse practitioner.

        d. Cultures per guidelines

    2. Induction of labor

        a. Per routine orders after consult with physician

        b. Obtain patient's temperature every two hours.

    c. Antibiotics: Guidelines differ. Many give 1 to 2 g of ampicillin IV or 1 to 2 g of Mefoxin IV every six hours prophylactically. Others monitor maternal temperature and FHT rate and use that information to determine when antibiotics may be needed.

 PREMATURITY

I.   **Definition.** Premature labor is that which occurs after the 20th week and before the 37th week of gestation.

II.   **Incidence.** 7% of all pregnancies

III.   **Etiology**

    A. In 66% of cases, the cause is never determined.

    B. Maternal factors

        1. Debilitating medical disorders

            a. Cardiovascular disease

            b. Renal disease

            c. Severe hypertension

            d. Poorly controlled diabetes

            e. Any other serious disease

        2. Abdominal surgery involving uterine displacement and/or manipulation when pregnant

        3. Maternal injury

        4. Pre-eclampsia or eclampsia

        5. Uterine anomalies

        6. Pelvic sepsis or tumors

        7. Infections

            a. Viral

                (1) Cytomegalovirus

                (2) Herpes simplex

                (3) Hepatitis

            b. Bacterial

                (1) Group B-Strep

                (2) Bacterial Vaginosis

            c. Pyelonephritis

            d. Chorioamnionitis caused by infection

        8. Cervical incompetence

        9. Two or more previous abortions

    C. Placental factors-abruption

    D. Fetal factors

        1. Multiple gestation

        2. Polyhydramnios

   3. Large baby
   4. PROM
   5. Infection (rubella, toxoplasmosis, etc.)
IV. Management
   A. If previous history of premature labor:
      1. Explore possible causative factors.
      2. Consider obtaining screening cultures especially if:
         a. History of more than one previous premature labor
         b. History of any of the associated infections
         c. History of previous unexplained stillbirth
      3. Cervical exams in office each antepartal visit
   B. If patient presents in labor:
      1. Determine if labor is true or false.
         a. If contractions are irregular, infrequent, or painless, probably Braxton-Hicks. Instruct patient to:
            (1) Increase fluid intake.
            (2) Lie down.
            (3) Call back if contractions increase in regularity, frequency, or pain.
         b. If contractions are regular, frequent, or uncomfortable, instruct patient to come into office or to labor and delivery for external monitoring.
      2. Fetal fibronectin (fFN) may be assessed by sterile speculum exam and cervico-vaginal swab.
         a. Normally present in cervico-vaginal fluid after 20 weeks EGA.
         b. It is released as a result of compromise in the fetoplacental membrane structure or strength.
         c. Eighty-seven percent of those with a positive test will deliver within seven days.
         d. Ninety-nine and one half percent of those with a negative fFN will deliver over seven days after the test; 97% will deliver over 14 days after a negative test.
      3. If patient is in true labor, consult with physician. Usual treatment:
         a. Labor will usually not be stopped if any of the following conditions are present.
            (1) Before 20 or after 35 weeks' gestation
            (2) Three to four centimeters dilation and 50% to 75% effaced
            (3) Maternal complications, such as hypertension or diabetes
            (4) Fetal complication, such as IUFGR
            (5) Placental complications, such as abruption
            (6) Premature rupture of membranes: May want to stop labor for 24 hours to mature fetal lungs
            (7) Chorioamnionitis

    b. If chance of delivery is high and patient is less than 32 weeks, she should be transferred to a hospital with level III nursery due to need of neonatal intensive care for infant.

    c. If labor is to be stopped, follow standard hospital guidelines for terbutaline or magnesium sulfate as ordered by the co-managing physician.

    d. Factors to be considered if delivery is inevitable.

        (1) If there is a chance that at least 24 hours might elapse before delivery, and patient is less than 33 weeks' gestation, consider Betamethasone therapy to increase surfactant production and mature the fetal lungs.

        (2) Keep analgesia to a minimum. Narcotic depression is exaggerated in the premature baby.

        (3) Electronic fetal monitoring is indicated.

        (4) Cut a large episiotomy; avoid trauma to the fetal head.

        (5) The pediatrician or neonatal nurse practitioner should be called to be present for the delivery.

 PRURITUS IN PREGNANCY

I. **Definition.** Pruritus in pregnancy is a generalized body itching with or without accompanying jaundice.

II. **Etiology**

    A. Not definite but could possibly be caused by:

        1. Obstetric cholestasis

        2. High estrogen levels

        3. Elevated serum bile salts

    B. More common in multiple gestations

    C. See Skin Conditions in Pregnancy later in Part V.

III. **Clinical Features**

    A. Generalized or local body itching especially the abdomen and feet

    B. Mild jaundice

    C. Elevated serum bilirubin levels

    D. Rash usually beginning on the trunk and abdomen and spreading to include the entire body

    E. Usually begins after 28 weeks of pregnancy

    D. Subsides soon after delivery

    F. See Table 5-3 for additional characteristics.

IV. **Differential Diagnosis**

    A. Hepatitis

        1. Previous history of hepatitis, jaundice

        2. Family member with hepatitis

        3. Working/living in a high exposure area

        4. IV drug use

B. Liver disease

    1. Rare with no previous history or history of hepatitis

    2. Get SMAC-20 plus CBC to test liver function if any doubt.

C. Scabies

    1. Look for rash or papules in skin folds.

    2. Ask if other family members have same symptoms.

D. Allergic reactions, poison ivy topical medication, etc.

    1. Look for accompanying hives and/or rash

    2. History of recent exposure to allergen

    3. Itching is in area exposed, which is not usually the abdomen or feet

E. Skin disease

    1. Previous history

    2. Lesions not characteristic of simple excoriation from scratching

F. Cholestasis of pregnancy

    1. Recurs in each pregnancy (familial)

    2. High level of alkaline phosphate and serum bile acids

    3. Pruritus, jaundice may be present. No anorexia or malaise

    4. Last trimester

V. **Management**

A. When a patient presents with pruritus, make differential diagnosis

B. Consult if any doubt about diagnosis.

C. Simple pruritus gravidarum is managed symptomatically.

    1. Avoid scratching; it may lead to secondary infection due to excoriation of the skin.

    2. Try antipruritic lotion, such as Calamine or Benadryl.

    3. Try anesthetic ointment or spray, such as Americaine.

    4. Apply ice packs to affected area.

    5. In severe cases, may try Benadryl 25 to 50 mg orally every four to six hours as necessary; use sparingly.

    6. Mild excoriation may respond to hydrocortisone 1% cream.

D. In severe skin excoriation, probable allergic response or skin disease, refer to dermatologist.

E. See sections on Skin Conditions in Pregnancy (Part V) and Skin Conditions (Part IV) for further information.

 PUERPERAL INFECTION

I. **Definition.** A puerperal infection is any infection of the genital tract during the puerperium, accompanied by a temperature of 100.4°F or higher on any two of the first ten days postpartum exclusive of the first 24 hours.

Table 5-3. Skin Disorders Unique to Pregnancy

Disorder	Frequency	Clinical Characteristics	Histopathology
Pruritus Gravidarum			
	Common (1%–2%)	Onset third trimester; intense pruritus; generalized itching; excoriations common	Noncharacteristic; excoriations common
Pruritic Urticarial Papules and Plaques of Pregnancy (PUPPS)			
	Common (0.25%–1%)	Onset second or third trimester; intense pruritus; patchy or generalized itching on the abdomen, thighs, arms, and buttocks; erythematous papules and urticarial papules, and plaques	Lymphocytic perivascular infiltrate; negative immuno-fluorescence
Papular Eruptions (Prurigo Gestations and Papular Dermatitis)			
	(1:300–1: 2400)	Onset second or third trimester; localized or generalized itching; 1- to 5-mm pruritic papules; excoriations common	Lymphocytic perivascular infiltrate; parakeratosis, acanthosis, and negative immuno-fluorescence
Herpes Gestations			
	Rare (1:50,000)	Onset second or third trimester, sometimes 1–2 wk postpartum; severe pruritus; generalized itching or localized to the abdomen or extremities; urticarial papules, erythematous vesicles, and bullae	Edema; infiltrate of lymphocytes, histocytes, and eosinophils
Impetigo Herpetiformis			
	Rare	Onset third trimester; localized, then generalized rash; erythema with marginal sterile pustules; involved mucous membranes; systemic symptoms	Microabscesses

Perinatal Outcome	Treatment	Comments
Increased perinatal morbidity	Antipruritics, cholestyramine	Possibly a mild form of cholestatic jaundice; recurrence in subsequent pregnancies
No adverse effects	Antipruritics, emollients, topical steroids, oral steroids if severe	Common in nulliparas; infrequent recurrence in subsequent pregnancies
Possibly unaffected	Antipruritics, topical steroids, oral steroids if severe	Prurigo gestations localized to forearms and trunk; generalized papular dermatitis; no recurrence in subsequent pregnancies
Possible increased preterm birth; transient neonatal lesions (5%–10%)		Also associated with gestational tropho-blastic disease; exacerbations and remissions during pregnancy common; postpartum exacer-bations very common; recurrence in subsequent pregnancies in more severe form
Maternal sepsis common	Antibiotics, oral steroids	Possible pustular psoriasis; duration of weeks to months postpartum; possible recurrence with subsequent pregnancies

II. **Clinical Features**

    A. Predisposing factors

        1. Length of labor

        2. Duration of ROM

        3. Retained products of conception

        4. Abdominal delivery

        5. Number of vaginal exams during labor

        6. Anemia

    B. Symptoms

        1. Fever

        2. Malaise

        3. Abdominal pain

        4. Uterine tenderness

        5. Purulent or foul-smelling lochia

    C. Differential diagnosis

        1. Dehydration

            a. Occurs in the first 24 hours after delivery.

            b. Should not last more than 24 hours.

            c. Temperature should not go over 100°F.

        2. Breast engorgement

            a. Occurs on the third to fifth day postpartum; when milk is coming in, breasts feel warm, full, and uncomfortable.

            b. Should not last more than 12 hours.

            c. Temperature should not go over 100.4°F

III. **Management**

    A. Physical exam

        1. Check temperature and pulse.

        2. Possible upper respiratory infection or pneumonia

            a. Inspect throat for infection, swelling, and drainage.

            b. Palpate lymph nodes of the head and neck for adenopathy.

            c. Auscultate lungs for rales, rhonchi, and wheezes.

        3. Possible mastitis: Observe breast for localized redness, tenderness.

        4. Possible wound infection: observe perineal or abdominal wound for redness, tenderness, warmth, swelling, purulent drainage, abscess formation.

        5. Possible endometritis

            a. Palpate uterus for tenderness.

            b. If other findings suggestive of endometritis, do speculum and bimanual exam, get endocervical cultures, and assess lochia for odor and characteristics.

        6. Possible UTI or pyelonephritis

            a. Check for costovertebral angle tenderness (CVAT).

      b. Question regarding signs and symptoms of UTI.

      c. Obtain clean catch or catheterized urine.

   7. Possible thrombophlebitis

      a. Presence of Homans sign

      b. Observe calves for any reddened areas that are warm to touch, and swelling.

B. Lab tests: Do as indicated by history and physical.

   1. Usual standard workup for most common causes

      a. Urinalysis and culture and sensitivity. Postpartum UTI is often asymptomatic, so this is fairly routine.

      b. Endometrial cultures

      c. Blood cultures

      d. CBC with sedimentation rate and differential

   2. Other lab work that may be done if history and physical indicate:

      a. Culture of perineal or abdominal wound

      b. Culture of breast milk

      c. Culture of sputum, throat, or both

C. Treatment

   1. Avoid use of antipyretics unless fever is over 101°F.

   2. If fever under 101°F in first 24 hours, force fluids at 200cc/hr (orally or IV) and retake temperature in two to three hours. If still elevated, do workup.

   3. If fever under 100°F at time milk is coming in, encourage frequent breast-feeding and warm compresses to breasts. Monitor temperature every two to three hours. If fever gets higher and/or persists longer than 12 hours, do work-up.

   4. If tests are normal, treat as indicated. Otherwise, consult physician for IV/PO antibiotics.

 ROUND LIGAMENT PAIN

I. **Etiology**

   A. The round ligaments attach on either side of the uterus just below and in front of the insertion of the fallopian tubes, cross the broad ligament in a fold of peritoneum, pass through the inguinal canal, and insert in the anterior (upper) portion of the labia majora on either side of the perineum. They are supporting structures for the uterus.

   B. As the uterus grows in pregnancy, the ligaments become stretched and often contract, resulting in sharp pain along the side of the abdomen, just above the groin area, usually accentuated by sudden movements, coughing, lifting, etc.

II. **Differential Diagnosis**

   A. PID

    B. Appendicitis

    C. Kidney stone

    D. Gallbladder or other GI disease

    E. UTI

    F. Placental abruption

    G. Labor

III. Management

    A. Explain reason for pain and reassure patient.

    B. Comfort measures

        1. Avoid sudden movement, turn slowly to side and push up rather than trying to sit straight up from lying down.

        2. Apply local heat.

        3. Try a change of activity.

        4. Maternity belt or girdle may be helpful.

        5. Support uterus with a pillow when sitting or lying down.

        6. May take acetaminophen 500 mg every four to six hours as necessary for pain

    C. If no relief with above measures, obtain pelvic ultrasound.

    D. Instruct patient to call if sharp abdominal pain does not subside within 30 minutes; it may be something besides round ligament pain.

    E. If all tests are negative and discomfort continues, refer to physician, physical therapist, or chiropractor as needed.

 SKIN CONDITIONS IN PREGNANCY

I. Physiologic

    A. Definition. Physiologic alterations in the skin common in pregnancy

    B. Etiology. Hormonal changes during pregnancy, such as fetoplacental production, stimulation or changes in metabolism may increase the availability of estrogens, progesterone, androgens, and other hormones in the mother's body.

    C. Clinical Features

        1. Hyperpigmentation

            a. Incidence: 90%

            b. Stimulated by estrogen, progesterone, melatonin-stimulating hormone

            c. Darkening of linea nigra, genitalia areolae, nipples, freckles, nevi, recent scars

            d. Regresses after delivery

        2. Chloasma, mask of pregnancy

            a. Seen frequently in pregnant women

b. Seen in 5% of nonpregnant women on BCPs

c. Consists of blotchy, irregular hyperpigmentation on cheeks, forehead, upper lip, and neck. Exacerbated by sun and wind.

d. Regresses after delivery. Type caused by BCPs may persist

3. **Hirsutism/alopecia**

 a. During pregnacy, hair growth is stimulated.

 b. Postpartum hair re-enters resting phase.

 c. Many hairs shed within three to six months causing thinning hair and dandruff looking scalp.

 d. Patient education consists of reassurance, shampoo for dandruff.

4. **Striae**

 a. Appear in 90% of patients

 b. Probably caused by increased adrenocortical activity

 c. No clear correlation with abdominal girth

 d. Appear as pink or purple atrophic bands, which fade to white

 e. Pruritus at site is a frequent complaint. Antipruritic ointment and lotions help.

5. **Vascular distention, proliferation, and instability**

 a. Congestion of the vestibule and vagina

 b. Palmar erythema

 c. Varicosities, involve saphenous, vulval, hemorrhoidal veins

 d. Arterial spiders (65% of Caucasians, 11% of African American)

 e. Pallor, facial flushing, hot and cold sensations, are secondary to vasomotor instability.

 f. Hyperemia and hypertrophy of gums

 g. Most vascular changes regress postpartum.

II. **Skin Disorders Unique to Pregnancy—see Table 5-3.**

III. **Skin Manifestations of Diseases That Affect Pregnancy**

 A. Coxsackie B Enterovirus

  1. Rash is typically maculopapular exanthema that resembles rubella.

  2. Diagnosis

   a. Viral culture of throat and rectum

   b. Acute and convalescent IgM, IgG

  3. Fetal problems

   a. Main concern is maternal infection in third trimester, resulting in neonatal exposure. The risk to the neonate is less if the interval to delivery is four to six weeks. This allows the mother to develop immunity, which is passively transmitted to her fetus.

   b. Rare cases of congenital cardiac defects have been reported.

 B. Fifth disease: "Slapped face" syndrome

1. Caused by parvovirus B-19
2. Epidemic late winter and spring
3. Spread by nasal droplets
4. Incubation 4 to 14 days
5. Signs and symptoms are general malaise, fever, URI. Infection wanes as rash appears. Rash starts on the face and resembles slapped cheeks. It then spreads to the trunk and extremities.
6. Diagnosis
   a. B-19 parvovirus antibody. IgM can be detected three days after symptoms. Starts to fall in 30 to 60 days, may persist at low levels four to six months.
   b. Parvovirus B-19 IgG can be detected after seven days of illness, persists for year.
   c. Since labs report both IgM and IgG, need only draw blood once between four days and four weeks of the onset of symptoms.
7. Management of positive infection during pregnancy
   a. Serial hemoglobin and hematocrit to detect aplastic anemia resulting from bone marrow suppression
   b. Serial ultrasound to watch for fetal hydrops. The virus destroys fetal erythroid precursors. Fetal death, usually 1 to 12 weeks after infection, is caused by severe anemia, congestive heart failure. Babies treated in utero for severe anemia often do well with no lasting problems.

C. Varicella (chickenpox, varicella-zoster)
1. Clinical features
   a. Varicella-zoster virus causes both chickenpox and herpes zoster.
   b. Chickenpox: Incubation period for primary infection is 10 to 20 days. Lesions begin on trunk and spread. Lesions progress from macules to vesicles and crust over. New lesions appear for three to five days, causing severe itching.
   c. Herpes zoster recurrent form. Lesions develop along nerves.
2. Fetal effects
   a. Maternal illness: 5 to 21 days before delivery results in mild chickenpox in newborn.
   b. Maternal illness four days before to 48 hours after delivery may result in severe disseminated disease in baby, 30% fatal.
   c. Maternal infection earlier in pregnancy may cause fetal skin scarring, muscle atrophy, hypoplastic extremities, clubfeet, cortical atrophy, encephalitis.
3. Maternal effects-watch for maternal pneumonia.
4. Lab tests
   a. Isolation of virus from lesion first four days
   b. Fluorescent antibody membrane antigen (FAMA) or enzyme-linked immunosorbent assay (ELISA) to determine immune status

    c. Antibody found two weeks following illness. Increase in titer over previous value indicates recent infection. Antibody disappears over time.

    d. Check to see if IgG present.

5. Prevention

    a. Avoid exposure to persons with known active disease if immunity uncertain.

    b. If negative history of disease or not immune can give immunity within 96 hours of exposure. Give VLIG, varicella/zoster immune globulin IM. One vial of 125 units/10kg of weight (maximum = 625 units).

PART 6

Complementary
Therapies

Geri Morgan, CNM, ND

The terms "complementary therapies" and "alternative therapies" are becoming interchangeable. Webster's dictionary defines "complementary" as anything that complements or helps to fill out, mutually making up what is lacking. "Alternative" is defined as that which may be chosen or omitted as one of several things; when one is chosen, the other choices are eliminated.[1]

Complementary or alternative therapies have assumed a place alongside conventional medicine in the U.S. health care system. It is estimated that at least 40% of those needing assistance in the last year have turned either to alternative practices, such as acupuncture, homeopathy, and Ayurveda, or to complementary therapies, such as herbals, diet, lifestyle changes, manual healing (e.g., chiropractic, massage, therapeutic touch, reflexology), or mind/body control such as Reiki, guided imagery, meditation, prayer, counseling, yoga, music, humor, and art.

Although cost may be a factor in the choices made, it is very likely that complementary or alternative therapies are chosen because they tend to empower the individual to play an integral role in his or her own recovery. A balanced lifestyle is stressed, and the whole person is treated rather than just the symptoms or illness.

Increasing use of complementary therapies makes it important for everyone working in health care to have a basic knowledge and awareness of the possible impact these therapies may have on patients. A thorough history should include other treatments used now or in the past. There should also be a specific place on any history form to list current over-the-counter (OTC) medications. Many patients do not consider OTC products as medications and, therefore, may not mention them unless asked.

All complementary therapies are based on a holistic health model of self-care and personal responsibility for wellness. The emphasis is on the "wholeness" of a person, prevention of disease, and maintenance of health.[2]

 TRADITIONAL CHINESE MEDICINE

Traditional Chinese Medicine (TCM) does not recognize illness in terms of cause and effect, but rather in terms of relationships. Yin and yang represent a duality of opposing forces or energies that when joined form a whole. When yin and yang are in balance, harmony and health exist.

The life force (chi, qi, vital essence) that circulates throughout the body is complementary to yin and yang. This energy flows throughout the body through a system of meridians or channels in a given pattern to form a network, which governs all parts of the body. Everything in life affects chi, from our emotions and stress to diet, exercise, and weather. If chi is interrupted or unable to flow freely, disharmony and illness can result. TCM uses acupuncture, acupressure massage, and Chinese herbs to restore balance. It is the patient's responsibility to take proper care of herself and maintain a balance and hence health.

I. **Acupuncture.** Acupuncture points on the body are areas of decreased electrical resistance on the skin that, when stimulated, affect the increased production of endorphins. For TCM, the points are loci beneath the skin along the meridians that each have a unique ability to

---

[1]Merriam-Webster's Collegiate Dictionary, 1998

[2]Kass-Annese, 1999, p. 198

affect the flow of chi. A certain point stimulated by a needle can enhance, reverse, or draw energy from one meridian to another. The yin and yang are again balanced.[3]

A. The World Health Organization of the United Nations considers acupuncture appropriate for the following conditions:

1. Infections: Cold, flu, bronchitis
2. Dermatologic: Eczema, acne, herpes
3. Emotional or mental: Anxiety, depression, insomnia
4. Reproductive: Premenstrual syndrome (PMS), irregular periods with cramps, infertility
5. Internal: High blood pressure, indigestion
6. Musculoskeletal: Sciatica, back pain, sprains
7. Neurologic: Headache (migraine, sinus, tension)
8. General: Weight control

B. Acupuncture is not recommended in the following circumstances:

1. Under 6 years of age
2. In the third trimester of pregnancy when it might induce labor

C. Treatments have a cumulative effect. The longer the problem occurs, the longer it will take to return to harmony.

II. **Acupressure massage** uses pressure and massage along meridian lines to affect and balance chi. Sea-bands used by pregnant women, as well as sailors and others to prevent motion sickness, are an example. The band, with its mushroom-shaped button, is placed 1 to 2 inches above the crease of the inner wrist between the two tendons.

III. **Chinese herbs** assist in the correction of imbalances.

A. Ginseng (Asian) contains phytohormones, which are naturally occurring chemicals derived from plants. Phytohormones create effects in the body similar to those of estrogen, progesterone, and testosterone.

B. Dong quai has many uses. It lowers blood pressure and blood lipid levels and has a regulator effect on uterine contractions, making it helpful in treating PMS and dysmenorrhea.[4] This same effect makes it contraindicated in pregnancy.

CHIROPRACTIC

According to chiropractic, the spine is the center of a person. All physiologic function depends on normal transmissions between the nervous system and all other systems. Because the root of most diseases results from misalignment of the spine, adjusting the spinal column can restore normal function to organs, muscles, joints, and tissues. Chiropractors do not perform major surgery or prescribe medications. They successfully treat headaches, neck, shoulder, back, and leg pain. Insomnia and backaches that result from pregnancy can be treated with varying degrees of success. The further along the pregnancy is, the shorter the duration of relief an individual treatment will provide.

[3]Stampe, 1998

[4]Kass-Annese, 1999, p. 206

HERBAL MEDICINE

Illness occurs when the body is stressed beyond its capacity to respond. The stressors may be internal or external and of short duration or chronic. Herbal medicines attempt to regenerate health by eliminating toxins and by nourishing, building up, and stimulating the body.

In the United States, 25 % of prescription drugs are derived from plants. Another 25% are modeled to mimic actual plant constituents. These medications are carefully studied and rigorously controlled prescription drugs.[5] The rest of the herbs in use are classified as dietary supplements in the United States. They fall into two categories. The medicines in the first category are OTC phytomedications, which are therapeutics based on plant material from either the whole plant or its extracts. These are equivalent to OTC pharmaceuticals. The second category is traditional herbal medicines. These have been used effectively for years without evidence of serious side effects and hence are judged safe without having undergone extensive clinical studies. These two categories contain a multitude of active ingredients whose interactions are extremely complex, making them difficult and costly to study.

Herbal medicines are unlikely to cause adverse reactions because of the low concentrations of active ingredients, unless someone has an idiosyncratic reaction,[6] is pregnant, is taking other medications, or is taking an excess dose of the herbal medication.

Perhaps the greatest concerns regarding herbs are quality control and use.[7] Herbs used may be of poor quality; contaminated by pesticides, microbial toxins, or metals; or prepared in a way that affects the potency and the amount contained in the product. Use issues are the same as those for prescription medications. The full course of treatment may not be completed, and medications may be skipped or taken in excess with the thought that "if one works, two will work better or faster."

See Table 6-1 for herbal classifications and Tables 6-2 and 6-3 for more information on herbals. For more information on soy, see Osteopenia and Osteoporosis in Part 4.

MIND/BODY CONTROL

Mind/body control can empower a person to effectively deal with the stressors encountered in daily life. With relaxation, endorphins and enkephalins are released. The immune system receives a boost. The person feels more peaceful and in control. Mind, spirit, and body come into balance. When stressors in the form of life changes, illness, pain, and so on are present, these can be more effectively handled. See Display 6-1 for examples of mind/body control therapies.

REIKI

Reiki is the channeling (bringing in and passage) of spiritually guided life-force energy. It reduces stress, promotes relaxation, and in turn speeds the

---

[5]Schirmer, 2000, p. 1

[6]Weil, 1998

[7]Kass-Annese, 1999, p. 223

Table 6-1. Herbal Classifications by Botanical Safety[1]

Class 1	Herbs that can be safely consumed when used appropriately
Class 2	Herbs for which the following use restrictions apply, unless otherwise directed by an expert qualified in the use of the described substance:
	(2a) For external use only
	(2b) Not to be used during pregnancy
	(2c) Not to be used while nursing
	(2d) Other specific use restrictions as noted
Class 3	Herbs for which significant data exist to recommend the following labeling: "To be used only under the supervision of an expert qualified in the appropriate use of this substance." Labeling must include proper use information: dosage, contraindications, potential adverse effects, and drug interactions, as well as any other relevant information related to the safe use of this substance.
Class 4	Herbs for which insufficient data are available for classification
Caution:	Herbs are dilute drugs. Herbal medicine has a greater risk of adverse affects and interactions with conventional therapy than any other complementary or alternative therapy.
Evaluation:	The website *www.consumerlab.com* evaluates herbals by name.
Tea preparation:	Mix tea and cold water, bring to a boil, simmer tea 5 to 10 minutes or pour boiling water over tea and let it stand for 5 to 10 minutes.

[1]Classified by the American Herbal Products Association

healing process. Reiki works by balancing energies on all levels: body, mind, spirit, and emotion. It is compatible with medical and psychologic treatment. In addition, it works well with other complementary therapies, such as acupressure massage, aromatherapy, guided imagery, meditation, massage therapy, music, prayer, and reflexology. Reiki is increasingly being offered to patients in hospitals and hospice care facilities. A website has been developed for practitioners who are and who would like to provide Reiki in hospitals: http://www.srpt.org.

MASSAGE AND THERAPEUTIC TOUCH

Massage and therapeutic touch relaxes tense muscles and improves circulation, which have the overall effect of promoting healing and decreasing pain. Because of the release of endorphins, the person feels good and has more energy to deal with life's stressors.

Table 6-2. Herbs for Women's Health

Herb	Class[1]	Actions	Clinical Applications	Dosage	Comments
Black cohosh (*Cimicifuga racemosa*) Synonyms: Black Snakeroot Cohosh Bugbane	2b	Phytoestrogen Antispasmodic— possible opposing effect as a uterine stimulant Sedative	Perimenopausal signs and symptoms PMS Dysmenorrhea Anxiety reduction	200 to 400 mg daily	Has the same contra-indications as estrogen OTC—Remifemin, NewPhase: Black cohosh plus chaste tree
Bugleweed	2b	Unknown	Breast pain and tenderness	0.02 to 2 g per day	Should be decreased slowly when stopping
Caster Oil	2b 2d	Water retained in bowel	Constipation Bowel preparation Initiation of labor in a term pregnancy (not recommended)	1 to 2 tsp (5 to 10 g) Maximum dose is 6 tsp at one time	Can cause potassium depletion Is contraindicated in bowel obstruction, breast-feeding, and pregnancy
Chamomile	Class 1	Antispasmodic Antiinflammatory Sedative	Nausea of pregnancy Nausea and vomiting Ulcers Insomnia	Tea: 4 to 8 g (2 to 4 tsp) of flower heads in 8 oz of water or equivalent in tincture form Half hour before bed	May cause allergic reaction if allergic to ragweed

(continued)

Table 6-2. Herbs for Women's Health (*Continued*)

Herb	Class[1]	Actions	Clinical Applications	Dosage	Comments
Chaste tree (*Vitex agnus-castus*)	2b	Phytoprogesterone Increase of luteinizing hormone and mild inhibition of follicle-stimulating hormone	Perimenopausal signs and symptoms Regulation of menses—give last 14 days of cycle		Decreases the effectiveness of birth control pills (BCPs) Has the same contra-indications as estrogen OTC—*NewPhase:* Chaste tree and black cohosh
	2d	Modulation of the secretion of prolactin, which increases breast milk production	Problems with lactation		
Cinnamon (ubiquinone-10)	1	Flavoring, digestive aid	Pregnancy, lactation		
Coenzyme Q10 (ubiquinone-10)		Supplementation—found naturally in the human body Immune system boost	Breast cancer—reduction of or elimination of metastasis to liver and other organs	Breast cancer: 400 mg per day Capsules: 50 mg once or twice daily	Decreases the effectiveness of anticoagulants OTC—Q10 plus Soy by Sundown
Cranberry	Class 1	Prevention of bacteria from attaching to wall of urinary tract Increase in urine acidity	Urinary tract infections (UTIs)	500 mg tablet every 4 to 6 hours Juice	
Dandelion root (*Taraxacum officinalis*)	2b	Liver tonic that increases bile flow High in calcium	Digestion Prevention of osteopenia and osteoporosis Pregnancy and lactation	375 mg one to two times daily	Has more calcium in the leaf; tea is recommended

Dong quai (*Angelica sinensis*)	2b	Phytohormone Uterus effects—can cause relaxation or contractions Lowers blood pressure Mild antiinflammatory Mild sedative	Perimenopause (hot flashes) Osteoporosis prevention PMS Dysmenorrhea Protection against heart disease, colon cancer	4.5 to 9 g daily 500-mg tablets twice/day for dysmenorrhea	Is a good phytoestrogen to use if have, or have had, breast cancer Promotes menses Serves as an abortive in early pregnancy Has the same contra-indications as estrogen May have drug interactions with anticoagulants OTC—*Rejuvex:* Dong quai, magnesium, and boron
Echinacea (Of nine Types, three are used most: *Echinacea purpurea, Echinacea angustifolia, Echinacea pallida*)	Class 1	Immune system stimulant Antibacterial Antiviral Antiinflammatory Antipyretic Appetite stimulant	Colds, flu, upper respiratory infections (URIs), UTIs—at onset or in early stages Poorly healing wounds, ulcers, burns, eczema, psoriasis, and herpes simplex	Capsules: 300 mg three times daily Juice, tincture, powder, cream, salve, and freeze—dried herbs follow label directions	Should be cautious if have asthma allergies Does *not* prevent disease Should not take tablets more than 2 to 3 weeks May intensify the effects of warfarin
Evening primrose oil (*Oenothera biennis*)	Class 1	Estrogen and progesterone balance Mild sedative	Perimenopause, PMS, premenstrual breast tenderness Aromatheraphy, massage	3 g daily, 14 days before menses	Should not use if taking phenothiazines or medications for schizophrenia
Feverfew (*Tanacetum parthenium*)	2b	Inhibition of prostaglandins Antiinflammatory	Migraine headaches	Capsules: 125 mg daily	Is contraindicated if allergic to it or to ragweed, chamomile, or yarrow Is not recommended in pregnancy May cause gastrointestinal (GI) upset, mouth ulcers *(continued)*

Table 6-2. Herbs for Women's Health (*Continued*)

Herb	Class[1]	Actions	Clinical Applications	Dosage	Comments
Garlic (*Allium sativum*)	2c	Antioxidant, antiviral, antibacterial, antimycotic Hypotensive Reduction of cholesterol Antiinflammatory Prolongation of bleeding and clotting time	URIs and other infections High blood pressure High cholesterol Arteriosclerosis	1 to 2 cloves daily 500 µg Allicin/day (check tablet label) 2.5 mg garlic oil daily	Is GI irritant—may cause nausea, vomiting, gas, and diarrhea May interact with anticoagulant drugs
Ginger root (*Zingiber officinale*)	Fresh, Class 1 Dried, 2b, 2d	Antinauseant Antispasmodic Antioxidant Cholesterol lowering	Nausea of pregnancy[2] or after surgery Dysmenorrhea, cramps, gas	2 to 4 500-mg tablets daily Tea: 1 tsp dried ginger in 8 oz water two to three times daily Fresh ginger as needed (PRN)	Should not be taken with aspirin or Coumadin Should use fresh ginger, if patient is pregnant
Ginkgo biloba	2d	Improved circulation to brain Enhanced memory and alertness Antioxidant Diuretic	Cerebral vascular insufficiency Dementia Aging—decreases free radicals, slowing damage and hence aging Edema in feet and ankles, claudication	2 to 4 60-mg tablets daily	May cause bleeding when used with nonsteroidal antiinflammatory drugs (NSAIDs) and anticoagulants May cause GI irritation, headaches, allergic reactions

		Actions	Uses/Indications	Dosage	Notes
Ginseng-Asian (*Panax*)	2d	Phytoestrogen Immune stimulant Appetite stimulant Mild diuretic	Perimenopausal and menopausal signs and symptoms Poor appetite during illness and convalescence Edema	1 to 2 g dry root chewed Tincture: 1 to 3 mL daily	Has the same contra-indications as estrogen Is contraindicated with acute illness, hypertension, or other stimulants
Green tea (*Camellia sinensis*)	2d	Cholesterol reduction—Lowers low-density lipoproteins (LDLs), increases high-density lipoprotein (HDL) cholesterol Antitumor activity—Stops progression of cancer Antioxidant	High cholesterol Chemoprevention	Tea: 1 oz per 8 oz of water	Should limit amount to a maximum 10 cups per day
Kava kava (*Piper methysticum*)	2b 2d	Sedative Antianxiety Topical antifungal Mild analgesic Mild muscle relaxant	Insomnia Anxiety Candidiasis	Herb: 60 to 120 mg kava pyrones Standardized extract (70% kava lactones): 100 mg 2–3 times daily Insomnia: 200 mg at bedtime	Works better taken PRN than daily Is not recommended during pregnancy or lactation or with other sedatives or antidepressants
Lavender external use	1	Mood elevator—aromatherapy, massage Mild sedative	Insomnia Pregnancy, lactation		

(continued)

Table 6-2. Herbs for Women's Health (Continued)

Herb	Class[1]	Actions	Clinical Applications	Dosage	Comments
Licorice (*Glycyrrhiza glabra*)	2b 2c 2d	Active ingredient glycyrrhizin; Estrogenlike; Smooth muscle affected; Increased cortisol—increased sodium and water retention, which elevates blood pressure	Hot flashes (decreases); Peptic ulcer, gastritis, colic, bronchitis; Use as a flavoring agent	5 to 15 g or root (equals 200 to 600 mg glycyrrhizin); Tincture: 1 to 3 mL three times daily	Is *toxic* in large doses; Is contraindicated for diabetes, hypertension, kidney disease, liver disease, hypokalemia; May potentiate laxatives, cortisol, cardiac glycosides, potassium depletion of thiazide diuretics
Mint	1	Flavoring, digestive aid, high in calcium and magnesium	Pregnancy, lactation		
Passion Flower (*Passiflora incarnata*)	Class 4	Antispasmodic; Smooth muscle relaxer; Sedative	PMS; Insomnia	Tea: ½ tsp (0.5 to 7 g) in 8 oz water	
Peppermint (*Mentha piperita*)	Class 1	Antispasmodic—affects GI smooth muscle; Antinauseant	Abdominal distention, gas, pain; irritable bowel syndrome (IBS); Nausea	IBS: 0.6 mL enteric-ecoated capsule; Tea: 3 to 6 g daily; Oil: 0.2-mL single use	May cause heartburn
Psyllium Seed	Class 1	Bulk-forming agent	Constipation		Is recommended in pregnancy; Is contraindicated in bowel obstruction
Red Raspberry	Class 1	Antiabortive; Toning of uterus and smooth muscle; Antiseptic; Antioxidant	Early pregnancy; Irregular menstrual cycle (balances cycle)	Tea: 1 oz per 8 oz water, two to three times daily; Tincture: 2 to 4 mL three times daily	

	Class	Actions	Dosage	Indications	Notes
Shepherd's Purse		Antispasmodic Mild analgesic	5 to 15 g daily	History of heavy periods and cramping	
Soybeans (*Glycine max*) and Soy-based Products	Class 1	Phytoestrogen: the major isoflavone with estrogen activity Antioxidant Anticancer activity Maintenance of bone density Lowering of total serum lipids: Increased HDLs Lowered LDLs Coronary artery dilation	200 to 400 mg daily	Perimenopausal and menopausal signs and symptoms (decreases) Removal of free radicals from system; prevention of aging and damage to DNA and lysosomes Breast cancer Osteoporosis Cholesterol-lowering agent Preventive—heart disease	Has the following approximate isoflavone content: Soy milk 40 mg Tofu 40 mg Miso 40 mg Soy protein, textured and cooked 35 mg Soy flour 35 mg Many OTC products— *Estroven:* Soy, B$_6$, B$_{12}$, E, calcium *Healthy Woman:* 320 mg soybean, 55 mg isoflavone genistin *Promensil:*40 mg of isoflavone
St. John's wort (*Hypericum perforatum*)	2d	Antidepressant— Increase in brain serotonin levels Sedative Antiviral	300 mg three times daily	Anxiety, apathy, and depression Medication substitute—Prozac Wound and burn healing Fibromyalgia, multiple sclerosis (some success)	*Decreases effectiveness and should not be used with*[3] *warfarin.* cyclosporin, digoxin, theophylline, BCPs Do not use with other antianxiety or antidepressant medications May try folic acid, vitamins B$_6$ and B$_{12}$, thiamin, and niacin for mild depression before trying St. John's wort, or use them concurrently

(continued)

Table 6-2. Herbs for Women's Health *(Continued)*

Herb	Class[1]	Actions	Clinical Applications	Dosage	Comments
Valerian (*Valeriana officinalis*)	Class 1	Sedative—Blocks arousal centers of the brain Mild pain relief	Insomnia Anxiety (decreased) Stomach cramps	Insomnia: 300 to 400 mg root extract standardized to equal 0.5% essential oil Anxiety: 200 to 300 mg twice daily Tea: 1 oz tea to 8 oz water, 2–3 times/day	Should not use with other OTC or prescription sleeping pills
Willow bark (*Salix alba*)	2b 2d	Active ingredient salicin (aspirin) Antipyretic Antiinflammatory	Pain Fever Inflammation	6 to 12 g twice daily (equals 60 to 120 mg salicin)	Has been used in TCM for more than 2500 yrs Is contraindicated in those with aspirin sensitivity, children, and pregnant women

[1]See Table 6-1 for a description of safety classifications. [2]Vutyavanich, T., et al. (2001). Ginger reduces nausea and vomiting of pregnancy. *Obstetrice and Gynecology, 97*, 577–582. [3]Yue, O.Y., Berquist, C., & Gorden, B. (2000). Safety of St. John's wort. *Lancet, 355*, 576–577.

Table 6-3. Herbs, Pregnancy, and Lactation

Recommended	Rationale
Chamomile	Antispasmodic—nausea relief
	Sedative—insomnia
Chaste tree	Use for increasing breast milk production
Cinnamon	Flavoring, digestive aid
Cranberry	Use for UTI signs and symptoms
Dandelion root	Digestion aid, high in calcium
Evening primrose oil	Mild sedative—good for massage, aromatherapy
Ginger	Antinausea medication
Lavender, External Use	Mood elevator—aromatherapy, massage
	Mild sedative—sleep aid when placed on pillow
Mint	Flavoring, digestive aid, high in calcium and magnesium
Peppermint	Antispasmodic—nausea, heartburn relief
Psyllium seed	Bulk-forming agent used for constipation relief
Red raspberry	Antiabortive
	Use for toning the uterus and smooth muscles
Rose hips	Flavoring and vitamin C
Valerian	Sedative—insomnia
	Mild pain relief—insomnia

Not Recommended	Rationale
Angelica	Risk for promoting menstruation
Black cohosh	Abortive—may act as uterine stimulant
Coltsfoot	Risk to liver of fetus
Comfrey	Risk because contains toxic alkaloids—liver damage
Ephedra (ma huang)	Risk because increases heart rate—stroke
	Abortive—causes uterine contractions
Feverfew	Risk because promotes menstruation
Ginseng	Potential to increase general discomfort
Golden seal	Abortive—stimulates uterine contractions
Kava kava	Inadequate studies
Licorice	Toxic in large doses
Pennyroyal—European (*mentha pulegium*)	Potential to cause death

(continued)

Table 6-3. Herbs, Pregnancy, and Lactation (Continued)

Not Recommended	Rationale
Rue (*Ruta graveolens*)	Risk for causing uterine contractions
	Risk for lowering blood pressure
Tansy	Risk to liver of fetus
Willow Bark	Mild anticoagulant
	Risk for prolonging pregnancy
Yarrow	Risk for decreasing blood pressure
	Risk for promoting menstruation

Special Cases	Rationale
Castor Oil	Water retained in bowel—*not* recommended in pregnancy; may cause electrolyte imbalance, dehydration
	Potential cramps, diarrhea in infant—*never use* in breast-feeding with castor oil, 3 to 4 tsp in 8 oz of cold orange juice
	Induction of labor—in a term or postterm pregnancy is *not* recommended.
Chaste Tree	Phytoprogesterone—not recommended in pregnancy
	Use in lactating women—modulates the secretion of prolactin and increases production of breast milk
Dong Quai	Early pregnancy—not recommended; is abortive
	Term or postterm pregnancy—may induce labor by causing the uterus to contract; short-term use only

 AROMATHERAPY

Aromatherapy is the enhancement of body, mind, and spirit with aromatic botanical essential oils. The essential oil of each plant is its life force. It is readily absorbed through the skin and, when inhaled, affects the brain to release neurochemicals. Specific oils can soothe, relax, increase mental alertness and energy, and so on.

I.   **Oils.** Commonly used oils are grapefruit (reduces cellulite, balances fluids, prevents obesity), lavender (improves sleep, reduces aches and pains, serves as a disinfectant), sandalwood (uplifts the mood, calms, moisturizes the skin), spearmint (cools, improves digestion, opens sinuses, relieves aches and pains), bergamot (reduces stress, increases mental alertness), tangerine (calms, uplifts the mood), patchouli (prevents sleep, serves as a stimulant and aphrodisiac).

DISPLAY 6-1   Examples of Mind/Body Control Therapies

Mind/body control therapies are many and varied, and include the following:

Biofeedback	Prayer
Counseling	Meditation
Psychotherapy	Healing essence
Hypnotherapy	Guided imagery
Support groups	Relaxation techniques
Yoga	Music
Tai Chi	Dance
Chi' kong	Art
Humor	

II. **Recommended Aromatherapies During Pregnancy**

   A. Sleep: Lavender on pillow

   B. Relaxation: Three drops of tangerine, three drops of sandalwood and 1 tsp of carrier oil

   C. Energizing: Three drops of spearmint, three drops of patchouli, and 1 tsp of carrier oil

III. **Recommended Massage Oils During Pregnancy**

   A. Aches and pains: Three drops of lavender, two drops of spearmint, and 1 tsp of a carrier oil

   B. Mental clarity: Three drops of spearmint, two drops of bergamot, and 1 tsp of carrier oil

 NUTRITION, EXERCISE, AND LIFESTYLE

Nutrition, exercise, and lifestyle changes affect women throughout their life cycle. These are discussed in individual sections throughout this book.

PART 7

Drug Index

Geri Morgan, CNM, ND

Carole Hamilton, BSN, MA, CNM

This drug index provides a quick reference to the commonly used drugs suggested in the other sections of this book. The description of each drug includes its generic name, class of drug, pregnancy category, indications, dosages, contraindications, precautions, interactions, adverse reactions, and the forms in which the drug is supplied. It is especially important, when caring for pregnant women, to be aware of the effects of a drug on the fetus and on the baby when the patient is lactating. To that end, each drug described has an FDA classification indicating its safety in pregnancy. An explanation of those classifications follows.

Drug Classifications

Category A: Well-controlled human studies have not disclosed any fetal risks.

Category B: Animal studies have not disclosed any fetal risk or suggested some risk that is not confirmed in controlled studies in women; or there are no adequate studies in women.

Category C: Animal studies reveal adverse fetal effects; or there are no adequate controlled studies in women.

Category D: Some fetal risk exists. The benefits may outweigh the risks (e.g., life-threatening illness, no safer effective drug available). The patient should be warned of the risks.

Category X: Fetal abnormalities occurred in animal and human studies. The risk does not outweigh the benefit. This drug is contraindicated in pregnancy.

ACTIFED

TRIPROLIDINE HCL AND PSEUDOEPHEDERINE HCL

Drug class: Antihistamine, sympathomimetic

Pregnancy Category B

Indications:

- Rhinitis
- Congestion

Adult dosage: Take one tablet orally every 4 to 6 hours for a maximum of four doses a day. Also 12-hour capsules: Take one capsule every 12 hours.

Contraindications: If taken during or within 14 days of taking monoamine oxidase inhibitors, patients may experience severe hypertension, coronary disease, or gastrointestinal or urinary obstruction.

Precautions: Thyroid disease, diabetes

Interactions: Hypertensive crisis may occur with monoamine oxidase inhibitors; beta-blockers may increase the pressor effects of sympathomimetics. Alcohol and other central nervous system depressants are potentiated.

Adverse reactions: Drowsiness, anticholinergic effects, gastrointestinal upset, dizziness, anxiety, weakness, insomnia, thickening of the bronchial secretions, hypotension, respiratory depression or difficulty, palpitations

How supplied: Tablets, 12-hour capsules, syrup: 4 oz or pint

ACYCLOVIR

ZOVIRAX

Drug class: Antiviral, purine nucleoside analogue

Pregnancy Category B

Indications:

- Genital herpes
- Herpes zoster (shingles)
- Varicella (chickenpox)

Adult dosage: For genital herpes, take an initial dose of 400 mg five times a day for 10 to 14 days. For recurring genital herpes, take 400 mg twice a day for 5 to 7 days. For chronic genital herpes, take 400 mg daily for up to 12 months. For herpes zoster, take 800 mg every 4 hours (maximum five times per day) for 7 to 10 days. For Varicella, initiate dosage at the earliest sign, taking 20 mg/kg, four times a day for 5 days. The maximum dose is 800 mg/kg. Start suppression at 36 weeks' gestation to reduce the risk of a cesarean section at term. For ointment application, see Part 8, Topical Agents.

Precautions: Early pregnancy, lactation

Contraindications: Allergy to acyclovir, renal disease, seizures, congestive heart failure

Interactions: Probenecid decreases urinary excretion of acyclovir.

Adverse reactions: Nausea, vomiting, headache, central nervous system disturbances, diarrhea, vertigo, arthralgias, rash, malaise, fatigue, viral resistance

How supplied: Tablets: 200 mg, 400 mg; 5% ointment

AMERGE

NARATRIPTAN HCL

Drug class: Selective 5-HT receptor agonist

Pregnancy Category C

Indications: Acute migraines

Adult dosage: Take 1 mg to 2.5 mg; consider repeating dose once after 4 hours for a maximum of 5 mg/day.

Contraindications: Ischemic cardiac, cerebral, or peripheral vascular disease; hypertension; renal or hepatic dysfunction

Precautions: Confirm the diagnosis; exclude cardiovascular disease, elderly, pregnancy, lactation

Interactions: Serotonin syndrome develops with administration of selective serotonin reuptake inhibitors (SSRIs).

Adverse reactions: Fatigue, pain, pressure or tightness in the throat, serious cardiac event (rare)

How supplied: Tablets: 1 mg, 2.5 mg

Amoxicillin (TRIMOX, AMOXIL)

AMPICILLIN (OMNIPEN, PRINCIPEN)

Drug class: Broad-spectrum penicillin

Pregnancy Category B

Indications: Amoxicillin-sensitive infections, including those of the ear, respiratory or genitourinary tract, skin, and soft tissue; acute uncomplicated gonorrhea

Adult dosage: Take 250 to 500 mg orally every 8 hours.

Contraindications: Allergy to penicillins, cephalosporins, or other allergens. Use caution in the presence of renal disorders, lactation.

Precautions: Allergy to cephalosporins or other allergens, lactation. Monitor blood, renal, and liver function in long-term use. Continue therapy for 2 to 3 days after symptoms improve.

Interactions: Probenecid potentiates amoxicillin and ampicillin.

Adverse reactions: Superinfection, anaphylaxis, urticaria, gastrointestinal upset, blood dyscrasias, hyperactivity

How supplied: Capsules: 100, 250, and 500 mg; chewable tablets: 125, 250 mg; suspension: 80, 100, 180 mL; drops: 50 mg/mL

Aygestin

NORETHINDRONE ACETATE

Drug class: Progestin

Pregnancy Category X

Indications:

- Abnormal uterine bleeding secondary to hormonal imbalance
- Endometriosis
- Secondary amenorrhea

Adult dosage: For amenorrhea or abnormal uterine bleeding, take 2.5 to 10 mg daily for 5 to 10 days; for endometriosis, take 5 mg daily for 2 weeks, followed by 7.5 mg for 2 weeks and then increase the dose by 2.5 mg every 2 weeks to a maximum of 15 mg per day for 6 to 9 months.

Contraindications: Renal and hepatic dysfunction, migraines, undiagnosed vaginal bleeding, breast and genital cancer, any thromboembolic disorder

Precautions: Cardiac, renal, or hepatic dysfunction. Discontinue if vision loss, migraine headache, or thrombophlebitis occurs.

Adverse reactions: Rash, menstrual and cervical changes, edema, decreased glucose tolerance

How supplied: Tablets: 2.5, 5, 10 mg

Bactrim DS

SULPHAMETHOXAZOLE-TRIMETHOPRIM

Drug class: Sulfa

Pregnancy Category C

Indications:

- Urinary tract infections
- Traveler's diarrhea
- Chronic bronchitis

Adult dosage: For urinary tract infections, take 1 tablet orally twice a day for 3 to 10 days; for traveler's diarrhea, take 1 tablet twice a day for 3 to 5 days or as a prophylaxis, use 1 tablet daily.

Contraindications: Anemia, folic acid deficiency

Precautions: Hepatic and renal dysfunction, glucose-6-phosphate dehydrogenase (G6PD) deficiency

Adverse reactions: Stomach, colon, and renal problems; lupuslike syndromes; depression

How supplied: Tablets: One tablet consists of 800 mg of sulfamethoxazole and 160 mg of trimethoprim.

Bellergal-S

Drug class: Barbiturate, ergot alkaloid, anticholinergic

Pregnancy Category X

Indications: Menopausal disorders with hot flashes, sweats, restlessness, or insomnia

Adult dosage: Take 1 tablet twice daily.

Contraindications: Coronary or peripheral vascular disease, hypertension, impaired hepatic or renal function, glaucoma, pregnancy, or lactation. Paradoxical reactions result from phenobarbital administration.

Precautions: Gastrointestinal problems, myasthenia gravis, asthma

Interactions: Avoid other vasoconstrictors (e.g., dopamine). Concomitant antacids may inhibit absorption. Bellergal-S may antagonize anticoagulants. Monitor patients on concomitant beta-blockers. Additive anticholinergic effects occur with tricyclic antidepressants.

Adverse reactions: Drowsiness, nausea, vomiting, local edema, itching, vasoconstrictive complications, tachycardia or bradycardia, paresthesia of extremities, anticholinergic effects, paradoxical excitement

How supplied: Tablets

Benadryl

DIPHENHYDRAMINE HCL

Drug class: Antihistamine
Pregnancy Category B in Third Trimester
Indications:

- Allergic and vasomotor rhinitis, conjunctivitis, pruritus, reactions to blood
- Adjunct in anaphylaxis
- Sleep aid

Adult dosage: Take 25 to 50 mg orally every 4 to 6 hours for a maximum of 300 mg daily. Take 25 to 50 mg intramuscularly (IM) every 4 to 6 hours.

Contraindications: Allergy to any antihistamines, lactation

Precautions: Asthma, lower respiratory disorders, glaucoma, hyperthyroidism, hypertension, cardiovascular disease, and gastrointestinal or urinary obstruction

Interactions: Benadryl potentiates central nervous system depression with alcohol and other central nervous system depressants. Benadryl potentiates anticholinergic effects with monoamine oxidase inhibitors.

Adverse reactions: Drowsiness, dizziness, anticholinergic effects, gastritis, paradoxical excitement, blood dyscrasias, hypotension

How supplied: Capsules: 25, 50 mg; elixir: 12.5mg/5mL IM and 10 or 50 mg/mL intravenously (IV)

Betamethasone SODIUM PHOSPHATE/BETAMETHASONE ACETATE

CELESTONE SOLUSPAN

Drug class: Corticosteroid, glucocorticoid, and hormonal agent
Pregnancy Category C
Indications: Maturation of fetal lungs in premature labor

Adult dosage: Take 12.5 mg IM. Repeat dose in 24 hours. Consider repeating dose 1 week later.

Contraindications: The Food and Drug Administration (FDA) has not currently approved betamethasone for premature labor. *Do not* give the medication to patients taking anticonvulsant drugs or those who are allergic to betamethasone.

Adverse reactions: Burning, itching, irritation at injection site, sweating, tachycardia

How supplied: 12.5 mg/mL IM

BICILLIN L-A

PENICILLIN G BENZATHINE

Drug class: Antibiotic

Pregnancy Category B

Indications: Moderately severe infections, including respiratory, skin, and soft tissue.

Adult dosage: For a group A streptococcal respiratory infection, take 1.2 million units IM in a single dose; for syphilis of less than 1 year's duration, take 2.4 million units IM in a single dose; for syphilis of more than 1 year's duration, take 2.4 million units IM weekly for three successive weeks.

Contraindications: *Never* give Bicillin IV; inadvertent IV administration has caused cardiac arrest and death. Use cautiously in patients with other drug allergies, especially allergies to cephalosporins.

Interactions: Probenecid potentiates Bicillin.

Adverse reactions: Anaphylaxis, seizures, nausea, hemolytic anemia, exfoliative dermatitis

How supplied: Injection: 300,000 or 600,000 units/mL

CHOLESTYRAMINE

QUESTRAN LIGHT

Drug class: Bile acid sequestrant

Pregnancy Category B

Indications:

- Hypercholesterolemia alone or with hypertriglyceridemia resistant to dietary management for the reduction in the risk of coronary heart disease
- Pruritus caused by partial biliary obstruction, induced by pregnancy

Adult dosage: Initially mix one packet or scoop with fluid or food one to two times daily. For maintenance, divide two to four packets or scoops into two doses for a maximum of six daily packets or scoops. Increase this amount at 4-week intervals, as needed.

Contraindications: Complete biliary obstruction, lactation

Precautions: Obtain baseline serum cholesterol, low-density lipoprotein (LDL) cholesterol, and triglyceride levels and monitor these levels during therapy. Consider supplementation of vitamins A, D, K, and folic acid with long-term therapy. Exclude secondary causes of hypercholesterolemia. A favorable trend in cholesterol reduction usually occurs within 1 month; continue therapy to sustain reduction. Use cautiously with patients who have phenylketonuria, constipation, or hemorrhoids.

Interactions: Cholestyramine inhibits the absorption of phenylbutazone, warfarin, cholorothiazide, propranolol, tetracycline, penicillin G, phenobarbital, thyroid drugs, digoxin, and many others; give other drugs 1 to 2 hours before or 4 to 6 hours after giving cholestyramine.

Adverse reactions: Constipation; aggravation of hemorrhoids; gastrointestinal disturbances; vitamins A, D, K, or folic acid deficiencies; rash

How supplied: Light 5-g packet-60; 9-g packet-60; 210-g can-1 (with scoop)

CHROMAGEN

Drug class: Hermatinics
Pregnancy Category—None
Indications: Iron deficiency
Adult dosage: Take one capsule orally daily.
Contraindications: Hemochromatosis, hemosiderosis
Precautions: Hepatitis, pancreatitis, achlorhydria, peptic ulcer, or gastrointestinal inflammation. Monitor hematocrit.
Interactions: Chromagen inhibits tetracycline absorption. Antacids inhibit iron absorption.
Adverse reactions: Nausea, rash, vomiting, diarrhea, black stools, flushing
How supplied: Capsules

CLEOCIN/CLEOCIN VAGINAL

CLINDAMYCIN PHOSPHATE AS INJECTION OR VAGINAL PREPARATION

Drug class: Lincosamide antibiotic
Pregnancy Category B
Indications:

• Systemic administration: Serious infections caused by susceptible strains of anaerobes, streptococci, staphylococci, pneumococci
• Reserve use for penicillin-allergic patients
• Treatment for acne vulgaris
• Treatment for bacterial vaginosis, vaginal preparation

Adult dosage: Take 150 to 300 mg orally every 6 hours, up to 300 to 450 mg every 6 hours in more severe infections. For vaginal preparation, insert one Cleocin Vaginal Ovule every night for 3 days or one 100-mg clindamycin phosphate preparation intravaginally at bedtime for 7 consecutive days.

Contraindications: Allergy to clindamycin or tartrazine, history of asthma, hepatic or renal dysfunction, lactation.

Adverse reactions: Systemic administration: nausea, vomiting, diarrhea, abdominal pain, esophagitis, anorexia, and rash. Vaginal preparation: Cervicitis, vaginitis, contact dermatitis.

How supplied: Tablets: 75, 150, and 300 mg; IV and injection: 150, 300 mg/mL; 2.5% cream; vaginal ovules.

Climara

ESTRADIOL

Drug class: Hormone—estrogen
Pregnancy Category X
Indications:

* Estrogen replacement therapy
* Moderate to severe vasomotor symptoms of menopause
* Vulvar or vaginal atrophy

Adult dosage: Apply one 0.1-mg/day patch once per week to trunk (avoid the breasts and waistline).

Contraindications: Undiagnosed abnormal genital bleeding, thromboembolic disorders, breast or estrogen-dependent carcinomas

Precautions: Familial hyperlipoproteinemia; cardiovascular disease; hepatic, renal, or cardiac insufficiency; uterine leiomyomatas; diabetes; thromboembolic disease. Discontinue if hypertension or jaundice occurs.

Adverse reactions: Increased risk of endometrial cancer or hyperplasia, gallbladder disease, thromboembolic disorders, breakthrough bleeding, mastodynia, nausea, abdominal cramps, headache, increased size of uterine fibromyomata, irritation at application site

How supplied: Patch: 0.05, 0.1 mg

Colace

DOCUSATE SODIUM

Drug class: Laxative
Pregnancy Category C
Indications: Short-term relief of constipation

Adult dosage: Take 50 to 200 mg orally every day, twice a day or 200 mg at bedtime.

Contraindications: Acute abdominal disorders, appendicitis, diverticulitis, and ulcerative colitis

Adverse reactions: Excessive bowel activity, perianal irritation, abdominal cramps, weakness, dizziness, and electrolyte imbalance

How supplied: Tablets: 50, 100, 240, 300 mg

DARVOCET-N 100

PROPOXYPHENE NAPSYLATE AND ACETAMINOPHEN

Drug class: Opioid

Pregnancy Category C

Indications: Mild to moderate pain

Adult dosage: Take one tablet orally every 4 hours as necessary.

Contraindications: Suicidal or addiction-prone patients

Interactions: Alcohol and other central nervous system depressants potentiate Darvocet-N 100.

Adverse reactions: Dizziness, sedation, nausea, vomiting, constipation, rash, respiratory depression

How supplied: Capsules or tablets consist of 100 mg of propoxyphene napsylate with 650 mg of acetaminophen

DEMEROL

MEPERIDINE HCL

Drug class: Opioid

Pregnancy Category C

Indications: Moderate to severe pain

Adult dosage: For pain, take 50 mg orally; 50 to 100 mg IM or subcutaneously every 3 to 4 hours, as necessary; or 25 to 50 mg IV every 3 to 4 hours, as necessary.

Contraindications: Administration within 14 days of taking monoamine oxidase inhibitors

Precautions: Increased intracranial pressure; acute abdomen; convulsive disorders; impaired respiratory, renal, hepatic, thyroid, or adrenocortical function; supraventricular tachycardias; drug abusers

Interactions: Toxicity occurs with monoamine oxidase inhibitors, which may be fatal. Alcohol, central nervous system depressants, phenothiazines, and tricyclics potentiate Demerol.

Adverse reactions: High abuse potential, sedation, dizziness, sweating, dry mouth, nausea, vomiting, constipation, urinary retention, hypotension, rash, convulsions with large doses, respiratory depression

How supplied: Tablets: 25, 50 mg; injection: 1 mL; syrup: 25, 50, 75, 100 mg/ 1 mL

DEPO-PROVERA

MEDROXYPROGESTERONE ACETATE

Drug class: Progesterone derivative

Pregnancy Category X

Indications: Injectable contraception

Adult dosage: Take 150 mg IM every 12 weeks. A dosage adjustment for body weight is not necessary.

Contraindications: Undiagnosed vaginal bleeding, thromboembolic disorders, cerebrovascular disease, hepatic dysfunction, lactation

Precautions: Asthma, epilepsy, migraines, diabetes, cardiac or renal dysfunction, or depression. Discontinue if jaundice, visual disturbances, migraines, or thrombotic disorders occur.

Interactions: Aminoglutethimide may antagonize Depo-Provera.

Adverse reactions: Irregular bleeding, edema, weight or cervical changes, cholestatic jaundice, thromboembolic events, depression, insomnia, nausea, breast tenderness, galactorrhea, hirsutism, alopecia, rash

How supplied: Injection: 100, 400 mg/mL

DETROL/DETROL LA

TOLTERODINE TARTRATE

Drug class: Anticholinergic and smooth muscle relaxant

Pregnancy Category C

Indications: Overactive bladder

Adult dosage: For Detrol, take 2 mg orally twice a day; for Detrol LA, 4 mg daily in an extended-release tablet.

Contraindications: Urinary retention, uncontrolled glaucoma, hypersensitivity

Precautions: Renal or hepatic dysfunction, controlled narrow-angle glaucoma

Adverse reactions: Dry mouth, headache, abdominal pain, constipation

How supplied: Extended-release tablets: 2, 4 mg

DIFLUCAN

FLUCONAZOLE

Drug class: Antifungal

Pregnancy Category C

Indications: Candidiasis

Adult dosage: Take 150 mg orally in a single dose; repeat the dose in 4 to 5 days if the condition is not completely resolved. Take 200 to 400 mg orally the first day, followed by 100 to 200 mg every day for 2 weeks for oropharyngeal and systemic candidiasis, respectively. For suppression, take 100 to 200 mg orally once a month.

Contraindications: Patients with hypersensitivity to fluconazole, caution in patients with underlying hepatic dysfunction

Precautions: Lactation

Adverse reactions: Headache, nausea, vomiting, diarrhea, skin rash

How supplied: Tablets: 50, 100, 150, 200 mg

DITROPAN/DITROPAN XL

OXYBUTYNIN CHLORIDE

Drug class: Anticholinergic and smooth muscle relaxant

Pregnancy Category B

Indications: Overactive bladder

Adult dosage: For Ditropan, take 2.5 to 5 mg, three or four times daily. For Ditropan XL, take 5 to 15 mg daily in extended-release tablets.

Contraindications: Urinary retention, uncontrolled glaucoma, hypersensitivity

Precautions: Renal or hepatic dysfunction, controlled narrow-angle glaucoma

Adverse reactions: Dry mouth, headache, abdominal pain, constipation

How supplied: Extended-release tablets: 5, 10, 15 mg

DOXYCYCLINE

VIBRAMYCIN

Drug class: Antibiotic
Pregnancy Category D
Indications:

- Pelvic inflammatory disease
- Sexually transmitted diseases (STDs) when penicillin is contraindicated
- Traveler's diarrhea prophylaxis

Adult dosage: Take 100 mg orally twice a day for 5 to 10 days. For traveler's diarrhea prophylaxis, take 100 mg orally every day. Begin 2 to 3 days before the trip.

Contraindications: Pregnancy, lactation, allergy to tetracyclines

Precautions: Monitor blood, renal, and liver function in long-term use; limit exposure to sunlight or ultraviolet light.

Interactions: Antacids, iron, zinc, calcium, magnesium. Urinary alkalinizers reduce absorption. Monitor prothrombin time with oral anticoagulants.

Adverse reactions: Superinfection, photosensitivity, gastrointestinal upset, enterocolitis, rash, blood dyscrasias, hepatotoxicity

How supplied: Capsules: 50, 100 mg

EFFEXOR XR

VENLAFAXINE HCL

Drug class: Antidepressant
Pregnancy Category C
Indications:

- Anxiety or depression
- Hot flashes for breast cancer survivors

Adult dosage: For anxiety or depression, take 75 mg to 150 mg; For hot flashes, take 75 mg daily.

Contraindications: Concomitant taking of monoamine oxidase inhibitors

Precautions: Monitor blood pressure; reduce dosage if hypertension occurs. Use medication cautiously if renal or hepatic abnormalities exist. Take it with food.

Adverse reactions: Nausea, vomiting, hypertension, dry mouth, anorexia, constipation, flatulence, visual disturbances, emotional changes

How supplied: Tablets and capsules: 37.5, 75, 150 mg

ENTEX LA (PHENYLPROPANOLAMINE AND GUAIFENESIN)

ENTEX PSE (PSEUDOEPHEDRINE AND GUAIFENESIN)

Drug class: Decongestant and expectorant

Pregnancy Category C

Indications: Nasal congestion associated with sinusitis, bronchitis

Adult dosage: Take one tablet every 12 to 24 hours; *do not* crush or chew the tablets.

Contraindications: Severe hypertension, coronary artery disease, administration within 14 days of taking monoamine oxidase inhibitors

Precautions: Hypertension, diabetes, cardiovascular disease, glaucoma, elderly, hyperthyroidism

Interactions: A hypertensive crisis may occur with monoamine oxidase inhibitors. Beta-blockers may increase the pressor effects of sympathomimetics. Antihypertensives may be antagonized.

Adverse reactions: Headaches, nervousness, dizziness, insomnia, convulsions, central nervous system depression, tachycardia, palpitations, urinary retention, gastrointestinal upset

How supplied: Capsules

EPINEPHRINE

ADRENALIN

Drug class: Adrenergic bronchodilator and vasopressor

Pregnancy Category C

Indications: Anaphylaxis, cardiac arrest, and prolongation of local anesthetic effect

Adult dosage: For anaphylaxis, give 0.1 to 0.5 mL of a 1:1000 solution subcutaneously or IM; repeat every 10 to 15 minutes as necessary, or give 0.1 to 0.25 mL of a 1:1000 solution IV. For cardiac arrest, give 0.5 to 1 mg IV or endotracheally. Doses may be given up to 5 mg, especially in patients who do not respond to the usual IV doses. For a local anesthetic effect, give 1:500,000 to 1:50,000 mixed with a local anesthetic.

Contraindications: Glaucoma, shock, organic brain damage, cardiac dilatation, coronary insufficiency, and patients in labor

Interactions: Beta-blockers may cause hypotension. β-blockers may cause vasoconstriction and reflex bradycardia.

Adverse reactions: Palpitations, tachycardia, nervousness, headache, apnea, hypertension, tachyarrhythmias, ventricular fibrillation, cerebrovascular accident

How supplied: Injection—various strengths

ERYTHROMYCIN BASE FILM TABS, E.E.S./E-MYCIN/ERY-TABS

ERYTHROMYCIN

Drug class: Macrolide antibiotic

Pregnancy Category B

Indications: Susceptible infections including respiratory, skin and soft tissue, genitourinary

Adult dosage: Take 250 to 500 mg orally every 6 hours, 1 hour before meals; take a maximum of 4 g daily for 7 to 10 days.

Contraindications: Allergy to medication, irritable bowel syndrome, colitis, bowel diseases

Precautions: Hepatic dysfunction

Interactions: Erythromycin may potentiate carbamazepine, methylprednisolone, cyclosporine, digoxin, theophylline, warfarin, ergotamine, terfenadine, triazolam, and others.

Adverse reactions: Hepatotoxicity, superinfection, gastrointestinal upset, rash, reversible hearing loss

How supplied: Capsules: 250, 500 mg; cream: 42.5 g

ESTRACE/ESTRACE 0.01% VAGINAL CREAM

ESTRADIOL

Drug class: Hormone—estrogen

Pregnancy Category X

Indications:

- Moderate to severe vasomotor symptoms associated with menopause
- Vulvar or vaginal atrophy
- Osteoporosis prevention

Adult dosage: Take 1 to 2 mg orally daily, cyclically. Apply cream vaginally every day for 1 week, every other day for 1 week, and then one to two times a week for a maintenance dose.

Contraindications: Breast or estrogen-dependent carcinoma, undiagnosed abnormal genital bleeding, thrombophlebitis; thromboembolic disorders, or history of associated disorders with previous estrogen use

Precautions: Increased risk of endometrial carcinoma; if medication is used in a patient with a uterus, a progesterone product will counter this effect. Impaired renal, hepatic, or cardiac function; immobilized patients; epilepsy; migraines; asthma; diabetes; depression

Adverse reactions: Breast tenderness and enlargement, uterine bleeding, dysmenorrhea, amenorrhea, vaginal candidiasis, gastrointestinal upset, depression, endometrial carcinoma, gallbladder or thromboembolic disease, hepatic carcinoma, skin changes

How supplied: Tablets: 1, 2 mg; cream

Estraderm

ESTRADIOL TRANSDERMAL PATCH

Drug class: Hormone—estrogen
Pregnancy Category X
Indications:

- Atrophic vaginitis
- Moderate to severe vasomotor symptoms of menopause
- Postmenopausal osteoporosis prophylaxis

Adult dosage: Initially apply one 0.05 to 0.1-mg/day patch twice a week to the trunk (avoid the breasts and waistline). Rotate application sites.

Contraindications: Undiagnosed abnormal genital bleeding, thromboembolic disorders, breast or estrogen-dependent carcinoma

Precautions: History of breast cancer; cardiovascular disease; hepatic, renal, or cardiac insufficiency; asthma; epilepsy; migraines; endometriosis; depression; gallbladder disease; diabetes. Discontinue if hypertension or jaundice occurs, if immobilization is necessary, or at least 4 weeks before surgery is performed that is associated with a risk of thromboembolism.

Adverse reactions: Increased risk of endometrial cancer or hyperplasia (add progesterone), thromboembolic disorders; increase in uterine fibromyomata size, breakthrough bleeding, mastodynia, abdominal cramps, headache, migraines, dizziness, fluid retention, intolerance to contact lenses

How supplied: Patch: 0.05, 0.1, 0.2 mg/d

Estratest/Estratest H.S.

ESTERIFIED ESTROGENS AND METHYLTESTOSTERONE

Drug class: Hormone—estrogen and testosterone
Pregnancy Category X
Indications:

- Moderate to severe menopausal vasomotor symptoms not improved by estrogens alone
- Decreased libido

Adult dosage: Take one tablet orally every day with progesterone if the patient has a uterus. Or take the medication cyclically (3 weeks on, 1 week off) with a progesterone on days 14 to 25 of the cycle if the patient is still having periods.

Contraindications: Breast or estrogen-dependent carcinoma, undiagnosed abnormal genital bleeding, thrombophlebitis, thromboembolic disorders or history of associated disorders with previous estrogen use, hepatic dysfunction

Precautions: Cardiovascular disease, asthma, migraines, epilepsy, diabetes, renal dysfunction, gallbladder disease, bone disease associated with hypercalcemia, depression, uterine leiomyomata; discontinue medication if jaundice or hypertension occur.

Interactions: Estratest may potentiate oral anticoagulants and insulin.

Adverse reactions: Nausea, breakthrough bleeding, weight changes, mastalgia, hypertension, depression, hair loss or hirsutism, changes in libido, virilization, polycythemia, increased risk of endometrial carcinoma, gallbladder disease, thromboembolic disorders, hepatic tumors

How supplied: Estratest: One tablet consists of 1.25 mg of estrogen and 2.5 mg of methyltestosterone. Estratest H.S.: One tablet consists of 0.625 mg of estrogen with 1.25 mg of methyltestosterone.

ESTRING

ESTRADIOL

Drug class: Hormone replacement therapy

Pregnancy Category X

Indications: Vaginal, urethral, and vulvar atrophy

Adult dosage: Insert one ring high into the vagina; change every 90 days.

Contraindications: Pregnancy, breast or estrogen-dependent cancer, abnormal undiagnosed uterine or vaginal bleeding, vaginal stenosis, uterine prolapse; the ring should be removed while treating vaginal infections.

Precautions: Liver dysfunction, vaginal irritation or infection

Adverse reactions: Vaginal discharge, skeletal pain, headache, vaginitis, urinary tract discomfort, pain or hemorrhage, insomnia, hot flashes

How supplied: Vaginal ring

FAMVIR

FAMCICLOVIR

Drug class: Antiviral

Pregnancy Category C

Indications: Management of acute herpes

Adult dosage: For cold sores and genital lesions, take 125 mg twice a day orally for 5 days. For shingles (herpes zoster), take 500 mg every 8 hours orally for 7 days.

Contraindications: Contraindicated in the presence of hypersensitivity to famciclovir or acyclovir. Use caution in the presence of cytopenia and impaired renal function. Use extreme caution with cytotoxic drugs, because the accumulation effect could cause severe bone marrow depression as well as gastrointestinal and dermatologic problems. Lactation not recommended.

Adverse reactions: Headaches, diarrhea, fever, rash, cancer, sterility

How supplied: Tablets: 125, 500 mg

FERROUS SULFATE

FEOSOL, FER-IRON DROPS, FEROSPACE, FERO-FOLIC-500

Drug class: Iron

Pregnancy Category A

Indications: Iron supplement

Adult dosage: Take one to three tablets orally daily. For pregnancy, take 325 to 600 mg orally daily in divided doses.

Contraindications: Hemochromatosis, gastrointestinal disease

Precautions: Hepatitis, pancreatitis, peptic ulcer. Monitor hemoglobin, hematocrit, and reticulocyte levels.

Interactions: Ferrous sulfate inhibits tetracycline absorption. It is best absorbed when taken between meals.

Adverse reactions: Nausea, abdominal discomfort, constipation, and black stools; it masks occult bleeding.

How supplied: Fero-folic-500 tablets: 525 mg of ferrous sulfate plus 500 mg of ascorbic acid and 1 mg of folic acid in controlled-release form. Fumarate tablets: 63, 195, 200, 325 mg; controlled-release: 300 mg. Gluconate tablets: 300, 350 mg; elixir: 300 mg/5mL. Sulfate tablets: 300, 325 mg; extended-release capsules: 525 mg.

FIORICET (BUTALBITAL, ACETAMINOPHEN, AND CAFFEINE)

FIORINAL (BUTALBITAL, ASPIRIN, CAFFEINE)

Drug class: Barbiturate, analgesic

Pregnancy Category C

Indications: Tension headache

Adult dosage: Take one to two tablets every 4 hours for a maximum of six daily.

Contraindications: Allergy to ingredients, Fiorinal during pregnancy.

Precautions: Drug abusers, impaired hepatic or renal function, mental depression, suicidal tendencies, lactation

Adverse reactions: Drowsiness, dizziness, paradoxical excitement, gastrointestinal disturbances, mental depression, hepatotoxicity

How supplied: Tablets

FLAGYL

METRONIDAZOLE

Drug class: Antiprotozoal
Pregnancy Category B
Indications:
- Bacterial vaginosis
- Trichomoniasis
- Pelvic inflammatory disease

Adult dosage: For trichomoniasis or bacterial vaginosis, take 500 mg orally twice a day for 5 to 7 days. If not pregnant, take 2 g orally at one time or 1 g in the morning and 1 g in the evening (divided dose) on the same day. For pelvic inflammatory disease, take 500 mg orally twice a day for 7 to 10 days.

Contraindications: Use with caution in first trimester of pregnancy.

Interactions: Avoid alcohol during use and for three days after use. Flagyl may potentiate oral anticoagulants, phenytoin, and lithium. Flagyl is antagonized by phenobarbital, phenytoin, and other hepatic enzyme inducers.

Adverse reactions: Seizures, peripheral neuropathy, gastrointestinal upset, anorexia, constipation, headache, metallic taste, *Candida* overgrowth

How supplied: Tablets: 250, 375, 500 mg

FLOXIN

OFLOXACIN

Drug class: Antibacterial
Pregnancy Category C
Indications:
- Susceptible infections including genitourinary tract infections, cystitis
- Acute pelvic inflammatory disease

Adult dosage: Oral: Take on an empty stomach with a full glass of water; take 200 to 400 mg every 12 hours for 7 days.

Contraindications: Do not use (contraindicated) in the presence of allergy to fluoroquinolones. Use caution in the presence of renal dysfunction, seizures, and lactation.

Adverse reactions: Headache, dizziness, insomnia, nausea, fever, rash

How supplied: Tablets: 200, 300, 400 mg

Folic acid

Drug class: Vitamin
Pregnancy Category A
Indications:

- Treatment of megaloblastic anemias caused by sprue, nutritional deficiencies, and pregnancy
- Prevention of neural tube defects in the fetus

Adult dosage: All women of childbearing age should take 400 μg daily to reduce risk of neural tube defects by 70%. Therapeutic dose of folic acid in prenatal vitamins is 1 mg daily.

Contraindications: Allergies to folic acid preparations and pernicious, aplastic, and normocytic anemias

Precautions: Therapy may mask signs of pernicious anemia.

Adverse reactions: Hypersensitivity, allergic reactions

How supplied: Tablets: 0.1, 0.4, 1 mg

Fosamax

ALENDRONATE SODIUM

Drug class: Aminobisphosphonate

Pregnancy Category C

Indications: Postmenopausal osteoporosis—can increase bone density by up to 7% per year

Adult dosage: Take in the morning with a full glass of plain water at least 30 minutes before any other beverage, food, or medication; avoid recumbency for at least 30 minutes afterward. For postmenopausal osteoporosis, take 10 mg/day or 70 mg/week; reevaluate periodically.

Contraindications: Hypocalcemia

Precautions: Fosamax is not recommended with upper gastrointestinal disease, renal dysfunction, and lactation. Ensure the patient has an adequate intake of vitamin D and calcium.

Interactions: Absorption of food, calcium, and iron will probably decrease.

Adverse reactions: Gastrointestinal upset, musculoskeletal pain, headache

How supplied: Tablets: 10, 35, 40, 70 mg

Hemabate

CARBOPROST TROMETHAMINE

Drug class: Prostaglandin

Pregnancy Category C

Indications: Postpartum hemorrhage caused by uterine atony, which has not responded to conventional methods

Adult dosage: For refractory postpartum uterine bleeding, give 250 mg IM. The dosage may be repeated in 5 to 15 minutes two times.

Contraindications: Allergy to prostaglandin preparations; active cardiac, hepatic, pulmonary, renal disease

Adverse reactions: Hypotension, nausea, flushing, dyspnea, diarrhea

How supplied: IM injection of 250 mg from a single-dose vial

Hepatitis A Vaccine

HAVRIX

Drug class: Vaccine

Pregnancy Category C

Indications:

- Hepatitis A immunization in persons 2 years of age and older
- Travelers visiting or working in high-risk areas
- People exposed to hepatitis A—immunoglobulin may be given concomitantly

Child dosages: Give children age 2-18 years an injection of 360 EL.U./0.5 mL IM. Repeat the dose at 1 month and 6 months.

Adult dosage: Give adults an injection of 720 EL.U./0.5 mL IM. Repeat the dose 6 to 12 months after the primary dose.

Contraindications: Known hypersensitivity to any component of the vaccine

Precautions: Pregnancy, lactation. Have an epinephrine injection available.

Adverse reactions: Local reactions, malaise, nausea, diarrhea, rash, anaphylaxis

How supplied: Single-dose vials of 360 EL.U./0.5 mL; single-dose vials and prefilled syringes of 720 EL.U./0.5 mL.

HEPATITIS B VACCINE

ENGERIX-B, HEPTAVAX

Drug class: Vaccine

Pregnancy Category C

Indications:

- Hepatitis B immunization
- Medical and other personnel who have a potential for exposure
- People with high-risk behaviors
- People who have been exposed to hepatitis B virus—newborn of infected mother

Adult dosage: Give 20 μg IM in the deltoid muscle. Repeat 1 and 6 months later.

Contraindications: Yeast hypersensitivity

Precautions: Pregnancy, lactation. Have an epinephrine injection available.

Adverse reactions: Local reactions, malaise, nausea, diarrhea, rash, anaphylaxis

How supplied: Injection: 10 mg/0.5 mL; 20 μg/mL

IBUPROFEN

ADVIL, EXCEDRIN IB, IBUPRIN, MOTRIN, NUPRIN, PAMPRIN-IB

Drug class: Nonsteroidal anti-inflammatory drug (NSAID) and nonnarcotic analgesic

Pregnancy Category B

Indications: Mild to moderate pain

Adult dosage: Take 200 to 400 mg every 4 hours. Take 600 mg every 6 hours or 800 mg every 8 hours.

Contraindications: Aspirin allergy, pregnancy

Precautions: Gastrointestinal disease, impaired renal or hepatic function, lactation

Interactions: Avoid aspirin. Ibuprofen may increase bleeding with anticoagulants, toxicity with methotrexate, and serum lithium levels.

Adverse reactions: Gastrointestinal problems, vision disorders, dizziness, rash, jaundice, hepatitis

How supplied: Capsules: 200, 400, 600, 800 mg

IMITREX

SUMATRIPTAN

Drug class: Selective 5-HT receptor agonist

Pregnancy Category C

Indications:

- Acute migraines
- Cluster headaches

Adult dosage: Take 25 to 100 mg orally; repeat the dose every 2 hours, as needed, for a maximum of 200 mg/day; Take 6 mg subcutaneously; repeat the dose every 2 hours, as needed, for a maximum of 12 mg/day. Use 5, 10, or 20 mg of nasal spray; repeat the spray every 2 hours, as needed, for a maximum of 40 mg/day.

Contraindications: Ischemic cardiac, cerebral or peripheral vascular disease; hypertension; renal or hepatic dysfunction

Precautions: Confirm the diagnosis; exclude cardiovascular disease, the elderly, pregnancy, lactation

Interactions: Serotonin syndrome develops with administration of SSRIs.

Adverse reactions: Tingling; flushing; chest, neck, sinus or jaw discomfort; serious cardiac event (rare); and taste disturbance with nasal spray

How supplied: Tablets: 25, 50, 100 mg; prefilled syringe; nasal spray: single dose

ISONIAZID

INH

Drug class: Antitubercular

Pregnancy Category C

Indications: Prophylaxis and treatment of susceptible tuberculosis

Adult dosage: For prophylaxis, take 300 mg orally daily. For active disease, take 5mg/kg daily. The maximum dose is 300 mg every day; a multiple drug therapy may be necessary.

Contraindications: Previous Isoniazid-associated hepatic injury, acute hepatic disease

Precautions: Impaired renal and hepatic function, diabetes, increased risk of liver damage with increasing age. Give pyridoxine concomitantly to decrease risk of neuropathy.

Interactions: Alcohol increases the risk of hepatitis.

Adverse reactions: Hepatitis, peripheral neuropathy, gastrointestinal distress, blood dyscrasias, pyridoxine deficiency, hyperglycemia, rheumatic and lupus-like syndrome

How supplied: Tablets: 300 mg

KEFLEX

CEPHALEXIN

Drug class: Antibiotic—first-generation cephalosporin

Pregnancy Category B

Indications: Susceptible infections including otitis media, skin, bone, respiratory, or genitourinary tract infections

Adult dosage: Take 250 to 500 mg orally every 6 hours for 5 to 7 days.

Contraindications: Allergy to cephalosporins or penicillins, renal failure

Precautions: Impaired liver function, epilepsy, asthma, migraines, depression, cardiac or renal insufficiency

Adverse reactions: Anaphylaxis, diarrhea, rash, gastrointestinal upset, blood dyscrasias

How supplied: Capsules or tablets: 250, 500 mg

LUNELLE

MEDROXYPROGESTERONE ACETATE AND ESTRADIOL CYPIONATE

Drug class: Contraceptive

Pregnancy Category X

Indications: Contraception

Adult dosage: Take 0.5 mg IM every 28 to 30 days—no earlier than 23 days and not to exceed 33 days between injections.

Contraindications: Allergy to components of Lunelle, pregnancy, breast or estrogen-dependent carcinoma, undiagnosed abnormal genital bleeding, thrombophlebitis, thromboembolic disorders, or history of associated disorders with previous estrogen use

Precautions: Breast-feeding, smoker older than age 35, elevated serum lipids, epilepsy, asthma, migraine headaches

Adverse reactions: Abdominal pain, acne, amenorrhea, fluid retention, breast tenderness, decreased libido, depression and anxiety, thromboembolic events, hypertension, headache, heavy bleeding, nausea, monilia vaginitis

How supplied: Injections (monthly): 25 mg of medroxyprogesterone and 5 mg of estradiol cypionate in a 0.5-mg injectable dose

Macrobid

NITROFURANTOIN

Drug class: Antibiotic

Pregnancy Category B

Indications: Susceptible urinary tract infections

Adult dosage: Take 100 mg every 12 hours with meals for 5 to 10 days.

Contraindications: Oliguria, pregnancy at term, lactation

Adverse reactions: Hemolytic anemia, nausea, headache, flatulence, dizziness, gastrointestinal disturbances, anorexia

How supplied: Capsules: 100 mg

Macrodantin

NITROFURANTOIN MACROCRYSTALS

Drug class: Antibiotic

Pregnancy Category B

Indications: Susceptible urinary tract infections

Adult dosage: Take 50 to 100 mg with food twice a day or four times a day for at least 7 days. For long-term suppressive use, take 50 to 100 mg at bedtime.

Contraindications: Oliguria, lactation

Adverse reactions: Nausea, headache, flatulence, dizziness, gastrointestinal disturbances, anorexia, anaphylaxis

How supplied: Capsules: 25, 50, 100 mg

Magnesium Sulfate

Drug class: Electrolyte, anticonvulsant

Pregnancy Category A

Indications:

- Inhibition of premature labor
- Treatment of toxemia and eclampsia

Adult dosage: Give a loading dose of 4 g/250 mL in 5% dextrose in sterile H2O (D_5W) IV in 15 minutes. Follow with 1 to 4 g every hour.

Contraindications: Allergy to magnesium products, heart block, myocardial damage abdominal pain, nausea, vomiting, or other symptoms of appendicitis. There is a risk of magnesium toxicity in the neonate if magnesium sulfate is used in labor and delivery.

Precautions: Administer magnesium sulfate only after calcium gluconate is available for magnesium toxicity.

Adverse reactions: Hypocalcemia with tetany, fetal depression, magnesium intoxication; Measure magnesium level 2 to 4 hours after initiating treatment and every 4 to 6 hours, as necessary.

How supplied: Premixed bag of Hg in 100 cc or 40 g in 1000 cc

Maxalt

RIZATRIPTAN

Drug class: Selective 5-HT receptor agonist

Pregnancy Category C

Indications: Treatment of acute migraines

Adult dosage: Take 5 or 10 mg; consider repeating dose after 2 hours for a maximum of 30 mg/day.

Contraindications: Ischemic cardiac, cerebral, or peripheral vascular disease; hypertension; renal or hepatic dysfunction

Precautions: Confirm diagnosis; exclude cardiovascular disease, the elderly, pregnancy, lactation

Interactions: Serotonin syndrome develops with administration of SSRIs

Adverse reactions: Fatigue, pain, pressure or tightness in the throat, serious cardiac event (rare)

How supplied: Tablets: 2.5 mg

Mefoxin (CEFOXITIN FOR INJECTION)

Drug class: Antibiotic
Pregnancy Category B
Indications:

- Respiratory and urinary tract infections
- Pelvic inflammatory disease
- Prophylaxis prior to surgery

Adult dosage: For infections, give 1 to 2 g IV every 6 to 8 hours. For a pre-operative antibiotic, give a 2-g loading dose.

Contraindications: Hypersensitivity to cefoxitin or cephalosporins

Precautions: History of colitis, diarrhea

Adverse reactions: Rash, hypotension, anemia, diarrhea, abnormal liver function test, elevation in serum creatinine and blood urea nitrogen

How supplied: Vials of powdered drug that must be reconstituted

Metamucil

PSYLLIUM

Drug class: Laxative (bulk)

Pregnancy Category C

Indications: Constipation

Adult dosage: Dilute one tablespoon in 8 oz of water or juice and take 1 to 3 times a day for 2 to 3 days.

Contraindications: Allergy to bulk-forming laxatives. Symptoms of appendicitis, inflamed bowel, or intestinal blockage

Adverse reactions: Excessive bowel activity, abdominal cramps, cathartic dependence

How supplied: Bulk, wafers

METHERGINE

METHYLERGONOVINE MALEATE

Drug class: Oxytocic

Pregnancy Category C

Indications: Postpartum hemorrhage, uterine atony, subinvolution

Adult dosage: Take 0.2 mg orally every 4 hours for six doses. Get 0.2 mg IM every 2 to 4 hours after delivery, as needed.

Contraindications: Hypertension

Interactions: Vasoconstrictors and other ergot alkaloids potentiate Methergine.

Adverse reactions: Hypertension or hypotension, stroke, nausea, vomiting, chest pain, dyspnea, dizziness, headache, hematuria, diarrhea, diaphoresis, palpitations

How supplied: Tablets: 0.2 mg; ampules for injection: 0.2 mg/mL

MICRONOR

NORETHINDRONE

Drug class: Contraceptive

Pregnancy Category X

Indications: Oral contraception—preferred for nursing mothers because there is less effect on the amount of milk production compared to combination birth control pills

Adult dosage: Take one tablet orally daily without interruption. Start this continuous regimen 4 to 6 weeks postpartum.

Contraindications: Thrombophlebitis of thromboembolic disorders, cerebrovascular or cardiovascular disease, undiagnosed abnormal genital bleeding

Interactions: Micronor is antagonized by hepatic enzyme-inducing drugs, including anticonvulsants. Antacids and antibiotics may inhibit absorption.

Adverse reactions: Hypertension, nausea, vomiting, cramps, breakthrough bleeding, menstrual irregularities, changes in weight, mental depression, headaches

How supplied: Tablets: 28-day pack of 0.35 mg

MIFEPREX (RU 486)

MIFEPRISTONE

Drug class: Abortifacient; progesterone blocker

Pregnancy Category X

Indications: Medical abortion of early pregnancy (up to 49 days)

Adult dosage: Take 600 mg orally on day 1 as a single dose, followed by 400 mg of misoprostol orally on day 3 if abortion has not occurred.

Contraindications: Ectopic pregnancy, intrauterine device in place, chronic adrenal failure, anticoagulant therapy, hemorrhagic disorders, and long-term corticosteroid therapy

Precautions: Accurate gestational dating is mandatory. The patient must be willing to complete the abortion surgically if medical abortion is unsuccessful because of reports of fetal malformations after administration of this drug.

Adverse reactions: Nausea, vomiting, chills, fever, diarrhea, cramping, and heavy bleeding, most of which have a short duration

How supplied: Tablets: 200 mg

MILK OF MAGNESIA

MAGNESIUM HYDROXIDE

Drug class: Laxative, antacid

Pregnancy Category C

Indications:

- Upset stomach caused by hyperacidity
- Hyperacidity caused by a peptic ulcer, gastritis, peptic esophagitis, gastric hyperacidity, hiatal hernia
- Prophylaxis of gastrointestinal bleeding, stress ulcers, aspiration pneumonia
- Constipation

Adult dosage: Take 5 to 15 mL of antacid liquid or 650-mg to 1.3-g tablets orally four times a day. Take 15 to 60 mL of laxative medication orally with liquid.

Contraindications: Allergy to magnesium products; use caution in the presence of renal insufficiency.

Adverse reactions: Diarrhea, nausea, perianal irritation

How supplied: Tablet or liquid

Monistat 7/Monistat 3

MICONAZOLE

Drug class: Antifungal
Pregnancy Category B
Indications:

• Vulvovaginal candidiasis
• Fungal skin infections

Adult dosage: For Monistat 7, insert one applicator of cream at bedtime for 7 days. For Monistat 3, insert one suppository vaginally daily at bedtime for 3 consecutive days. For external relief, apply cream to affected areas twice a day. If prescribed for skin infection, continue treatment for 5 to 7 days after sores have healed.

Contraindications: Allergy to miconazole.

Adverse reactions: Allergic reactions with local swelling and increased discharge

How supplied: Vaginal suppositories: 100, 200 mg of 2% cream. Monistat 3 combination pack: Suppositories plus 0.32 oz of vulvar cream

Monurol

FOSFOMYCIN

Drug class: Antibiotic
Pregnancy Category B
Indications: Urinary tract infections
Adult dosage: Mix 3-g sachet in water and drink immediately after mixing.
Contraindications: Hypersensitivity to fosfomycin
Precautions: Do not retreat with Monurol if single dose is not effective.
Adverse reactions: Diarrhea, headaches, vaginitis
How supplied: Single-dose sachets: 3 g

Nonoxynol 9

SEMICID

Drug class: Contraceptive spermicide
Pregnancy Category X
Indications: Contraception
Adult dosage: Insert vaginally at least 15 minutes and up to 1 hour before intercourse.
Contraindications: Discontinue if irritation occurs.
How supplied: Suppository, VCF (vaginal contraceptive film), coating in some condoms

Noroxin

NORFLOXACIN

Drug class: Antibiotic
Pregnancy Category C
Indications

- Urinary tract infections
- Gonorrhea

Adult dosage: For urinary tract infections, take 400 mg orally every 12 hours for 3 days; for gonorrhea, take 800 mg orally in a single dose.

Contraindications: Hypersensitivity to quinolones

Precautions: Phototoxicity, hemolytic reactions in patients with G6PD

Adverse reactions: Dizziness, nausea, cramping, headaches, anorexia, colitis, hepatitis

How supplied: Tablets: 400 mg

Ogen

ESTROPIPATE

Drug class: Hormone—estrogen
Pregnancy Category X
Indications:

- Hormone replacement therapy
- Atrophic vaginitis and moderate to severe vasomotor symptoms of menopause
- Osteoporosis prevention

Adult dosage: For menopause, take 0.625- to 1.25-mg tablets orally daily or in a cycle of 3 weeks on and 1 week off; apply 2 to 4 g of cream vaginally daily; give medication daily at bedtime for 1 week, every other day for 1 week, and a maintenance dose one to two times per week. Ogen administration requires progesterone for long-term use in women with a uterus.

Contraindications: Breast or estrogen-dependent carcinoma, undiagnosed abnormal genital bleeding, thromboembolic disorders, thrombophlebitis

Precautions: Cardiovascular disease, asthma, migraines, epilepsy, hepatic or renal dysfunction, gallbladder disease, uterine leiomyomatas

Adverse reactions: Nausea, vomiting, breakthrough bleeding, weight changes, swollen and tender breasts, hypertension, mental depression, increased size of uterine fibroma. The risk of an estrogen-dependent carcinoma increases if Ogen is given without progesterone in a woman with a uterus, gallbladder disease, thromboembolic disorders, or hepatic tumors.

How supplied: Tablet: 0.625, 1.25 mg; cream

Oscillococcinum

Drug class: Homeopathic

Indications: Flu symptoms such as fever, chills, body aches, and pains

Adult dosage: At the first sign of infection, take the entire contents of one tube, preferably sublingually for optimal absorption. Repeat every 6 hours as needed. Do not take with food.

Contraindications: None known

How supplied: Three tubes of absorbable pellets

Phenergan/Phenergan VC

PROMETHAZINE

Drug class: Antipertussis, Phenergan VC: Narcotic

Pregnancy Category C

Indications:

- Cough
- Nasal congestion
- Symptoms associated with the common cold

Adult dosage: Take 1 teaspoon orally every 4 to 6 hours, as necessary.

Contraindications: Diabetes, peptic ulcer, pregnancy, lactation, and allergy to ingredients. Use caution with a history of alcohol or drug dependence.

Adverse reactions: Drowsiness, dizziness

How supplied: Liquid Phenergan: 0.625 mg of promethazine plus 15 mg dextromethorphan; liquid Phenergan VC: 0.625 mg promethazine plus 15 mg dextromethorphan plus 10 mg codeine

Pitocin

OXYTOCIN

Drug class: Oxytocic, hormonal agent

Pregnancy Category C

Indications:

- Initiation of contractions or improvement in their consistency
- Production of uterine contractions during the third stage of labor and control of postpartum bleeding

Adult dosage: For induction or stimulation of labor, begin initial dose of no more than 1 to 2 mU/min (0.001 to 0.002 U/min) by IV infusion through an infusion pump. Increase dose in increments of no more than 1 to 2 mU/min at 15- to 30-minute intervals, until a contraction pattern similar to normal labor is established. Discontinue in the event of uterine hyperactivity or fetal distress. To control postpartum uterine bleeding with an IV drip, add 10 to 40 units to 1000 mL of nonhydrating diluent; run it at a rate to control uterine atony. For IM administration, inject 10 units after delivery of placenta.

Contraindications: Significant cephalopelvic disproportion, unfavorable fetal positions or presentation, hypertonic uterine patterns, induction or augmentation of labor when vaginal delivery is contraindicated

Adverse reactions: Nausea, vomiting, cardiac arrhythmias, postpartum hemorrhage, fetal bradycardia

How supplied: Ampules: 10 units in 1 mL

Ponstel

MEFENAMIC ACID

Drug class: NSAID

Pregnancy Category C

Indications: Mild to moderate pain

Adult dosage: Take 500 mg orally and then 250 mg every 6 hours.

Contraindications: Aspirin allergy, ulcers, gastric inflammation, renal dysfunction, late pregnancy

Interactions: Avoid aspirin, which may increase bleeding with anticoagulants; Ponstel may potentiate methotrexate. Do not take with magnesium antacids.

Precautions: Hepatic dysfunction, bleeding disorders, hypertension, elderly older than 65 years old

Adverse reactions: Gastrointestinal disturbances, anemia, headaches, rash, hepatic dysfunction

How supplied: Capsules: 250 mg

Prednisolone (DELTA-CORTEF, NOVOPREDNISOLONE [CANADIAN], PRELONE)

PREDNISONE (APO-PREDNISONE [CANADIAN], DELTASONE, PANASOL)

Drug class: Adrenal corticosteroid, hormonal agent

Pregnancy Category C

Indications:

- Short-term inflammatory allergic reaction, dermatologic diseases, status asthmaticus, and autoimmune disorders (systemic)
- Hematologic disorders such as thrombocytopenia purpura, erythroblastopenia (systemic)

Adult dosage: Take 5 to 60 mg/day orally, IM, or IV. Increase until the lowest effective dose is reached. Decrease slowly if therapy is long term; *Do not* suddenly stop medication administration.

Contraindications: Do not use in the presence of infections, especially tuberculosis, fungal infections, amebiasis, vaccinia, varicella, and antibiotic-resistant infections. Use cautiously with lactation, kidney or liver disease, hypothyroidism, active or latent peptic ulcer, inflammatory bowel disease, congestive heart failure, hypertension, thromboembolic disorders, osteoporosis, convulsive disorders, and diabetes mellitus. Prednisone suppresses skin-test reactions.

Adverse reactions: Vertigo, headache, increased appetite, weight gain with long-term therapy, sodium and fluid retention, immunosuppression, aggravation or masking of infections, and impaired wound healing. Toxic effects will increase if Prednisone is taken concurrently with estrogens (including oral contraceptives). Steroid blood levels will decrease when Prednisone is taken with barbiturates, phenytoin, or rifampin. Prednisone decreases the effectiveness of salicylates.

How supplied: Tablets 1, 2.5, 5, 10, 25, 50 mg; liquid

PREMARIN

CONJUGATED ESTROGENS

Drug class: Hormone—synthetic estrogen

Pregnancy Category X

Indications:

- Moderate to severe vasomotor symptoms associated with menopause
- Vaginal atrophy
- Osteoporosis prevention

Adult dosage: For hormone replacement therapy, take 0.625 or 1.25 mg once orally every day. Take a dose during days 1 to 25 of each menstrual cycle. It *must* be given with a progestin, unless the patient has had a hysterectomy. For atrophic vaginitis, insert one applicator vaginally daily at bedtime for 1 week then every other day for 1 week; then decrease application to two per week. For maintenance, use one to two for 1 week.

Contraindications: Breast or estrogen-dependent carcinoma, active thrombophlebitis or thromboembolic disorders; undiagnosed abnormal genital bleeding

Precautions: Asthma, epilepsy, migraines, diabetes, cardiac or renal dysfunction, and depression. Discontinue medication if jaundice, visual disturbances, migraines, or thrombotic disorders occur.

Adverse reactions: Thromboembolic events, edema, cholestatic jaundice, depression, pyrexia, insomnia, nausea, breast tenderness, galactorrhea

How supplied: Tablets: 0.3, 0.625, 0.9, 1.25, 2.5 mg; cream

PREMPHASE

CONJUGATED ESTROGENS AND MEDROXYPROGESTERONE ACETATE

Drug class: Hormone—estrogen and progestin

Pregnancy Category X

Indications:

- Moderate to severe vasomotor symptoms associated with menopause
- Vulvar and vaginal atrophy
- Osteoporosis prevention

Adult dosage: Take one tablet of 0.625 mg of Premarin orally every day for the first 14 days. Tablets for days 15 to 28 of a woman's cycle contain 5 mg of Cycrin as well.

Contraindications: Breast or estrogen-dependent carcinoma, active thrombophlebitis of thromboembolic disorders, undiagnosed abnormal genital bleeding, hepatic impairment

Precautions: Gallbladder disease, asthma, migraines, epilepsy, and cardiac or renal dysfunction; monitor blood pressure and discontinue medication if visual abnormalities occur.

Adverse reactions: Nausea, vomiting, cramps, abdominal swelling or tenderness, hepatic impairment, breast tenderness or enlargement, uterine fibroids, breakthrough bleeding or spotting, headache, migraines, dizziness, vision changes, depression, glucose intolerance

How supplied: First blister card: fourteen tablets of Premarin containing 0.625 mg; second blister card: fourteen tablets of Premarin containing 0.625 mg plus 5 mg of Cycrin

PREMPRO

CONJUGATED ESTROGENS AND MEDROXYPROGESTERONE ACETATE

Drug class: Hormones—estrogen and progestin

Pregnancy Category X

Indications:

- Moderate to severe vasomotor symptoms associated with menopause
- Osteoporosis prevention

Adult dosage: Take one tablet containing Premarin and Cycrin daily.

Contraindications: Breast or estrogen-dependent carcinoma, active thrombophlebitis of thromboembolic disorders, undiagnosed abnormal genital bleeding, hepatic impairment

Precautions: Gallbladder disease, asthma, migraines, epilepsy, hypercalcemia in breast cancer, and cardiac or renal dysfunction. Monitor blood pressure. Discontinue medication if visual abnormalities occur.

Adverse reactions: Nausea, vomiting, cramps, abdominal swelling or tenderness, hepatic impairment, breast tenderness or enlargement, uterine fibroids, breakthrough bleeding or spotting, headaches, migraines, dizziness, vision changes, depression, glucose intolerance

How supplied: Two blister cards containing 28 tablets of Premarin in 0.625-mg doses and Cycrin in 2.5-mg doses. Both medications are in each tablet.

PREPARATION H

Drug class: hemorrhoidal preparation

Pregnancy Category A

Indications: Hemorrhoids

Adult dosage: Apply freely to external surface three to five times daily. Insert one suppository rectally in the morning and afternoon and after each evacuation.

Adverse reactions: Discontinue the medication if local irritation occurs, including redness, pain, and swelling.

How supplied: Ointment, cream, suppository

PROBENECID

BENEMID

Drug class: Uricosuric, sulfonamide derivative

Pregnancy Category B

Indications: Adjunct in penicillin and cephalosporin treatment

Adult dosage: Take 1 g orally with 3.5 g of ampicillin or 1 g 30 minutes before an injection of 4 to 8 million units of ueous penicillin G procaine IM.

Contraindications: Hypersensitivity, hepatic disease, severe renal disease

Interactions: Benemid increases the activity of oral anticoagulants. Toxicity increases when sulfa drugs combine with Benemid. May potentiate para-aminosalicylic acid (PAS), rifampin, naproxen

Adverse reactions: Headache, drowsiness, bradycardia, glycosuria, and thirst

How supplied: Tablets: 0.5 g

PROCTOFOAM-HC

Drug class: Antipruritic and steroid

Pregnancy Category C

Indications: Steroid-responsive anogenital dermatoses

Adult dosage: Apply three to four times daily.

Precautions: Tuberculosis, diverticulitis, lactation. Treat infection if present. Significant systemic absorption may occur. Discontinue medication if there is no improvement in 2 to 3 weeks.

Adverse reactions: Adrenal suppression, dermal and epidermal atrophy, poor wound healing, local irritation, folliculitis, hypertrichosis, hypopigmentation, macerations, secondary infections, striae, miliaria

How supplied: Aerosol, cream

PROGESTERONE IN OIL

Drug class: Hormone—progestin

Pregnancy Category X

Indications: Treatment of secondary amenorrhea

Adult dosage: For amenorrhea, inject 100 mg IM. Expect withdrawal bleeding in 48 to 72 hours. Spontaneous normal cycles may follow.

Contraindications: Allergies to progestins, thromboembolic disorders, cerebral hemorrhage or history of these conditions, hepatic disease, and missed abortion. Use caution in the presence of epilepsy, migraines, asthma, and cardiac or renal dysfunction.

Adverse reactions: Dizziness, thrombophlebitis, breakthrough bleeding, spotting, change in menstrual flow

How supplied: Injection: 25, 50, 100 mg/mL IM

PROMETHAZINE HCL (PHENERGAN)

Drug class: Antiemetic

Pregnancy Category C

Indications:

- Nausea and vomiting
- Motion sickness

Adult dosage: Take 25 mg orally every 4 to 6 hours, as necessary. Inject 12.5 to 25 mg IM every 4 hours, as necessary. Insert a 25-mg suppository rectally; repeat this process in 4 to 6 hours, as needed. For motion sickness, take 25 mg orally twice a day.

Contraindications: Hypersensitivity to antihistamines or phenothiazines

Interactions: Phenergan potentiates central nervous system depression with alcohol and other central nervous system depressants. It may alter the results of human chorionic gonadotropin pregnancy tests.

Adverse reactions: Drowsiness, lowered seizure threshold, cholestatic jaundice, rash

How supplied: Tablets: 12.5, 25, 50 mg; injection: 25, 50 mg/mL IM

PROMETRIUM

MICRONIZED PROGESTERONE

Drug class: Hormone—progesterone

Pregnancy Category B

Indications:

- Prevention of endometrial hyperplasia when a woman is taking estrogen
- Secondary amenorrhea
- Prevention of spontaneous abortion in women with a luteal phase defect

Adult dosage: For prevention of endometrial hyperplasia, take 200 mg every day for 10 to 12 days each month. For secondary amenorrhea, take 400 mg every day for 10 nights. For prevention of spontaneous abortion, take 100 mg orally twice daily until the end of the 12th week of pregnancy.

Contraindications: Undiagnosed vaginal bleeding, breast or genital carcinoma, severe liver dysfunction, history of thrombophlebitis, allergy to peanuts

Precautions: Use caution with renal or hepatic dysfunction. Discontinue medication if vision loss, migraines, diplopia, or thrombophlebitis occurs. Monitor diabetes.

Adverse reactions: Breast pain and tenderness, headache, abdominal pain and bloating, emotional instability

How supplied: Tablets: 100, 100 mg

PROSTIN E₂, PREPIDIL

DINOPROSTONE

Drug class: Prostaglandin

Pregnancy Category C

Indications: Induction of labor, initiation of cervical ripening

Adult dosage: Insert one Prostin E_2 dose into the cervical os every 2 hours three times. Insert one dose of Prepidil gel into the cervical os. Repeat 6 hours later, as necessary.

Contraindications: Allergy to prostaglandin preparations; active cardiac, hepatic, pulmonary, or renal disease; malposition of the fetus; hypertonic contractions; fetal distress

Adverse reactions: Drowsiness, confusion, nervousness, epigastric distress, nausea, vomiting, diarrhea, hypotension, palpitations, tachycardia

How supplied: Prostin E_2 suppository: 20 mg; Prostin E_2 and Prepidil gel: premixed single dose in syringe with insertion catheter

Proventil

ALBUTEROL

Drug class: Beta-2 agonist
Pregnancy Category C
Indications:

- Bronchospasm
- Asthma

Adult dosage: Take one to two inhalations every 4 to 6 hours, as needed. For exercise-induced bronchospasm, take two inhalations 15 minutes before exercise.

Contraindications: Hypersensitivity to albuterol, heart disease, hypertension

Adverse reactions: Tachycardia, hypertension, tremors, nervousness, headaches, dizziness, hyperactivity, insomnia, nausea, muscle cramps, paradoxical bronchospasm, local irritation

How supplied: Inhaler: 17 g (200 inhalations)

Provera

MEDROXYPROGESTERONE ACETATE

Drug class: Hormone—progestogen
Pregnancy Category X
Indications:

- Secondary amenorrhea
- Abnormal uterine bleeding caused by hormonal imbalance without organic pathology
- Protection against endometrial cancer in hormone replacement therapy (used with estrogen)

Adult dosage: For amenorrhea, take 5 to 10 mg daily for 5 to 10 days. For cyclic hormone replacement therapy or abnormal bleeding, take 5 to 10 mg daily for 10 to 12 days, starting on days 14 to 16 of the menstrual cycle or the first 10 to 12 days of each month, to induce optimum secretory transformation or a primed endometrium. For hormone replacement therapy, take a continuous dose of 2.5 or 5 mg every day with estrogen.

Contraindications: Active thrombophlebitis or thromboembolic disorders, cerebral apoplexy, hepatic dysfunction or disease, undiagnosed abnormal vaginal bleeding, pregnancy

Precautions: Asthma, epilepsy, migraines, diabetes, cardiac or renal dysfunction, depression

Adverse reactions: Thromboembolic events, edema, depression, insomnia, nausea, acne, hirsutism, alopecia, rash

How supplied: Tablets: 2.5, 5, 10 g

Pyridium

PHENAZOPYRIDINE HCL

Drug class: Analgesic

Pregnancy Category B

Indications: Urinary tract infections

Adult dosage: Take 200 mg three times a day for a maximum of 3 days.

Contraindications: Renal insufficiency

Precautions: Liver disease, anemia. Urine will stain items orange; contact lenses may be stained as well.

Adverse reactions: Headache, rashes, anemia, renal or hepatic toxicity, gastrointestinal disturbances

How supplied: Tablets: 100 mg

Reglan

METOCLOPRAMIDE HCL

Drug class: Antiemetic

Pregnancy Category B

Indications:

- Gastroesophageal reflux
- Nausea and vomiting of pregnancy

Adult dosage: Take 10 mg orally four times a day, 10 to 30 minutes before each meal and at bedtime; inject 2 mg/kg IV every 2 hours for a maximum of five doses; may be given in a subcutaneous pump dosed to symptoms.

Contraindications: Hypersensitivity to drug, seizure disorders, gastrointestinal obstructions, breast cancer

Precautions: Lactation, gastrointestinal hemorrhage

Adverse reactions: Sedation, restlessness, headache, dry mouth, constipation, nausea, vomiting, diarrhea, supraventricular tachycardia (rare)

How supplied: Tablets: 5, 10, 15 mg; injection: 5 mg/mL

RHOGAM

RH$_o$(D) IMMUNE GLOBULIN, HUMAN

Drug class: Immunomodulators

Pregnancy Category C

Indications: Prevention of Rh$_o$(D) sensitization in nonsensitized Rh$_o$(D)-negative or Du-negative patients to the Rh factor, following pregnancy or accidental transfusion

Adult dosage: Each vial or syringe prevents sensitization to a volume of up to 15 mL of Rh-positive packed red blood cells. Administer IM at 28 weeks of gestation, within 72 hours of an Rh-incompatible delivery, miscarriage, abortion, or transfusion accident. Use MICRhoGAM for abortions performed at less than 12 weeks' gestation.

Contraindications: Rh$_o$(D)-positive patients

Adverse reactions: Local reactions

How supplied: Single-dose syringes, MICRhoGAM: single-dose syringes

ROCEPHIN

CEFTRIAXONE SODIUM

Drug class: Antibiotic—cephalosporin

Pregnancy Category B

Indications:

- Susceptible bacterial septicemia
- Lower respiratory or urinary tract infection
- Infections of the skin and skin structure, bones, and joints
- Gynecologic and intra-abdominal infections
- Meningitis
- Gonorrhea
- Surgical prophylaxis

Adult dosage: Inject 1 to 2 mg IM or IV daily or in two equally divided doses for a maximum of 4 g/day. For gonorrhea, follow STD guidelines.

Precautions: Penicillin or other allergy; concomitant renal and hepatic impairment

Interactions: Probenecid potentiates Rocephin.

Adverse reactions: Anaphylaxis, elevated liver enzymes, and local reactions, such as rash, diarrhea, nausea, vomiting

How supplied: Vials: 250, 500 mg; 1, 2 g

Rubella Virus Vaccine

MERUVAX II

Drug class: Vaccination

Pregnancy Category C

Indications: Rubella immunization

Child and adult dosage: For people age 12 months and older, give a single subcutaneous injection. The dose for any age is 0.5 mL.

Contraindications: Hypersensitivity to neomycin, active respiratory or other febrile infection, active untreated tuberculosis, immune deficiency, and pregnancy during and up to 3 months after vaccination

Precautions: Have epinephrine injection available. Defer vaccination for at least 3 months after blood or plasma transfusions or immune serum globulin, and for a least 1 month before or after other live virus vaccines. Lactation—may be transmitted in breast milk, so should be given with caution.

Adverse reactions: Malaise, rash, fever, headaches, local reactions, arthritic symptoms, thrombocytopenia purpura, encephalitis

How supplied: Injection: single-dose vial

Senokot

DOCUSATE SODIUM/SENNA

Drug class: Laxative (emollient)

Pregnancy Category C

Indications: Constipation

Adult dosage: Take one to eight tablets a day at bedtime.

Contraindications: Allergy to emollient laxatives, abdominal pain and fever related to appendicitis

Adverse reactions: Abdominal cramping and discomfort

How supplied: Tablets

Slow FE/ Slow FE Plus Folic Acid

FERROUS SULFATE

Drug class: Iron supplement

Pregnancy Category A

Indications: Prevention and treatment of iron deficiency anemias

Adult dosage: Take one tablet daily.

Contraindications: Hemochromatosis, hemosiderosis

Interactions: Slow Fe inhibits tetracycline absorption.

Adverse reactions: Nausea, abdominal discomfort and pain, constipation, diarrhea

How supplied: Time-release tablets, time-release tablets with folic acid

SPECTINOMYCIN

TROBICIN

Drug class: Antibiotic
Pregnancy Category B
Indications:
- Severe infections
- Gonorrhea

Adult dosage: Take 2 to 4 g as a single dose; follow STD guidelines (see Gonorrhea).

Contraindications: Lactation, allergy to spectinomycin

Caution: Pregnancy (safety not established)

Adverse reactions: Dizziness, chills, decreased urine output without documented renal toxicity, soreness at injection site

How supplied: Injection: 2, 4 g IM

STADOL

BUTORPHANOL TARTRATE

Drug class: Opioid (partial agonist)
Pregnancy Category C
Indications: Pain management when opioid analgesia is appropriate

Adult dosage: Inject 1 to 4 mg IM every 3 to 4 hours; inject 1 to 2 mg IV every 3 to 4 hours as needed.

Precautions: Impaired respiratory, cardiac, renal, or hepatic function; hypertension; drug users

Interactions: Alcohol and central nervous system depressants potentiate Stadol. It may precipitate withdrawal in narcotic addicts.

Adverse reactions: Sedation, dizziness, gastrointestinal upset, respiratory depression, diaphoresis, hypotension, hypertension, rash

How supplied: Injection (vials): 1, 2 mg/mL

SUDAFED/SUDAFED 12 HOUR

PSEUDOEPHEDRINE HCL

Drug class: Sympathomimetic
Pregnancy Category C
Indications: Nasal and eustachian tube congestion

Adult dosage: For Sudafed take one tablet orally every 4 to 6 hours; for Sudafed 12 Hour, take one tablet orally every 12 hours.

Contraindications: Severe hypertension, cardiovascular disease, during or within 14 days of taking monoamine oxidase inhibitors

Interactions: Hypertensive crisis with monoamine oxidase inhibitors. Beta-blockers increase the pressor effects of sympathomimetics. Arrhythmias may occur with epinephrine and isoproterenol. Stadol antagonizes methyldopa, reserpine, and guanethidine.

Adverse reactions: Central nervous system overstimulation, palpitations, headaches, hypertension, dizziness, gastrointestinal disturbances, nervousness, tremors, weakness, pallor, dysuria, insomnia, convulsions

How supplied: Tablets: 30, 60, 120 mg; extended-release capsules: 120 mg

TERAZOL 3/TERAZOL 7

TERCONAZOLE

Drug class: Antifungal

Pregnancy Category C

Indications:

- Vulvovaginal candidiasis
- Fungal infections of the skin

Adult dosage: Use one full applicator of vaginal cream at bedtime for 3 or 7 consecutive nights; insert one suppository vaginally at bedtime for 3 consecutive nights. Apply twice a day to affected skin area until all evidence of infection has been gone for 5 to 7 days.

Precautions: Confirm diagnosis with potassium hydroxide smears. Discontinue medication if fever, chills, irritation, or sensitization occurs.

Adverse reactions: Cream: headaches, fever, chills, itching, and body pain; suppository: localized burning, genital pain, and fever; Terazol 3 cream: dysmenorrhea

How supplied: Cream: 3 day, 7 day; suppository: 3 day

TERBUTALINE/BRETHINE

TERBUTALINE SULFATE

Drug class: Tocolytic

Pregnancy Category B

Indications: Inhibition of premature labor

Adult dosage: For premature labor, initiate IV administration at 10 mg/min. Titrate upward to a maximum of 80 mg/min. Maintain at a minimum effective dosage for 4 hours. Take 2.5 to 5 mg orally every 4 to 6 hours as a maintenance therapy. Not approved for tocylysis but generally used as noted above.

Contraindications: Hypersensitivity to terbutaline, tachyarrhythmias, unstable vasomotor system disorders, hypertension

Interactions: Terbutaline increases the likelihood of cardiac arrhythmias when given with halogenated hydrocarbon anesthetics or cyclopropane.

Adverse reactions: Restlessness, apprehension, anxiety, fear, nausea, cardiac arrhythmias, palpitations, respiratory difficulties, pulmonary edema

How supplied: Tablets: 2.5, 5 mg; ampules: 1 mg/mL

TETRACYCLINE

Drug class: Antibiotic

Pregnancy: Not recommended

Indications: Tetracycline-sensitive infections

Adult dosage: Take 1 hour before or 2 hours after meals. Take 250 to 500 mg four times a day for 7 days.

Contraindications: Pregnancy, lactation, allergy to any of the tetracyclines. Use caution in the presence of hepatic or renal dysfunction.

Interactions: Tetracycline may increase digoxin levels. Food reduces tetracycline absorption.

Adverse reactions: Superinfections, photosensitivity, gastrointestinal upset, enterocolitis, rash, blood dyscrasias, increased blood urea nitrogen, hepatotoxicity

How supplied: Tablets: 250, 500 mg

TIGAN

TRIMETHOBENZAMIDE HCL

Drug class: Antiemetic

Pregnancy Category C

Indications: Nausea and vomiting

Adult dosage: Take 250-mg capsules three to four times a day; insert 200-mg suppository rectally three to four times daily; inject 200 mg IM three to four times daily.

Precautions: Pregnancy, lactation

Interactions: Tigan potentiates alcohol and other central nervous system depressants.

Adverse reactions: Extrapyramidal reactions, drowsiness, blood dyscrasias, blurred vision, coma, seizures, depression, diarrhea, dizziness, jaundice, hypotension (injection), headaches, muscle cramps, and opisthotonos; Tigan may mask emetic signs of disease.

How supplied: Capsules: 100, 200 mg; suppositories: 200 mg; ampules: 100 mg/mL

TYLENOL

ACETAMINOPHEN

Drug class: Analgesic
Pregnancy Category B
Indications:

- Mild to moderate pain
- Fever

Adult dosage: Take 325 to 1000 mg every 4 to 6 hours.
Contraindications: Allergy to acetaminophen. Use caution in the presence of impaired hepatic function and chronic alcoholism.
Adverse reactions: Rash, hepatotoxicity (overdose)
How supplied: Tablets: 325 mg; 500 mg

TYLENOL #3/TYLENOL #4

ACETAMINOPHEN WITH CODEINE PHOSPHATE

Drug class: Analgesics
Pregnancy Category C
Indications: Mild to moderately severe pain
Adult dosage: Take one to two tablets every 4 to 6 hours as necessary for pain.
Precautions: Head injury; acute abdomen; impaired renal, hepatic, thyroid, or adrenocortical function; asthma; drug abusers; and lactation
Interactions: Potentiation occurs with alcohol, central nervous system depressants, monoamine oxidase inhibitors, tricyclic antidepressants, and anticholinergics.
Adverse reactions: Dizziness, sedation, nausea, vomiting, constipation, urinary retention, rash, respiratory depression, hepatotoxicity (overdose)
How supplied: One tablet consists of 300 mg of acetaminophen and 30 mg of codeine phosphate. Tylenol #3 consists of 300 mg of acetaminophen and 30 mg of codeine. Tylenol #4 consists of 300 mg of acetaminophen and 60 mg of codeine.

Unisom

DOXYLAMINE SUCCINATE

Drug class: Antihistamine, mild sedative
Pregnancy Category C
Indications:
- Insomnia
- Nausea aid in pregnancy when used with vitamin B6
- Hay fever, hives, rash, or itching

Adult dosage: For insomnia, take one to two tablets orally at bedtime; for nausea, take 1/2 Unisom tablet with 25 mg of vitamin B_6 orally four times a day as necessary; for hay fever, take 25 mg orally four times a day.
How supplied: Tablets: 25 mg

Valtrex

VALACYCLOVIR HYDROCHLORIDE

Drug class: Antiviral
Pregnancy Category B
Indications:
- Genital herpes
- Herpes zoster (shingles)
- Varicella (chickenpox)

Adult dosage: For treatment, take 1 g orally two times a day for 10 days; for suppression, take 500 mg to 1 g orally daily; for episodic treatment, take 500 mg twice a day for 5 days; for herpes zoster, take 1 g three times a day for 7 days.

Precautions: Use with extreme caution with preexisting renal conditions.

Contraindications: Hypersensitivity to the drug or any component of the formulation

Adverse reactions: Nausea, vomiting, headaches, central nervous system disturbances, diarrhea, vertigo, arthralgias, rash, malaise, fatigue, viral resistance

How supplied: Tablets: 500 mg

VISTARIL, ATARAX, ANXANIL

HYDROXYZINE HYDROCHLORIDE

Drug class: Antihistamine, antianxiety, antiemetic

Pregnancy Category C

Indications:

- Anxiety
- Management of pruritus caused by allergic conditions
- Preoperative and postoperative anxiety and nausea

Adult dosage: Take 25 to 100 mg orally two to four times a day. Inject 25 to 100 mg IM every 4 to 6 hours.

Contraindications: Early pregnancy

Precautions: Therapy for more than 4 months

Interactions: Vistaril potentiates central nervous system depression with alcohol and other central nervous system depressants.

Adverse reactions: Drowsiness, dry mouth, tremors, convulsions

How supplied: Tablets: 10, 25, 50, 100, 500 mg; injection: 50 to 100 mg; syrup consists of 10 mg/5 mL of hydroxyzine hydrochloride and 0.5% alcohol

ZANTAC

RANITIDINE

Drug class: Histamine antagonist

Pregnancy Category B

Indications:

- Active duodenal or benign gastric ulcer
- Gastroesophageal disease

Adult dosage: Take 150 mg orally twice a day; take 300 mg orally at bedtime.

Contraindications: Allergy to ranitidine

Interactions: Zantac increases the effects of warfarin and tricyclic antidepressants. It decreases the effectiveness of diazepam if they are taken concurrently.

Adverse reactions: Headaches, gastrointestinal disturbances, jaundice, hepatitis, rashes, central nervous system disturbances, arrhythmias, arthralgias, myalgias, blood dyscrasias, anaphylaxis

How supplied: Tablets and capsules: 150, 300 mg; injection: 25 mg/mL IM

ZITHROMAX

AZITHROMYCIN

Drug class: Antibacterial, macrolide antibiotic

Pregnancy Category B

Indications: Mild to moderate susceptible infections, including those of the respiratory tract and uncomplicated skin and skin structures; nongonococcal urethritis; chlamydia; cervicitis

Adult dosage: Take 500 mg on day 1, either 1 hour before meals or 2 hours after, and then 250 mg daily for 4 days. For nongonococcal urethritis and chlamydia. take 1 g as a single dose. The oral suspension (Zithromax cocktail) comes in a single-dose packet. Mix the entire contents of the packet with 2 oz of water. Drink the entire contents immediately and add an additional 2 oz of water. Mix and drink all of that liquid. The Zithromax cocktail can be taken with or without food.

Precautions: Renal or hepatic impairment; monitor for superinfection and hypersensitivity.

Interactions: *Avoid concomitant antacids*

Adverse reactions: Gastrointestinal upset, abdominal pain, vaginitis, cholestatic jaundice

How supplied: Capsules: 250 mg; Z-pack (six capsules); oral suspension: one-dose pack

ZOMIG

ZOLMITRIPTAN

Drug class: Selective 5-HT receptor agonist

Pregnancy Category C

Indications: Treatment of acute migraines

Adult dosage: Take 2.5 mg orally, repeated every 2 hours as needed for a maximum dose of 10 mg/day.

Contraindications: Ischemic cardiac, cerebral, or peripheral vascular disease; hypertension; renal or hepatic dysfunction

Precautions: Confirm diagnosis; exclude cardiovascular disease, elderly patients, pregnancy, and lactation.

Interactions: Serotonin syndrome develops with administration of SSRIs.

Adverse reactions: Fatigue, pain, pressure or tightness in the throat, serious cardiac event (rare)

How supplied: Tablets: 2.5 mg

PART 8

Topical Agents

Geri Morgan, CNM, ND

Table 8-1.

Drug	Brand Name	Recommended Dosage	Considerations
Adrenocorticoids			
	Medrol	Apply small amount and gently rub into skin.	Use to relieve redness, swelling, and itching caused by hemorrhoid discomfort, insect bites, poison ivy, oak, sumac, soaps, cosmetics, and jewelry.
Anesthetics			
Benzocaine	Hurricane topical	Use only enough to cover irritation.	Apply anesthetic for minor surgical procedures.
Dibucaine	Americaine anesthetic Nupercainal ointment		Relieves pain and itch of sunburn, insect bites, scratches, hemorrhoids, and other minor skin irritations.
Lidocaine hydrochloride	Lidocaine	Use lowest dose possible to achieve desired results. Comes in a viscous solution: 1%, 2% (1–2 mg/mL). Dose varies with area to be anesthetized.	Use to relieve burning, stinging, tenderness, and tissue irritations.
Antibiotics			
Mupirocin	Bactroban	Apply small amount to affected area three times a day. Can be covered with gauze dressing.	Use to treat impetigo caused by *Staphylococcus aureus*, streptococci, and *pyogenes*. Monitor for signs of superinfection; reevaluate if no response in 3 to 5 days.
	Neosporin	Apply small amount every 3 to 4 hours for 7 to 10 days.	Use to prevent infection caused by minor cuts, scrapes, and burns.

(continued)

Table 8-1. (*Continued*)

Drug	Brand Name	Recommended Dosage	Considerations
Antifungals			
Clotrimazole	Lotrimin; Mycelex	Gently massage into affected area twice a day.	Cleanse area before applying; use for up to 4 weeks. Discontinue if irritation occurs or condition worsens.
Econazole nitrate	Spectazole	Apply locally twice a day.	Use for athlete's foot; change socks and shoes at least once a day. Cleanse area before applying; treat for 2 to 4 weeks. Discontinue if irritation or burning occurs or condition worsens.
Gentian violet		Apply locally twice a day.	Note that medication may stain skin and clothes; *do not* apply to active lesions.
Naftifine HCl	Naftin	Gently massage into affected area twice a day.	Avoid occlusive dressings; wash hands thoroughly after application. *Do not* use longer than 4 weeks.
Oxiconazole	Oxistat	Apply twice every day.	Consider that patient may need medication for up to 1 month.
Terbinafine	Lamisil	Apply to area twice a day until clinical signs of improvement, usually 1 to 4 weeks.	*Do not* use occlusive dressings; report local irritations. Discontinue if local irritation occurs.
Tolnaftate	Tinactin; Genaspor; Ting; Aftate	Apply small amount twice a day for 2 to 3 weeks; 4 to 6 weeks may be necessary if skin is thick.	Cleanse skin with soap and water before application; dry thoroughly. Wear loose, well-fitted shoes; change socks at least four times a day.

Antipsoriatics

| Ammoniated mercury | Emersal | Apply twice every day. | Protect skin from light; potential sensitizer, provoking severe allergic reactions. |
| Anthralin | Anthra-Derm; Lasan; Drithocreme | Apply every day only to psoriatic lesions. | Note that medication may stain fabrics, skin, hair, nails; use protective dressing. |

Antiseborrheics

| Selenium sulfide | Selsun Blue; Exsel | Massage 5–10 mL into scalp; allow to sit 2 to 3 minutes, then rinse. | Remove jewelry before use to avoid damaging it. Discontinue if irritation occurs. |

Antiviral

Acyclovir	Zovirax	Apply 5% ointment in 40-g tube to affected areas every 4 hours.	Apply prior to voiding to decrease discomfort. Use to decrease pain and help dry sores of herpes simplex virus.
Imiquimod	Aldara	Apply to infected areas every other night. Leave on 6 to 10 hours before washing. Reassess if warts are not gone by 16 weeks.	Use to enhances cell-mediated immunity to human papilloma virus. Expensive self-treatment involves single-use packets containing 250 mg cream, 12 packets/box. Local irritation is reduced by every-other-night treatment schedule.
Podofilox	Condylox	Apply every 12 hours for 3 consecutive days, stop application for 4 days, then repeat cycle as necessary. Reassess in 4 to 6 weeks.	Use this keratolytic agent for self-treatment of genital warts. Allow area to dry before usage. Dispose of used applicator; reuse may cause burning and discomfort.

(continued)

Table 8-1. (*Continued*)

Drug	Brand Name	Recommended Dosage	Considerations
Emollients			
Boric acid ointment	Borofax	Apply as needed.	Use to relieve burning, itching, and irritation.
Dexpanthenol glycerin	Panthoderm	Apply twice every day.	Use to relieve itching and aid in healing mild skin irritations.
Eucerin		Apply as needed.	Use to relieve dry skin and pruritus.
Lanolin		Combine with other ingredients, such as rose water.	Use for its moisturizing effect.
		Apply generously ointment based.	Exercise caution if allergic to sheep or sheep products; provides base for many ointments.
Vitamin A acid, tretinoin derivative	Retin-A	Initially apply to cleansed and completely dry skin once daily at bedtime. Adjust strength of frequency as tolerated and needed.	Use for acne vulgaris.
Vitamins A and D		Apply locally with gentle massage two to four times a day.	Use to relieve minor burns, chafing, skin irritations. Refer to specialist if no improvement within 7 days.
Zinc oxide		Apply as needed.	Use to relieve burns, abrasions, diaper rash.
Keratolytics			
Benzoyl peroxide	Persa-Gel; Benzagel 14% gel	Apply to cleansed area one to two times per day. Avoid mouth and mucous membranes.	Use to relieve acne vulgaris.

Desquam	Massage into cleansed area one to two times per day. Avoid mouth, eyes, and mucous membranes.	Use to relieve mild to moderate acne.

Lotions and Solutions

Burow's solution aluminum acetate	Bluboro Powder; Boropak Powder; Domeboro Powder; Pedi-Boro Soak Paks	Dissolve one packet in a pint of water; apply four times a day for 30 minutes.	Apply astringent wet dressing for relief of inflammatory conditions, insect bites, athlete's foot, and bruises; do not use occlusive dressing.
Calamine lotion	Calamox; Resinol; Calamatum	Apply to affected areas three to four times a day.	Use to relieve itching and pain of poison ivy, sumac, and oak; insect bites; and other minor skin irritations.
Hamamelis water	Witch Hazel; Tucks; A-E-R	Apply locally up to six times a day.	Use to relieve itching and irritation of vaginal infections, hemorrhoids, postepisiotomy discomfort, posthemorrhoidectomy.

Pediculicide and Scabicides

Crotamiton	Eurax	Thoroughly massage onto entire body; repeat in 24 hours. Take cleansing bath or shower 48 hours after application.	Use externally only. Shake well before using. Change bed linens and clothing the next day. Dry-clean or wash contaminated clothes in hot cycle.
Lindane	Kwell; Scabene; G-Well	Apply thin layer to entire body and leave 8 to 12 hours; then wash thoroughly. Shampoo 1 to 2 oz into hair and leave for 4 minutes.	Apply externally only. A single application is usually sufficient. Reapply after 7 days if any sign of live lice. Ensure all contacts are treated; the disease is readily communicated. Teach patient hygiene and prevention.

(continued)

Table 8-1. (*Continued*)

Drug	Brand Name	Recommended Dosage	Considerations
Permethrin	Nix, Elimite	Thoroughly massage into skin (30 g/adult); wash off after 8 to 14 hours. Shampoo into freshly washed, rinsed, and towel-dried hair. Leave on 10 minutes and rinse.	Use externally only. Single application is usually curative. Notify health care provider if rash or itching worsens.

NOTES

Bibliography

Abramowicz, M. (1995). *The medical letter* (37th ed., p. 964). New Rochelle, NY: The Medical Letter Inc.

Aikins, M. P. (1992). Periconceptional supplementation with folic acid: Does it prevent neural tube defects? *Journal of Nurse-Midwifery, 37*(1), 25-32.

American Academy of Pediatrics, American College of Obstetricians and Gynecologists. (1992). *Guidelines for perinatal care* (3rd ed.). Elk Grove Village, IL: American Academy of Pediatrics.

American Cancer Society. (2000). *Cancer facts and figures*, (p. 9). Brochure. Washington, DC. Author.

American College of Nurse-Midwives. (1978). *Philosophy*. Washington, DC: Author.

American College of Obstetricians and Gynecologists. (1992). *Women's health: The menopause years*. Washington, DC: Author.

American College of Obstetricians and Gynecologists. (1998, April). ACOG Educational Bulletin No. 246. Washington, DC: Author.

American College of Obstetricians and Gynecologists. (1994). *Management of hypertension in pregnancy* (ACOG Technical Bulletin). Washington, DC: Author.

American Health Consultants. (2001, January). *Contraceptive Technology Update, 22*(1), 1-12.

American Health Consultants. (2001, February). *Contraceptive Technology Update, 22*(2), 14-24.

American Health Consultants. (2001, April). *Contraceptive Technology Update, 22*(4).

American Society of Hospital Pharmacists. (1993). Contraceptives estrogen-progestin combinations. *American Hospital Formulary Service Drug Information, 68*, 1924-1929.

Andolina, V. F., Lille, S., & Willison, K. M. (1992). *Mammographic imaging*. Philadelphia: JB Lippincott.

Apgar, V. (1953). A proposal for a new method of evaluation of the newborn infant. *Current Research in Anesthesia and Analgesia, 32*, 260-267.

Association of Reproductive Health Professionals. (2001, March). *ARHP Clinical Proceedings*. Washington DC.

Baines, C. (1992). Physical examination of the breasts in screening for breast cancer. *Journal of Gerontology, 47*, 63-67.

Baldwin, H. E. (2001). STD update: Screening and therapeutic options. *International Journal of Fertility and Women's Medicine, 46*(2), 79-88.

Basler, R., & Seraly, M. (2001). Common dermatologic problems in athletes. *Patient Care for Nurse Practitioners, 4*(6), 55-63.

Belen, C. (1999). Herbs and childbearing women. *Journal of Nurse-Midwifery, 44*(3), 231-248.

Benson, M. (2000). *Gynecological pearls* (2nd ed.). Philadelphia: FA Davis Company.

Bloom, K. C., & Ewing, C.A. (2001). Group B streptococcal (GBS) disease screening and testing during pregnancy: Nurse-midwives' consistency with 1996 CDC recommendations. *Journal of Nurse-Midwifery and Women's Health, 46*(1), 17-23.

Blumenthal, M. (2001). Asian ginseng: Potential therapeutic uses. *Advance for Nurse Practitioners, 9*(2), 26-33.

Bradshaw, L. (1995). Posthysterectomy Pap smears. *American Journal of Obstetric Gynecology, 173*, 424.

Byyny R. L., & Speroff, L. (1996). *A clinical guide for the care of older women*. Baltimore: Williams & Wilkins.

Cabaniss, C. D., & Cabaniss, M. L. (1987). Physiologic hematology of pregnancy. In D. Z. Kitay (Ed.), *Hematologic problems in pregnancy.* Oradell, NJ: Medical Economics Books.

Caro-Paton, T. et al. (1997). Is metronidazole teratogenic? A meta-analysis. *British Journal of Clinical Pharmacology, 44,* 179-182.

CCS Publishing. (1992). *Current clinical strategies: Gynecology and obstetrics.* Newport Beach, RI: Author.

Centers for Disease Control and Prevention. (1989). Sexually transmitted diseases treatment guidelines. *MMWR, 38*(Suppl. S-8).

Centers for Disease Control and Prevention. (1996, May). Prevention of perinatal group B streptococcal disease: A public health perspective. *MMWR, 45*(RR-7), 1-24.

Centers for Disease Control and Prevention. (1998, January). Sexually transmitted diseases treatment guidelines. *MMWR, 47*(Suppl. RR-1).

Chang, E. & Ramsey-Goldman, R. (2001, April). Antiphospholipid antibodies and RA. *Women's Health Gynecology Edition, 1*(2).

Clark-Coller, T. (1991). Dysfunctional uterine bleeding and amenorrhea: Differential diagnosis and management. *Journal of Nurse-Midwifery, 36*(1), 49-62.

Cook, M. J. (1993). Perimenopause: An opportunity for health promotion. *Journal of Obstetric Gynecology and Neonatal Nursing 2nd, 22*(3), 223-228.

Corbett, J. V. (1992). *Laboratory tests and diagnostic procedures with nursing diagnosis.* Norwalk, CT: Appleton & Lange.

Crandall, C. (2001, February). Osteoporosis: Update on prevention and treatment. *Consultant,* 259-266.

Crowell, D. T. (1995). Weight change in the postpartum period. *Journal of Nurse-Midwifery, 40,* 418-423.

Crum, C., & Newkirk, G. (1995). Abnormal Pap smears, cancer risk, and HPV. *Patient Care,* 35-61.

Cuccinelli, J. (1998). Alternative medicine: Echinacea. *Clinician Reviews, 9*(9), 101-104.

Cunningham, F. G, Grant, N. F., Leveno, K, Gilstrap III, L. C., Hauth, J., & Wenstrom, K. (2001). *Williams obstetrics* (25th ed.). Columbus, OH: McGraw-Hill.

Danco Laboratories. (2000, September). Mifeprex (mifepristone) tablets, 200 mg: The early option pill.

DeCherney, A. H., & Pernoll, M. L. (1994). *Current obstetric & gynecologic diagnosis & treatment* (7th ed.). Norwalk, CT: Appleton & Lange.

Diamond, S., & Vrban, G. (2001, July). *Consultant,* p. 1131.

Dickey, R. (2000). *Managing contraceptive pill patients* (10th ed.). New Orleans: EMIS Medical Publishers.

Eddy, D. M. (1991). *Common screening tests.* Philadelphia: American College of Physicians.

Eschenbach, D. A. (1993). History and review of bacterial vaginosis. *American Journal of Obstetrics and Gynecology, 169,* 441-445.

Felig, P., et al. (1987). *Endocrinology and metabolism* (2nd ed.). New York: McGraw-Hill.

Fishbach, F. (1992). *A manual of laboratory & diagnostic tests* (4th ed.). Philadelphia: JB Lippincott.

Gomel, V., Munro, M. G., & Rowe, T. C. (1990). *Gynecology: A practical approach.* Baltimore, MD: Williams & Wilkins.

Gray, M. (1992). *Genitourinary disorders.* St. Louis, MO: CV Mosby.

Haagensen, C. (1986). *Diseases of the breast* (3rd ed.). Philadelphia: WB Saunders.

Harris, J. R., et al. (1991). *Breast diseases*. Philadelphia: JB Lippincott.

Hatcher, R. A., Stewart, F., & Trussell, J. *Contraceptive Technology: 1990-1992* (15th ed.). New York: Irvington, 1992.

Hatcher, R. A, Trussell, J., Guest, F., Cates, W., Stewart, G., & Kowal, D. (1998). *Contraceptive technology* (17th ed.). New York: Ardent Media.

Houle, A., Pickard, C. G., Ouimette, R., Lohr, J., & Greenberg, R. (1995). *Patient guidelines for nurse practitioners* (4th ed.). Philadelphia: JB Lippincott.

Iams, J. D., Casal, D., & McGregor, J. A. (1995). Fetal fibronectin improves the accuracy of diagnosis of preterm labor. *American Journal of Obstetrics and Gynecology, 173*(1), 141-145.

Institute of Medicine. (1988). *Prenatal care: Reaching mothers, reaching infants*. Washington, DC: National Academy Press.

Institute of Medicine. (1990). *Nutrition during pregnancy: Summary*. Washington, DC: National Academy Press.

Joint American College of Obstetrics and Gynecology. (1990). *Guidelines for labor and delivery*. Washington, DC: Author.

Jonas, W. B., & Leven, J. S. (1999). *Essentials of complementary and alternative medicine*. Maryland: Lippincott Williams & Wilkins.

Karch, A. M. (1996). *Lippincott's nursing drug guide*. Philadelphia: JB Lippincott.

Kass-Annese, B. (1999). *Management of the perimenopausal and postmenopausal woman*. Philadelphia: Lippincott.

Kass-Annesse, B. (1998). *Management of the perimenopausal and postmenopausal woman - a total wellness program. Philadelphia: Lippincott*.

Keppel, K. G., Taffel, S. M. (1993). Pregnancy-related weight gain and retention: Implications of the 1990 Institute of Medicine guidelines. *American Journal of Public Health, 83*, 1100-1103.

Lash, A., Mertens, D., & Okumus, H. (2001, June). *Advance for nurse practitioners*, 59-65.

Lemke, D. P, Pattison, J., Marshall, L. A., Cowley, D. S. (Eds.). (1995). *Primary care of women*. Norwalk, CT: Appleton & Lange.

Lichtman, R., & Papera, S. (1990). *Gynecology well woman care*. Norwalk, CT: Appleton & Lange.

Long, P. (1995). Rethinking iron supplementation during pregnancy. *Journal of Nurse-Midwifery, 40*(1), 36-40.

Lossick, J. G., & Kent, H. L. (1991). Trichomoniasis: Trends in diagnosis and management. *American Journal of Obstetrics & Gynecology, 165*, 1217-1222.

Malasanos, L, Barkauskas, V, & Stoltenberg-Allen, K. (1990). *Health assessment* (4th ed.). St. Louis, MO: CV Mosby.

Mays, M. (1993). Tuberculosis: A comprehensive review for the certified nurse-midwife. *Journal of Nurse-Midwifery, 38*(3), 132-139.

McDonough, J. (Ed.). (1993). *Stedman's concise medical dictionary* (2nd ed.). Baltimore, MD: Williams & Wilkins.

Medical Economics. (1995). *The PDR family guide to nutrition and health*. Montvale, NJ: Author.

Merriam-Webster's collegiate dictionary (10th ed.). (1993). Springfield, MA: Merriam-Webster, Inc.

Myriad Genetic Laboratories. (1997, December). *BRAC analysis: Understanding genetic predisposition to breast and ovarian cancer*. Salt Lake City, UT: Author.

Nachtigall, L. (2000, June). Assessing alternative approaches to menopause. *Contemporary OB/GYN*, (Supple.).

Nelson, A., Hatcher, R., et al. (2000). *A pocket guide to managing contraception* (millennium ed. 2000-2001, 3rd ed.). Tiger, GA: Bridging the Gap Foundation.

Nelson, D. M. (1998, March). *Precontraceptive care: Key to improving pregnancy outcomes - What to ask, what to test, what to tell.* Lecture conducted at the Symposia Medicus in Cancún, Mexico.

Novey, D. W. (2000). *Clinician's complete reference to complementary and alternative medicine.* St. Louis: Mosby.

Olopade, O. F., & Cummings, S. (2000, September). Breast and ovarian cancer, Part 1. *Consultant*, 1809-1814.

PDR for herbal medicines (2nd ed.). (2000). Montvale, NJ: Medical Economics Company, Inc.

Pettit, J. (2001). Alternative medicine: Peppermint. *Clinician Reviews, 11*(3), 71-73.

Physicians' desk reference (55th ed.). (2001). Montvale, NJ: Medical Economics Company, Inc.

Pittit, J. (2001). Alternative medicine: Feverfew. *Clinician Reviews, 11*(2), 113-114.

Planned Parenthood of Central and Northern Arizona. (2001, January). Abortion. In *Manual of medical standards and guidelines* (Section VII-B1). Phoenix, AZ: Author.

Primary care update. Domestic violence: The silent epidemic. (2001, April 15). *Consultant*, pp. 686-687.

Redmond, G. P., Olson, W. H., Lippman, J. S., Kafrissen, M. E., Jones, T. M., Jorizzo, J. L. (1997). N.O. and E.E. in the treatment of acne vulgaris: A randomized placebo controlled trial. *Obstetrics and Gynecology, 89*, 615-622.

Roberts, R.G. (2001). Overactive bladder, a new clinical perspective. *A supplement to patient care for the nurse practitioner, Spring*, 22–30.

Roe v. Wade, 410 U.S. 113 (1973).

Schirmer, G. P. (2001, Spring). *Herbal medicine workshop* (p.1). Bedford, TX. MED/2000.

Sibai, B. M. (1988, May). Definitive therapy of pregnancy-induced hypertension. *Contemporary OB/GYN*, 51-66.

Sitruk-Ware, R., & Bardin, C. W. (1992). *Contraception: Newer pharmacological agents, devices, and delivery systems.* New York: Marcel Dekker.

Skidmore-Roth, L. (1995). *Mosby's 1995 nursing drug reference.* St. Louis, MO: CV Mosby.

Speroff, L., & Darney, P. D. (1998). *A clinical guide for contraception.* Baltimore, MD: Williams & Wilkins.

Spitz, I. M., & Bardin, L. et al. (1998). Early pregnancy termination with mifepristone and misoprostol in the United States. *New England Journal of Medicine, 338*, 1241-1247.

Stampe, S. (1998, May). Paper presented at the Integrative Medicine Workshop, sponsored by the Family Planning Council, Tucson, AZ.

Star, W., Shannon, M., Sammons, L., Lommel, L., & Gutierrez, Y. (1990). *Ambulatory obstetrics: Protocols for nurse practitioners/nurse midwives* (2nd ed.). San Francisco, CA: School of Nursing, University of California Press.

Stewart, F. H., et al. (2001, May). Clinical breast and pelvic examination requirements for hormonal contraception - Current practice vs. evidence. *JAMA, 285*(17), 2232-2240.

Stine, G. J. (1992). *The biology of sexually transmitted diseases*. Dubuque, IA: WC Brown.

Stumpf, S. (1998, May). Paper presented at the Integrative Medicine Workshop, sponsored by the Family Planning Council, Tucson, AZ.

Swaya, G. E., Grady, D., Kerlikoske, K., et al. (2000). The positive predictive value of cervical smears in previously screened postmenopausal women: The Heart and Estrogen/Progestin Replacement Study (HER). *Annals of Internal Medicine, 133*, 942-950.

Sweet, R. L., & Gibbs, R. S. (1990). *Infectious diseases of the female genital tract* (2nd ed.). Baltimore, MD: Williams & Wilkins.

Takanishi, G. (2001, February). Drug therapies for hot flashes in breast cancer survivors. *Women's Health, Gynecology Edition, 1*(1).

Tierney LM Jr, McPhee SJ, Papadakis MA, Schroeder SA, eds. *Current Medical Diagnosis & Treatment*. Norwalk, CT: Appleton & Lange, 1993.

United Health Foundation. (2000, December). *Clinical evidence* (Issue 4). Minneapolis, MN: BMJ Publishing Group.

Uphold, C. R., & Graham, M. V. (1998). *Clinical guidelines in family practice* (3rd ed.). Gainesville, FL: Barmarre Books.

U.S. Department of Health and Human Services, Public Health Service. (1989). *Caring for our future: The content of prenatal care*. Washington, DC: Author.

U.S. Department of Health and Human Services, Public Health Service. (1991). *Healthy people 2000: National health promotion and disease prevention objectives* (DHHS Publication No. 91-50212). Washington, DC: U.S. Government Printing Office.

Usha, V., & Gopalakrishnan, N. (2000). A comparative study of oral ivermectin and topical permethrin cream in the treatment of scabies. *Journal of the American Academy of Dermatology, 42*, 236.

Varney, H. (1986). *Nurse-midwifery*. Boston, MA: Blackwell Scientific.

Vutyavanich, T., et al. (2001). Ginger reduces nausea and vomiting of pregnancy. *Obstetrics and Gynecology, 97*, 577-582.

Weil, A. (1997). *Eight weeks to optimum health*. New York: Random House.

Weil, A. (1997). The joy of soy. *Self-healing, 1*, 6-7.

Weil, E. K., Murphy, J. L., & Burke, J., (Eds.). (1995). *Nurse practitioners prescribing reference*. New York: Prescribing Reference Inc.

Winkler, H. A., & Sand, P. K. (1998, April). Stress incontinence: options for conservative treatment. *Women's Health in Primary Care, 1*(3), 279–294.

Wright, V. C., & Lickrish, G. M., (Eds.). (1989). *Basic and advanced colposcopy*. Houston, TX: Biomedical Communications.

Yue, Q. Y., Bergquist, C., & Gorden, B. (2000). Safety of St. John's wort, *Lancet, 355*, 576-577.

WORLD WIDE WEB

Academy for Guided Imagery	www.healthy.net/agi
Advance for Nurse Practitioner	www.advanceforNP.com
American Association of Professional Hypnotherapists	www.aaph.org
American Botanical Council	www.herbalgram.org
American College of Nurse-Midwives	www.midwife.org
American College of Obstetricians and Gynecologists	http://www.acog.org/
American Dietetic Association	www.eatright.org

American Music Therapy Association www.musictherapy.org
Danco Laboratories http://www.earlyoptionpill.com/
    (Mifeprex)
Domestic Violence National http://www.ncjrs.org/victdv.htm
    Institute of Justice
End Abuse: Family Violence www.fvpf.org
    Prevention Fund
Food and Drug Administration http://www.fda.gov/default.htm
Herb Research Foundation www.herbs.org
Inventory of Services and Funding http://www.cdc.gov/ncipc/
    Sources for Programs Designed dvp/vawprograms
    to Prevent Violence Against
    Women
Menopause www.menopause.org
 www.newlifehealth.com
Mirena (intrauterine device [IUD]) http://www.mirena.com/
Myriad Genetics www.myriad.com
 e-mail: BRAC@myriad.com
National Certification Commission www.nccaom.org
    for Acupuncture and
    Oriental Medicine
Physicians' Desk Reference www.pdr.net
Planned Parenthood of Central www.ppcna.org
    and Northern Arizona
Reiki in Hospitals Support Group www.srpt.org
Women's Health . . . in the news www.womenshealthinthenews.
 com

INDEX

A

Abortion
  incomplete, 222, 229
  induced, 219–225
    complications of, 223–224
    counseling before, 219
    medical, 220–222
    physical examination before,
      219–220
    safety of, 219
    surgical, 222–223
    in United States, 219
  spontaneous
    under 20 weeks gestation, 230–231
    Rh immune globulin in, 232
    vaginal bleeding in, 229–230
    vs. ectopic pregnancy, 241
Abruptio placentae, 224–225, 226t
Abscesses, of breast, 169
Abstinence, for contraception, 8
Abuse, 97–100
  clinical manifestations of, 99
  definition of, 99
  incidence of, 99
  patient management in, 99–100
  reporting of, 100
Acetaminophen, 353
Acne, 183
  oral contraceptives and, 13t
Acquired immunodeficiency syndrome
    (AIDS). See Human immunodefi-
    ciency virus (HIV) infection
Actifed, 309
Actinomycosis, genital, intrauterine device
    and, 30–31
Activella, 73t
Acupressure massage, 292
Acupuncture, 291–292
Acyclovir, 310, 361t
  for herpes simplex virus infection, 158
Adenocarcinoma, cervical, 177t
Adrenalin, 321
Adrenocorticoids, 359t
Advil, 330
AFP (alfafetoprotein), serum, 137–138
Aftate, 360t
Age, maternal, and genetic screening, 136
AIDS (acquired immunodeficiency syn-
    drome). See Human immunodefi-
    ciency virus (HIV) infection
Albuterol, 346
Alcohol, fetal effects of, 39
Aldara, 164, 361t
Alendronate sodium, 327
Alfafetoprotein (AFP), serum, 137–138
Alfafetoprotein test, 53
Allergies, and contact dermatitis, 184–185
Alopecia, postpartum, 285

Alternative therapy. See Complementary
    therapy
Amenorrhea, 103–105
  clinical features of, 103–104
  definition of, 103
  etiology of, 103
  laboratory studies in, 104
  management of, 104–105
  oral contraceptives and, 19–20
Amerge, 310
Americaine spray, 359t
Ammoniated mercury, 361t
Amniotic fluid, excessive, 266–267
Amniotomy, 59
Amoxicillin, 311
Analgesia, for labor, 60
Anemia, 105–112
  acquired hemolytic, 108–109
  clinical features of, 106
  definition of, 105
  etiology of, 105–106
  iron deficiency, 109–110
  management of, 106–108
  megaloblastic, 110–111
  pernicious, 111
  sickle cell, 112
Anesthetics, topical, 359t
Antacids, for heartburn, 85t
Antepartum care, 42–48
  indications for referral in, 47–48
  initial visit for, 42–45
  laboratory studies in, 43–44
  objectives of, 42
  obstetric history in, 43
  patient education during, 45
  philosophy of, 42
  physical examination in, 43–44
  for return visit, 45–46
  ultrasonography in, 44–45
Anthralin, 361t
Antibiotics, 359t. See also specific drug
  and vaginitis, 209
Antibodies, to herpes simplex virus, 157
Anticholinergic drugs, for urinary inconti-
    nence, 206
Antidepressants, tricyclic, for urinary
    incontinence, 206
Antiepileptic medications, in pregnancy,
    39
Antifungal drugs, 360t
Antiphospholipid antibody syndrome,
    225–227
Antipsoriatic drugs, 361t
Antiseborrheic drugs, 361t
Antiviral drugs, 361t
Anxanil, 355
Appendicitis, vs. ectopic pregnancy, 241
Aromatherapy, 304–305

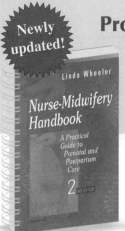
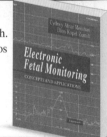
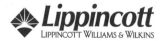